CURRENT GASTROENTEROLOGY®
Volume 16

CURRENT

GASTROENTEROLOGY®

VOLUME 16

Edited by

Gary Gitnick, M.D.
Professor of Medicine
Chief, Division of Digestive Diseases
UCLA School of Medicine
Los Angeles, California

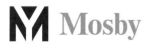 Mosby

St. Louis   Baltimore   Boston   Carlsbad   Chicago   Naples   New York   Philadelphia   Portland
London   Madrid   Mexico City   Singapore   Sydney   Tokyo   Toronto   Wiesbaden

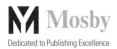

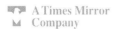

Vice President and Publisher, Continuity Publishing: Kenneth H. Killion
Director, Editorial Development: Gretchen C. Murphy
Acquisitions Editor: Shelley Scott
Developmental Editor: Miranda Jackson
Manager, Continuity—EDP: Maria Nevinger
Project Specialist: Denise Dungey
Assistant Project Supervisor: Sandra Rogers
Proofreading Manager: Barbara M. Kelly
Senior Marketing Manager: Eileen M. Lynch
Marketing Specialist: Lynn D. Stevenson

Printed in the United States of America
Composition by The Clarinda Company
Printing/binding by The Maple-Vail Book Manufacturing Group

Mosby–Year Book, Inc.
11830 Westline Industrial Drive
St. Louis, Missouri 63146

Editorial Office:
Mosby–Year Book, Inc.
200 North LaSalle St.
Chicago, Illinois 60601

International Standard Serial Number: 0198-8085
International Standard Book Number: 0-8151-3651-X

This book is dedicated to my family for their love, support, and tolerance—to my wife Cherna; to my children, Neil, Kim, Jill, and Tracy; to my mother Ann; and to my brother Jerry, his wife Saranne, and his daughters, Nan Marie and Andrea.

Contributors

Patricia L. Abbitt, M.D.
Associate Professor of Radiology
Chief, Division of Ultrasound
University of Florida College of Medicine
Gainesville, Florida

Stephan Böhm, M.D.
Postdoctoral Research Fellow
Departments of Surgery and Physiology
University of California, San Francisco, School of Medicine
San Francisco, California

Scott R. Brazer, M.D., M.H.S.
Assistant Professor of Medicine
Division of Gastroenterology
Department of Medicine
Duke University Medical Center
Durham, North Carolina

Nigel W. Bunnett, Ph.D.
Associate Professor
Departments of Surgery and Physiology
University of California, San Francisco, School of Medicine
San Francisco, California

Sharon S. Burton, M.D.
Associate Professor of Radiology
Chief, Division of Gastrointestinal Radiology
University of Florida College of Medicine
Gainesville, Florida

Joseph Cernigliaro, M.D.
Clinical Fellow of Radiology
Division of Body Imaging
University of Florida College of Medicine
Gainesville, Florida

Barry De Gregorio, M.D.
Division of Gastroenterology
Oregon Health Sciences University
Portland, Oregon

Martin Anthony Eastwood, M.B., Ch.B., M.Sc., F.R.C.P.E.
Consultant Gastroenterologist
Reader in Medicine
University of Edinburgh
Gastrointestinal Unit
Western General Hospital
Edinburgh, Scotland, United Kingdom

M. Brian Fennerty, M.D.
Division of Gastroenterology
Oregon Health Sciences University
Portland, Oregon

Eileen F. Grady, Ph.D.
Assistant Professor
Departments of Surgery and Physiology
University of California, San Francisco, School of Medicine
San Francisco, California

Felix W. Leung, M.D.
Acting Director
Division of Gastroenterology
UCLA—San Fernando Valley Program
Sepulveda Veterans Administration Medical Center and Olive View Medical
    Center
Professor of Medicine
UCLA School of Medicine
Los Angeles, California

Antony G. Maniatis, M.D.
Fellow, Division of Gastroenterology
Department of Medicine
Duke University Medical Center
Durham, North Carolina

S.J.D. O'Keefe, M.D., M.Sc., F.R.C.P., F.A.C.G.
Professor, Department of Gastroenterology
Groote Schuur Hospital
Cape Town, South Africa

Pablo R. Ros, M.D.
Professor and Associate Chairman of Radiology
Chief, Division of Body Imaging and Magnetic Resonance Imaging
University of Florida College of Medicine
Gainesville, Florida

J.A. Thompson, M.D.
Cell and Molecular Biology Collaborative Network in Gastrointestinal
    Physiology
Medical College of St. Bartholomew's Hospital
London, England

A.B.R. Thomson, M.D.
Cell and Molecular Biology Collaborative Network in Gastrointestinal
    Physiology
Nutrition and Metabolism Research Group
Department of Medicine
Division of Gastroenterology
University of Alberta
Edmonton, Canada

Gladys M. Torres, M.D.
Associate Professor of Radiology
University of Florida College of Medicine
Gainesville, Florida

G.E. Wild, M.D.
Cell and Molecular Biology Collaborative Network in Gastrointestinal
    Physiology
Department of Medicine
Division of Gastroenterology
McGill University
Montreal, Quebec, Canada

T.A. Winter, M.D., F.C.P.(S.A.)
Gastrointestinal Clinic
Department of Medicine
University of Cape Town and Groote Schuur Hospital
Cape Town, South Africa

Preface

The advances in the past year and our understanding of gastroenterologic problems, as well as the progress in our diagnosis of gastrointestinal diseases, have again been accompanied by a dramatic increase in medical and surgical approaches to these disorders. The volume of literature now available for our understanding of gastrointestinal disease is so great that it must be a burden to any physician who conscientiously tries to remain current. Unlike other reviews of medical literature, this text is not a compilation of abstracts, nor is it an encyclopedic review of the world's literature. Experts in each of the topics in this volume were asked to write a chapter about the advances in their field during the past year. They were also asked to reference the most important work and to discuss the interrelationships of studies, groups of studies, and scientific trends. Thus, their job was to review the literature, tell the reader what of importance was published, and relay how this information can affect clinical practice and research progress.

The authors of the chapters were chosen because of their knowledge regarding a specific subject and also because they are actively caring for patients and undertaking important research in the areas of review. I asked them to provide the reader with opinions regarding the quality of the work under review. As in past years, other experts in the same field were asked to review the chapters produced for this volume and to advise the editor and the authors of the acceptability of those chapters for publication. They were specifically asked to indicate areas of omission or areas in which works not necessarily of significance were included. Most important, they were asked to indicate any areas of prejudice that may have influenced the material submitted. Through such "peer review" it is hoped that a balanced review of the literature may result.

I am indebted to the following reviewers who generously participated in the peer review process: Lin Chang, M.D., Jonathan Kaunitz, M.D., Ronald Koretz, M.D., Thomas Kovacs, M.D., Rodger A. Liddle, M.D., and Charles Pope II, M.D. I am also indebted to Susan Dashe, whose expertise, experience, and efficiency brings this volume together each year.

Gary Gitnick, M.D.

Contents

Mosby Document Express

Copies of the full text of journal articles referenced in this book are available by calling Mosby Document Express, toll-free, at 1-800-55-MOSBY.

With Mosby Document Express, you have convenient 24-hour-a-day access to literally every journal reference within this book. In fact, through Mosby Document Express, virtually any medical or scientific article can be located and delivered by FAX, overnight delivery service, international airmail, electronic transmission of bitmapped images (via Internet), or regular mail. The average cost of a complete delivered copy of an article, including copyright clearance charges and first-class mail delivery, is $12.

For inquiries and pricing information, please call the toll-free number shown above.

CHAPTER 1

The Esophagus

Antony G. Maniatis, M.D.

Fellow, Division of Gastroenterology, Department of Medicine, Duke University Medical Center, Durham, North Carolina

Scott R. Brazer, M.D., M.H.S.

Assistant Professor of Medicine, Division of Gastroenterology, Department of Medicine, Duke University Medical Center, Durham, North Carolina

In the past year there have been significant advances in our understanding of the esophagus in the normal and disease states and in the treatment of esophageal disorders. This chapter will highlight the seminal advances rather than attempt to be an encyclopedic review.

PHYSIOLOGY

The action of the upper and lower esophageal sphincters as well as esophageal body peristalsis is coordinated by complex neuromuscular interactions. The esophageal musculature is divided into an outer longitudinal and an inner circular layer. The central nervous system (CNS) completely controls motility in the oropharynx and upper part of the esophagus. These structures are composed of striated muscle, in contrast to the mid and lower regions of the esophagus, which are composed of smooth muscle. Motility in the mid and lower sections of the esophagus is controlled by intrinsic neuromuscular mechanisms. Central innervation of the smooth muscle portion of the esophagus is via preganglionic parasympathetic neurons within the vagus nerve that synapse with postganglionic neurons, which then directly innervate esophageal smooth muscle. Central nervous system input appears to be essential for esophageal activity as demonstrated by the absence of primary and secondary esophageal contractions during deep sleep.[1]

At baseline, esophageal striated muscle maintains a constant tone, the disappearance of which facilitates swallowing. Striated esophageal muscle has less compliance and greater resistance than esophageal smooth muscle.[2] Esophageal smooth muscle tone appears to be mediated by nitrous oxide (NO). Combined NO synthase inhibition and muscarinic blockade completely inhibit neurogenic contraction in the smooth muscle of the opossum esophagus.[3] This implies that esophageal peristalsis is mediated by dual activation of cholinergic and nonadrenergic, noncholinergic (NANC) neurons. Mayrand and Diamant's results further suggest that NO is the neurotransmitter in NANC neurons that mediates the early inhibitory hyperpolarization as well as the excitatory depolarization seen with esophageal smooth muscle contraction.[2] Akbarali and Goyal[4] have shown that a NO donor, sodium nitroprusside (SNP), acts to inhibit the contraction of (relax) opossum esophageal circular muscle via membrane hyperpolarization. This is mediated by direct inhibition of calcium current influx and not by effects on the calcium-activated potassium channel. In opossum longitudinal muscle, SNP acts to induce initial relaxation via a cyclic guanine monophosphate (cGMP)-independent pathway, whereas subsequent contraction is cGMP dependent and mediated by eicosanoids in the cyclooxygenase pathway.[5] The role of additional neurotransmitters such as vasoactive intestinal peptide (VIP) in NANC transmission remains unclear; however, they would appear to play a secondary role.

Although the existence of cholinergic-mediated esophageal smooth muscle contraction has been appreciated for some time,[6] its pathway of action has not been fully defined. Sohn et al.[7, 8] have now demonstrated that the acetylcholine (ACh)-induced contraction of esophageal circular muscle in the cat is mediated by a protein kinase C (PKC)-dependent influx of extracellular calcium. This influx appears to activate phospholipase D to produce diacylglycerol (DAG) from phosphatidylcholine, which then acts independently of inositol trisphosphate (IP_3) and intracellular calcium.

Non–CNS-mediated or intrinsic mechanisms that affect esophageal contraction or relaxation are poorly understood. Huber et al.[9] have studied the role of the tachykinins (substance P, neurokinin A, and neurokinin B) in human distal esophageal circular muscle strips obtained at esophagectomy. They found that tachykinins contract esophageal circular muscle and the lower esophageal sphincter (LES)[10] via binding to the NK2 receptor. This has been confirmed by Sandler et al.[11] in a canine model using chemoreceptor activation by capsaicin. The tachykinin-mediated increase in LES pressure was dependent on cholinergic neurotransmission and muscarinic receptor excitation.

Gastroesophageal reflux (GER) is prevented by a zone of high pressure at the gastroesophageal junction (GEJ) that is in large measure due to the LES. Unlike the tone of the smooth muscle portion of the esophageal body, the LES resting

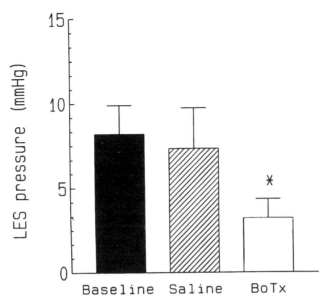

FIGURE 1.

The effect of intrasphincteric injection of botulinum toxin *(BoTx)* on resting lower esopha-geal sphincter *(LES)* pressure. After obtaining baseline LES pressure by using the station pull-through method *(filled bar,* baseline), normal saline was injected into the LES of five piglets (1 mL in each of four quadrants). One week later, LES pressure was again measured *(hatched bar,* saline), and BoTx (1 mL of a 10-unit/mL solution in each of four quadrants for a total of 40 units) was injected into the LES. After another week, the LES pressure was again measured *(open bar,* BoTx). Intrasphincteric BoTx caused a significant reduction in LES pressure when compared with baseline (*P < .01), whereas normal saline injection had no significant effect. (From Pasricha NJ, Ravich WJ, Raloo AN: *Gastroenterology* 105:1045–1049, 1993. Used by permission.)

tone is dependent on myogenic and cholinergic activity. Biancani et al.[12] have shown that cat LES tone is dependent on low-level production of IP_3 and DAG via a PKC-dependent pathway that results in submaximal calcium release insufficient for calmodulin activation. In contrast, ACh-induced maximal LES contraction oc-curs via the M3 receptor and results in maximal activation of phospholipase C, significant IP3 production, and calcium release sufficient to activate calmodulin.[8, 12] The technique of intrasphincteric botulinum toxin injection confirms the dominant role of cholinergic input in the maintenance of LES tone. Botulinum toxin inhibits the release of ACh from nerve terminals and, when injected into the LES of pig-lets, results in a 60% decrease in LES pressure (Fig 1).[13]

As in the esophageal body, relaxation of the LES is mediated at least in part by NANC neurons. To continue the parallel, NO appears to be an important mediator of NANC nerve effects in the LES. Nitric oxide synthase inhibition prevents LES relaxation in humans, which implies that NO mediates LES relaxation. Nitric oxide synthase inhibition has no effect on LES basal pressure.[14] Vasoactive intestinal peptide may act in concert with NO to achieve LES relaxation. Previous work has demonstrated that VIP can relax canine LES but does not reproduce membrane hyperpolarization as does NO.[15] For the first time, VIP receptors have been shown in high density in both the synaptosomal and smooth muscle plasma membranes of canine LES.[16] Therefore, VIP may mediate LES relaxation through NO-independent nerve pathways.

Although the LES has long been appreciated as the critical anatomic barrier for the prevention of GER, the role of other structures has been controversial. In particular, the contribution of the crural diaphragm to intraluminal pressure at the GEJ has been demonstrated by two recent studies. Mittal et al.[17] have shown that crural myotomy significantly increases spontaneous GER in anesthetized cats. Crural myotomy also abolished the increase in GEJ pressure seen during airway obstruction. Klein and coworkers[18] have elegantly demonstrated that the crural diaphragm can independently generate tone at the GEJ when they observed a high-pressure zone at the level of the diaphragm in nine of ten patients after esophagectomy (Fig 2). The role of crural diaphragm dysfunction in GER disease (GERD) remains speculative.

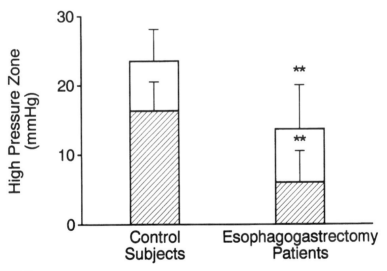

FIGURE 2.
Comparison of the high-pressure zone in ten control subjects and ten patients after esophagogastrectomy. The patient group has significantly lower midrespiratory pressure *(open area)* and good-expiratory pressure (EEP, *hatched area*). The difference in midrespiratory pressure is due to the significant decrease in tonic EEP pressure in the patient group. The phasic component is similar in both groups. Data are means ± SD. **$P < .01$. (From Klein WA, Parkman HP, Dempsey DT, et al: *Gastroenterology* 105:1362–1369, 1993. Used by permission.)

MOTOR DISORDERS OF THE ESOPHAGUS

Achalasia

Achalasia is the only esophageal motor disorder that is a true disease. Primary achalasia results from esophageal smooth muscle denervation and is characterized by aperistalsis of the esophageal body and incomplete LES relaxation. In resection specimens of 42 patients with achalasia, Goldblum et al.[19] found the following: (1) severe diminution if not an absence of myenteric ganglion cells, (2) lymphocytic and eosinophilic infiltrates of myenteric neurons, and (3) replacement of nerves by collagen. Barrett's mucosa with low-grade dysplasia was found in 4 specimens. Partial esophageal obstruction in cats or opossums by means of a Gore-tex band placed over the GEJ creates a clinical picture of achalasia that is characterized by (1) increased thickness, varicosities, and irregular angulations of nerve fiber bundles in the myenteric plexus; (2) ultrastructural changes in the mitochondria, endoplasmic reticulum, and lysosomes within neurons; and (3) collagen fibril infiltration.[20]

Although achalasia is a disorder of smooth muscle, abnormalities of proximal esophageal function have been identified. In a retrospective review of 156 consecutive achalasia patients,[21] 58% exhibited repetitive upper esophageal contractions. This finding may explain symptoms such as the globus sensation, inability to belch, and cervical dysphagia noted by some achalasia patients.

Therapy for achalasia has traditionally consisted of either balloon dilation or surgical myotomy. The technique of pneumatic dilation is not standardized. Kim et al.[22] randomized 14 patients to 30- or 35-mm-diameter balloons, 20-, 40-, or 60-second inflation duration, and one or two inflations in a $2 \times 2 \times 3$ factorial study. The mean LES pressure decreased from 43 to 26 mm Hg, and 75% of the patients noted relief of dysphagia. Although neither dilator size nor the frequency or duration of inflation had an impact on treatment effect, these results may be attributed to the small sample size (type II error). No complications of pneumatic dilation were reported.

The limiting factors for balloon dilation are the need for repeat dilation and the risk of perforation. Sharma and Achkar[23] reviewed 171 patients who underwent 215 pneumatic dilations over a 10-year period. Repeat dilation was necessary in 26% of the patients over the age of 60 as compared with 16% of those under 60 years of age. Perforation occurred in 7% of the patients overall; however, 86% of these perforations were in patients over the age of 60. At a mean follow-up of 62 months, 52% of the patients had an excellent or good result. In contrast to previous results, these investigators found that pneumatic dilation was more effective in patients under 60 years of age.

In a retrospective review of 178 patients who underwent 216 dilations for achalasia or diffuse esophageal spasm, Nair and coworkers[24] found 4 perforations (1.7%). None were fatal. All perforations were identified within 5 hours on the basis of symptoms or esophagrams, and the patients' course after surgical repair and myotomy was comparable to that of patients undergoing elective Heller myotomy. Multivariate analysis identified prior pneumatic dilation and inflation pressure greater than 11 psi as independent risk factors for perforation. Although these findings seem clinically appropriate, they may be spurious given the small sample size (n = 4). Schwartz et al.[25] retrospectively compared 7 patients with perforation after pneumatic dilation who underwent prompt (mean of 9.6 hours) emergency surgical repair and concomitant myotomy with 5 patients who underwent elective Heller myotomy during the same time period. The two groups had comparable postoperative outcomes, mean durations of surgery, hospitalizations, and intensive care unit stays.

The operative technique of Heller myotomy is also not standardized. The approach, length of myotomy, and addition of an antireflux procedure continue to be the subject of controversy. Ellis[26] reviewed his personal experience of 179 transthoracic, short myotomies without an antireflux procedure over a 22-year period. No operative deaths and only 16 (9%) minor complications were noted. At a mean 9-year follow-up, 20 patients (11%) reported dysphagia or GERD symptoms. Pellegrini et al.[27] treated 24 patients with myotomy via the thoracoscopic or laparoscopic approach. Two procedures were converted to an open technique because of esophageal perforation. Three myotomies were incomplete and required reoperations. The median hospital stay was 3 days. Twenty-one patients (88%) had good to excellent symptomatic results at early follow-up; however, 5 of 8 asymptomatic patients who underwent 24-hour pH monitoring had abnormal acid reflux.

Unrecognized GERD is a significant problem in both symptomatic and asymptomatic patients after Heller myotomy.[28] Of the 46 patients who underwent endoscopy and manometry at a mean of 13 years postoperatively, 21 patients reported reflux symptoms, 17 exhibited esophagitis, and 4 demonstrated Barrett's mucosa. Because of the significant incidence of GERD and Barrett's metaplasia in patients after myotomy, these investigators advocate regular endoscopic surveillance.

There is no concensus as to the optimal therapy for achalasia, especially with the recent addition of laparoscopic or thoracoscopic myotomy and botulinum toxin injection to the therapeutic armamentarium. We await randomized trials to define the respective roles of these treatments.

Scleroderma

Esophageal dysfunction is common in scleroderma. A decrease in esophageal propulsion as well as diminished LES pressure predisposes patients to GERD. Shoenut et al.[29] compared 11 symptomatic scleroderma patients with 11 sex- and age-matched controls. The mean acid contact time (ACT) for scleroderma patients was seven times that for controls (36% vs. 5%, $P < .01$). Omeprazole, 20 mg/day, normalized the ACT (mean ACT, 4%).

Given the significant incidence of esophageal abnormalities and GERD in asymptomatic patients with scleroderma, some investigators have proposed that all scleroderma patients be evaluated for GERD. Bhalla and coworkers[30] demonstrated that 20 of 25 (80%) asymptomatic patients with scleroderma had esophageal dilation by high-resolution computed tomography (CT). Miller et al.[31] evaluated 13 scleroderma patients and 13 controls with endoscopic ultrasound (EUS), pH monitoring, and manometry. Ten of 13 patients had hyperechoic abnormalities of the muscularis propria consistent with fibrosis, 6 of 13 had a prolonged total ACT, and 9 of 13 had abnormal manometry. There was a significant correlation among the three tests (0.70 to 0.89, $P < .02$).

Motor dysfunction may thus be the primary cause of esophageal injury in scleroderma patients. Basilisco and coworkers[32] evaluated 16 scleroderma patients with esophagogastroduodenoscopy (EGD), manometry, pH monitoring, and acid perfusion. Only the 8 patients with dysmotility were noted to have esophagitis, delayed acid clearance, and a prolonged ACT (30% vs. 6% in patients with normal motility). Esophageal dysfunction does not necessarily worsen in scleroderma. Dantas et al.[33] found no significant deterioration in motility or LES pressure in 16 of 17 patients undergoing repeat manometry after a median of 40 months.

Chest Pain of Undetermined Etiology

Fifteen percent to 20% of patients undergoing cardiac catheterization for chest pain have insignificant or no demonstrable coronary artery disease. These patients suffer from a heterogeneous group of gastrointestinal, musculoskeletal, and neuropsychiatric disorders, but a significant number will demonstrate an esophageal motor disorder, GERD, or both. Gignoux and colleagues[34] propose a high threshold for belching as an etiology for chest pain of undetermined etiology (CPUE). Chest pain reproduced by balloon distension may be related to nonpropagating proximal contractile activity and distal aboral traction force resulting in descending inhibition of contraction.[35] These results must be interpreted with caution. Uncovering manometric abnormalities in patients with CPUE does not necessarily imply that the abnormality is causing the chest pain.

Although GER is an accepted etiology of chest pain, differentiation of patients with both GER and chest pain from those with GER causing chest pain may be difficult. Singh et al.[36] found the chest pain symptom index to be of minimal utility in making this distinction. The authors divided 153 patients having undergone EGD and 24-hour pH monitoring with symptom index determination into 3 groups: (1) normal EGD and pH test, (2) normal EGD and abnormal pH test, and (3) abnormal EGD and pH test. A symptom index of greater than 50% was noted in 28%, 43%, and 45% of group 1, 2, and 3 patients, respectively, for a sensitivity of only 56% and a specificity of 68%. A simple and inexpensive technique for GER diagnosis in CPUE is to challenge patients with a single dose of omeprazole. Zierer et al.[37] demonstrated that the diagnostic yield of a single dose of 80 mg of omeprazole (82%) compared favorably with that of 24-hour pH testing with symptom index determination (86%), the Bernstein test (50%), and EGD with biopsy (86%). The utility of this technique may be limited in patients with infrequent episodes of chest pain.

Nonspecific Esophageal Dysmotility, Dysphagia, and Globus Sensation

In a normal esophagus, swallowing induces transient esophageal hyperpolarization during which time the muscle cannot contract. This latency period has been termed *deglutitive inhibition.* Sifrim and colleagues[38] have proposed a unifying theory for esophageal dysmotility: the spectrum of esophageal motility disorders is an expression of progressively failing deglutitive inhibition. These investigators evaluated 20 patients with achalasia, diffuse esophageal spasm, or nonspecific motility disturbance with manometry and intraesophageal balloon inflation. The high-pressure zone created was inhibited by 84% during normal contractions, by 41% during fast-propagating contractions, but only by 2.6% during simultaneous contractions. Progressive failure of deglutitive inhibition results in decreased latency and increased propagation velocity of esophageal smooth muscle contraction. Simultaneous contractions, a hallmark of manometric dysmotility, occur when there is an absence of inhibition. Behar and Biancani[39] have confirmed that there is a significantly decreased latency period for simultaneous contractions as compared with controls. Furthermore, consecutive swallows do not inhibit spontaneous contractions in patients with simultaneous contractions. The authors conclude that simultaneous contractions are explained by defective deglutitive inhibition, which appears to be associated with increased net excitation. The distinction between normal and disease states is blurred given Janssens and associates' discovery of bursts of nondeglutitive simultaneous contractions in 24 of 25 fasted normal volunteers.[40] These bursts of simultaneous contractions were temporally coincident with phase III of the migrating myoelectric complex (MMC) and not associated with LES relaxation. The authors conclude that simultaneous contractions represent the esophageal body component of the MMC.

Manometry remains the reference diagnostic standard for the evaluation of esophageal dysmotility. Johnston and colleagues[41] reviewed 276 consecutive manometric and patient records to determine the clinical utility of manometry. They found that manometry revealed dysmotility in 50% of cases, altered patient diagnosis in 25% of cases, and altered patient management in 50% of cases. Of course, the clinical utility of manometry will vary with patient selection. Computer modeling may serve as a useful adjunct to manometry. Li et al.[42] applied novel techniques of computer and mathematical modeling of manometric and videofluoroscopic data to case studies of liquid bolus propagation. They demonstrated that esophageal bolus retention can occur as a result of spatiotemporal discoordination of independent striated and smooth muscle peristaltic waves. Topographic analysis of conventional manometry tracings may also provide additional insight. Clouse and Staiano[43] created topographic plots from manometry records of patients with nutcracker esophagus and normal controls and were able to delineate separate components for each contraction: skeletal, proximal smooth muscle, distal smooth muscle, and LES. They found that nutcracker esophagus resulted from increased smooth muscle contraction (distal greater than proximal). Skeletal muscle and LES contractions were normal. Finally, the use of an intraluminal strain gauge may provide evidence of esophageal dysmotility in patients with normal manometry. Patients with dysphagia but normal manometry demonstrated decreased esophageal traction forces when compared with normal controls.[44]

Cervical dysphoria or globus sensation is a common patient complaint of unclear pathogenesis. Farkkila et al.[45] evaluated 21 such patients with previous normal otolaryngologic examinations by psychiatric evaluation, manometry, pH testing, EGD, and acid perfusion. Psychiatric diagnoses were made in 5 of 20 (25%) patients. Manometry revealed dysmotility in 66% of the patients, whereas esophagitis was detected in 14%. An abnormal Bernstein test was observed in 62%. When pH testing and EGD were combined, 33% of the patients were found to have GERD. Quite different results were obtained by Ott et al.,[46] who found that only a minority of patients with globus sensation had demonstrable pathology. Normal pH monitoring was noted in 18 of 22 patients, and videofluoroscopy and barium esophagrams were normal in 17 of 22.

Globus sensation may uncommonly result from an inlet patch of heterotopic gastric mucosa (IPHGM). This is typically observed as a small, sharply demarcated reddish mucosal patch in the upper part of the esophagus. Symptoms, if present, are thought to result from acid production and may respond to antisecretory therapy. Complications include stricture, cricopharyngeal spasm, polyp formation, tracheoesophageal fistula, development of adenocarcinoma, and the formation of a ring or web.[47] Nakajima et al.[48] described a prevalence of 3% in patients undergoing EGD and confirmed the ability of an IPHGM to produce acid.

It remains unclear whether esophagitis causes transient esophageal motor abnormalities or, conversely, whether esophageal dysmotility is a primary etiologic factor in the development of esophagitis. Kasapidis et al.[49] have demonstrated that the severity of esophagitis is directly correlated with the degree of esophageal acid exposure as determined by ambulatory pH monitoring and inversely correlated with esophageal peristaltic amplitude and duration. Likewise, Singh et al.[50] reported that the presence of Barrett's mucosa is strongly associated with increased acid exposure and esophageal motor dysfunction. The authors performed multivariate analysis on 94 patients with GERD and controls and concluded that there was a strong correlation between length of the Barrett's segment and the degree of acid exposure as measured by the ACT, as well as the degree of acid exposure and the presence of dysmotility.

Three studies have examined esophageal motility after healing of esophagitis and have found conflicting results. One[51] demonstrated no significant change in LES pressure, contraction amplitude, or distension threshold, but did note a significant increase in esophageal traction force. Another[52] reported that the percentage of peristaltic contractions significantly increased, with improvement in dyskinesia in 11 of 14 patients. The third study,[53] however, was unable to detect improvement in any parameter of esophageal motility. The inability to consistently demonstrate improvement in esophageal motility after healing of esophagitis may be due to insufficient length of antisecretory therapy, a type II study error, irreversible dysmotility after severe injury, or the presence of non–acid-related mediator(s) of dysmotility in GERD.

GASTROESOPHAGEAL REFLUX DISEASE

Pathogenesis

The pathogenesis of GERD is multifactorial: (1) incompetent LES, (2) abnormal GEJ barrier function, (3) impaired esophageal acid clearance or neutralization, (4) delayed gastric emptying, (5) altered esophageal mucosal resistance, or (6) enhanced potency of the gastroduodenal refluxate.

Multiple endogenous and exogenous substances affect LES pressure. Coben et al.[54] obtained LES pressures in subjects at the time of percutaneous gastrostomy and 24 hours later, before and after a feeding challenge. They observed that the mean LES pressure after continuous feeding was maintained at 14.3 mm Hg from a baseline of 16.6 mm Hg but fell to 2.1 mm Hg after bolus feeding. Gastroesophageal reflux was confirmed scintigraphically after bolus but not continuous feeding. They hypothesized that gastric distension after bolus feeding induces LES relaxation. Coffee may also induce reflux. Wendl et al.[55] demonstrated that although decaffeination of coffee significantly diminished GER, appreciable GER persisted. Caffeinated water, however, did not induce GER, which implies that components of coffee other than caffeine mediate GER. Cholestyramine stimulates cholecystokinin (CCK) release and decreases LES pressure. Cholecystokinin does not appear, however, to mediate LES basal tone.[56] Cholecystokinin induces transient LES relaxation in normal controls but not in patients with GERD.[57] Psychological stress created by cold, a math task, or a stressful interview also results in decreased LES pressure, which is in part compensated for by increased crural diaphragmatic contraction.[58]

Body positioning clearly affects esophageal clearance. Katz et al.[59] studied normal subjects after a refluxogenic meal and noted a significantly increased ACT with subjects in the right decubitus position vs. the left. The authors speculate that this may be due to straightening of the esophageal curve at the GEJ or, alternatively, may result from the anatomic position of the GEJ below the gastric pool.

The importance of supine reflux to the development of esophageal mucosal injury is an area of continued study. Orr et al.[60] compared upright and supine ACTs in GERD patients with and without esophagitis. The number of episodes of supine reflux lasting longer than 5 minutes was the best predictor of erosive mucosal damage. Saraswat et al.[61] found that patients with combined (both upright and supine) reflux or patients with supine reflux alone demonstrated increased acid exposure and more severe esophagitis than did patients with upright reflux alone.

The potency of the gastroduodenal refluxate, either acid or bile, affects the severity of esophageal injury. Gastric acid hypersecretion was demonstrated in fewer than 2% of the controls, 19% of the patients with pyrosis without esophagitis, 28% of the patients with esophagitis, and 35% of the patients with Barrett's metaplasia.[62] Acid hypersecretion is thus common in GERD, and its prevalence correlates with the severity of mucosal injury. Furthermore, acid hypersecretion is a predictor of treatment failure with standard-dose histamine receptor blocker (H$_2$RB) therapy.

Stein et al.[63] performed esophageal aspiration and pH monitoring after EGD on patients with GERD and controls. They found that patients with GERD, in particular those with Barrett's mucosa or a peptic stricture, had increased exposure to bile acids that correlated with alkaline contact time (pH > 7). These abnormalities were almost exclusively found in patients who had surgical disruption of the gastroduodenal barrier.

At a cellular level, the mechanisms of epithelial cell injury are poorly understood. One research focus has been acid injury in rabbit esophageal epithelial cells. Tobey et al.[64] have demonstrated that intracellular acidification occurs as a result of two mechanisms: (1) diminished extrusion of protons by Na$^+$/H$^+$ and Na$^+$-dependent Cl$^-$/HCO$_3^-$ exchangers, but more so by (2) increased proton loading mediated by the Cl$^-$ concentration–dependent, Na$^+$-independent Cl$^-$/HCO$_3^-$ exchanger. Another mechanism of cellular injury is cell volume regulation, an important mechanism of cell homeostasis. The regulatory volume decrease is K$^+$ and Cl$^-$ conduction dependent and inhibited by decreases in pH.[65]

Although the factors leading to esophageal injury have been well described, very little is known about the intrinsic mechanisms of the esophageal epithelium to protect itself and even less about what defects occur in GERD. Hills[66] has used techniques for the assessment of morphology and hydrophobicity on esophageal epithelium that were previously applied to gastric epithelium. He has postulated the existence of a bile salt–sensitive, surface-active phospholipid or surfactant layer on the esophageal epithelial surface similar but less dense than that associated with gastric epithelium by virtue of characteristic hydrophobicity and ultrastructural features. This has been confirmed by other investigators.[67]

In parallel, investigators at the University of Virginia have developed a new esophageal perfusion catheter equipped with two balloons that compartmentalizes a segment of esophageal lumen to allow analysis of the mucosa and esophageal secretions. They corroborate the existence of a superficial mucous layer characterized by indwelling prostaglandins, growth factors, and other proteins that constitutes the first layer of defense against gastric refluxate. Namiot et al.[68] demonstrated continuous basal esophageal mucus release, with a significant increase in mucus and protein release and decreased viscosity upon acid/pepsin exposure. The authors

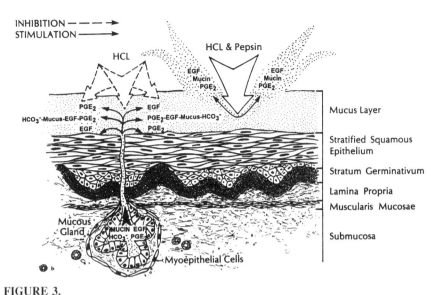

FIGURE 3.
Schematic outline of HCl and HCl/pepsin-related changes within the esophageal mucosal compartment leading to the luminal release of mucin, epidermal growth factor *(EGF)*, and esophageal prostaglandin E₂ *(PGE₂)*. (From Namiot Z, Sarosiek J, Rourk M, et al: *Gastroenterology* 106:973–981, 1994. Used by permission.)

believe that this is due to degradation of the mucous layer. Sarosiek et al.[69, 70] similarly described continuous esophageal prostaglandin E_2 (PGE_2) and epidermal growth factor (EGF) release that is significantly increased with acid/pepsin exposure. Again, this is thought to be due to degradation of the mucous layer with release of its indwelling proteins (Fig 3). Finally, via open perfusion of an esophageal segment, Brown et al.[71] have demonstrated esophageal bicarbonate secretion.

The contribution of esophageal bicarbonate to acid neutralization appears small, however, in comparison to the salivary component. Namiot et al.[72] have also suggested an important protective role for salivary secretion in the maintenance of esophageal epithelial integrity. The authors stimulated esophageal mechanoreceptors and chemoreceptors and observed an increase in the volume, pH, and viscosity of salivary secretions. The range of protective effects of the esophagosalivary reflex has yet to be established.

The University of Virginia group has also begun to investigate mucosal defense mechanisms in disease. Rourk et al.[73] demonstrated impaired salivary EGF release by esophageal mechanoreceptor and chemoreceptor stimulation in patients with reflux esophagitis. Edmunds et al.[74] demonstrated a profound decrease in esophageal EGF secretion in patients with reflux esophagitis. Moreover, this abnormality persists after healing of the esophageal mucosa, which may predispose the mucosa to recurrent injury.

Diagnosis

Assessment of acid exposure by esophageal pH monitoring is considered the gold standard for diagnosing GERD. Determination of the alkaline contact time, or the percentage of time with the pH greater than 7, during pH monitoring has been proposed as an index of alkaline reflux. Combined esophageal and gastric pH monitoring in ten normal subjects during salivary stimulation revealed simultaneous gastric and esophageal alkalinization in four of them.[75] This pattern mimics and can be mistaken for gastroduodenal reflux. Measurement of the bile acid concentration by esophageal aspiration is a more direct indication of alkaline reflux. Iftikhar et al.[76] noted that although bile acids were present in the esophagi of normal controls, increased concentrations were noted in patients with GERD and esophagitis, and this reached statistical significance in patients with Barrett's mucosa. The clinical importance of bile reflux in esophageal injury remains to be elucidated.

Barium radiography is inferior to pH monitoring for the detection of GERD. Using pH monitoring as the standard, Thompson et al.[77] found barium radiography to have a sensitivity of 26% for a diagnosis of GERD (specificity, 94%); this improved to 44% with the addition of stress maneuvers and to 70% with addition of the water-siphon test. Utilization of the water-siphon test, however, reduces the specificity to 74%.

Pulmonary Manifestations

Two main theories have been advanced to explain the pathogenesis of cough and reactive airway disease in some patients with GER: the aspiration theory and the esophageal-tracheobronchial reflux theory. Recent evidence supports the latter hypothesis. Ing et al.[78] challenged 22 patients with GERD and 12 controls with esophageal acid and saline perfusion. Acid perfusion triggered a significantly increased cough frequency in both groups. The cough frequency was higher in patients than controls. Acid-induced cough could be inhibited by esophageal instillation of a topical anesthetic and antagonized by ipratropium bromide. The authors conclude that cough is mediated by an esophageal-tracheobronchial reflex arc (rather than aspiration) involving esophageal mucosal receptors triggering an afferent sensory limb and a cholinergically mediated efferent limb. Irwin et al.[79] reached the same conclusion. They performed dual proximal and distal pH monitoring with symptom (cough) index determination on 12 patients with cough and suspected GER. Ten of 12 patients had a positive symptom index correlation with distal reflux, whereas no significant proximal reflux was noted. All patients' coughs resolved with antireflux therapy. The diagnostic yield of standard pH-metry and the Bernstein test was lower. This reflex arc has also been implicated in the pathogenesis of laryngospasm and may be an etiology of sudden infant death syndrome.

Bauman et al.[80] have shown that stimulation of canine distal esophageal mucosal chemoreceptors with capsaicin induces age-dependent, vagally mediated sustained laryngospasm.

Peptic Stricture

Peptic strictures occur in 2% to 5% of patients with GERD. Balloon dilation offers an alternative to traditional bougienage therapy. However, the bougie technique proved superior to balloon dilation in a recent randomized trial.[81] Thirty-nine percent of the patients in the balloon (Rigiflex) arm vs. 15% in the bougie (Celestin, Eder-Peustow) arm required redilation at the 1-year follow-up. Both treatments were extremely well tolerated, and no serious complications were reported.

Although antisecretory therapy has been successful in healing stricture-associated esophagitis, it has only recently been shown to have an impact on the need for dilation. Marks et al.[82] randomized 34 patients with esophagitis and peptic strictures to omeprazole, 20 mg/day, or standard-dose H_2RB after initial dilation. At the 6-month follow-up, the omeprazole group had a significantly higher rate of esophagitis healing (100% vs. 53%) and dysphagia relief (94% vs. 40%) and required fewer repeat dilations (31 vs. 11) than the H_2RB arm. A comparison between lansoprazole, 30 mg/day, and high-dose ranitidine, 600 mg twice daily, yielded similar results.[83]

Medical Therapy

Treatment of GERD should always include lifestyle and dietary modifications. When these fail, adjunctive pharmacologic therapy may be initiated. Histamine receptor blockers have been the mainstay of GERD therapy and have been proved to decrease reflux symptoms and improve esophagitis. The prokinetic agent cisapride has also been demonstrated to be effective in the treatment of GERD. Proton-pump inhibitors are the most powerful anti-secretory agents. Omeprazole has been extensively studied and proved to be the most effective medical therapy for GERD. Ducrotte et al.[84] have shown in an open crossover study that in esophagitis patients, omperazole, 20 mg/day, reduced the ACT from 6.5% at baseline to 0%, whereas famotidine, 40 mg twice daily, reduced the ACT to only 4%.

Standard practice is to administer omeprazole at 20 mg/day and either prolong the course of therapy or increase the dose for nonresponders. Bate et al.[85] randomized 313 patients with esophagitis to 8 weeks of omeprazole, 20 mg/day (group 1), or 4 weeks of omeprazole, 20 mg/day, followed by 4 weeks of omeprazole, 40 mg/day (group 2). Sixty-five percent of the patients in group 1 healed vs. 74% in group 2 (not significant), thus implying that the duration of therapy with omeprazole is more important than the dose for healing esophagitis.

Few data are available on the long-term outcome of treating patients medically for esophagitis. Kuster et al.[86] described the course of 107 patients primarily with mild esophagitis, 89 of whom had a 6-year follow-up. Twenty-three patients required surgery whereas 55% responded to conservative therapy and 20% depended on continuous antisecretory therapy. The initial therapeutic response predicted the continued long-term therapeutic response. Low LES pressure (<7 mm Hg), radiologic reflux, and esophagitis were independent predictors of the need for vigorous medical therapy.

Surgical Therapy

Despite the potency of the newer antisecretory agents, a minority of patients with GERD will prove refractory to medical therapy or require lifelong vigorous medical therapy and opt for surgical repair. The standard and by far most commonly performed operative procedure is the Nissen fundoplication (NF). It is well tolerated and no other open technique has to date proved more effective. Urschel[87] reviewed 355 antireflux procedures (349 NFs) and reported a 1% mortality and 17% morbidity rate, with prior hiatal dissection noted to be a significant risk factor for morbidity. Although several series by skilled surgeons have documented excellent results, concern has been raised as to the reproducibility of these results by less experienced surgeons. Dunnington et al.[88] reported a series of 58 patients who underwent NF performed by surgical residents supervised by their respective faculty members at eight Veterans Administration hospitals. There were no operative deaths, and the complication rate was 18%. Symptoms were relieved in 93% and the esophagitis was completely healed in 77% of the patients at the 2-year follow-up. Concern has also been raised regarding the advisability of performing NF or any antireflux surgery in patients with esophageal motility disorders. Bremner et al.[89] reported 100 patients who underwent NF, 44 of whom had a nonspecific motility disorder. At a 50-month median follow-up, they found no difference in postoperative success in this group as compared with those patients with normal motility. Clearly, however, a severe motility disturbance should still be considered a contraindication to NF. With longer follow-up, more frequent problems with NF may arise. At a mean follow-up of 11 years, Grande et al.[90] still noted excellent results, with 79% of their patients completely free of reflux symptoms and only 9% with disabling side effects. In contrast, in the longest follow-up to date, Luostarinen et al.[91] reported on 25 patients out of an initial cohort of 46. At a median follow-up of 20 years, the following were noted: 2 patients required repeat NF, 44% of the patients described GERD symptoms, 38% of those who underwent endoscopy demonstrated esophagitis, 6 defective wraps were noted at endoscopy, and an additional 32% of the patients noted gas bloating or dysphagia.

Since 1991 when the first NF was performed under laparoscopic guidance, the technique has become increasingly popular. Laparoscopic performance does not appear to compromise the procedure; in fact, better visualization may be achieved than via the open technique. Most patients can be discharged within 2 or 3 days, and the recovery period is considerably shortened. Early results indicate acceptable complication rates, low conversion rates, and comparable efficacy to the open procedure. Early postoperative dysphagia appears transient and resolves within 1 month in the majority of cases. Persistent reflux occurs in a minority of patients. In a review of 132 laparoscopic NF procedures, the mean hospital stay was 3 days.[92] No mortality and a 7.5% morbidity rate with 4 conversions to open procedures were reported. Within the first month, 9 patients required dilation for dysphagia, but by 3 months symptoms persisted in only 3 patients, 1 of whom required a reoperation. There were no cases of gas bloating and only 1 instance of recurrent GERD. Forty patients underwent follow-up EGD, and all had healed their esophagitis. Smaller series[93–95] have achieved similar results with excellent patient satisfaction. A nondisabling side effect frequently noted is persistent early satiety.[95] Longer follow-up is required, but there is no reason to expect that the laparoscopic approach will not supplant the open procedure as the mainstay of surgical antireflux procedures in the near future.

The laparoscopic Hill repair appears to be one viable alternative. In their series of 40 initial cases, Aye et al.[96] noted no serious complications; 5 conversions to open repair were required. Ninety-two percent of the patients thought their result to be good or excellent, although 6 patients required postoperative dilation. Concern remains, however, about the technical difficulty of the Hill technique and its general applicability to other centers.

Reoperation after failed fundoplication remains problematic. Collard et al.[97] have accumulated a series of 55 reoperations primarily for slipped or migrated wraps and noted a much higher complication rate; 5.4% mortality and 24% morbidity. Moreover, at a mean follow-up of 42 months after reoperation, 30% of the patients remained disabled. Twenty-one of the 55 patients undergoing reoperations were noted to have significant esophageal dysmotility, which underscores the need for careful patient selection before surgical referral.

Barrett's Metaplasia

With chronic esophageal injury in the setting of GERD, the normal squamous esophageal epithelium can be replaced by a metaplastic specialized intestinal epithelium, Barrett's epithelium (BE). The mechanism of replacement has been thought to be slow cephalad migration of the Z line representing progressive denudation of the squamous epithelium and replacement by BE (creeping substitution theory). This hypothesis has been challenged by a model of rapid loss of squamous epithelium whereby BE arises multifocally as islands from multipotential stem cells within esophageal glands of the squamous mucosa. In an elegant dog study, Li et al.[98] induced BE at the site of esophageal mucosal defects created surgically after GER was induced by cardioplasty and pentagastrin stimulation. Re-creation of the mucosal defect and removal of the acid stimulus resulted in a recurrence of BE, but interspersed among islands of normal squamous epithelium.

Cameron determined the clinically (endoscopically) diagnosed prevalence of BE to be 1.8 per 1,000 as compared with the autopsy prevalence of 37.6 per 1,000.[99] This is a sobering statistic: in only 1 in 20 patients is Barrett's esophagus diagnosed during their lifetime. Barrett's epithelium may be even more prevalent if one considers so-called short-segment Barrett's epithelium, defined as the presence of specialized intestinal epithelium within 2 cm of the GEJ. Zeroogian et al.[100] found short-segment BE in 20% of 102 patients undergoing EGD. The presence of esophageal symptoms did not correlate with the identification of short-segment BE.

Adenocarcinoma will develop in some patients with BE. Dysplasia is a crucial epithelial marker for neoplastic progression. Reid et al.[101] identified separate cell cycle abnormalities that distinguish BE and dysplasia. Barrett's epithelium is characterized by early mobilization of cells from G_0 and G_1 and increased cellular proliferation. Dysplasia correlates with loss of control of the transition between G_1 and S phase, a resultant accumulation in G_2, and genomic instability.

p53, a tumor suppressor gene on chromosome 17, has been identified as another biomarker for neoplastic progression. p53 is thought to mediate the G_1 checkpoint, so a lack of functional p53 gene expression allows cells to enter S phase inappropriately and also induces genomic instability.[102] p53 gene mutations lead to accumulation of the p53 protein intracellularly, thus allowing for its detection via antibody binding. Several studies have now demonstrated a parallel between increasing p53 immunoreactivity and neoplastic progression in BE.[103–105] p53 may thus be used to predict the development of cancer before the development of high-grade dysplasia or intramucosal carcinoma. The following remain unclear: (1) the percentage of patients with BE and p53 expression in whom adenocarcinoma will develop, (2) the time frame over which this progression may occur, and (3) the percentage of cancers that are not characterized by p53 expression.

Early, minimally invasive cancers are typically not visible endoscopically, and detection is based on periodic screening and random biopsy. Male sex, length of the BE segment, and smoking have been identified as risk factors for the development of adenocarcinoma in BE. These findings have not yet been incorporated into screening strategies.[106] Endoscopic ultrasonography unfortunately cannot differentiate between benign and malignant wall thickening.[107] Consequently, there is no role at present for EUS in BE screening.

Treatment of high-grade dysplasia (HGD) is controversial. Rice et al.[108] found that 6 of 16 (38%) patients who underwent esophagectomy for HGD harbored undetected intramucosal carcinomas. This would seem to justify the 6% mortality and 44% early and 73% late morbidity rates associated with esophagectomy. In contrast, only 1 undetected carcinoma was discovered in 13 patients undergoing esophagectomy for BE with HGD at the Mayo Clinic.[109] An alternative to prophylactic esophagectomy is endoscopic screening. The University of Washington group[110] has adopted an aggressive screening strategy for patients with BE and HGD that involves jumbo biopsy forceps, multiple biopsy specimens per endoscopy, and frequent procedures. Of 50 patients enrolled in such screening, 28 went to esophagectomy, thus allowing a correlation with endoscopic histology. Endoscopy correctly identified all 19 carcinomas and 7 of the 9 cases of HGD. Two patients thought to harbor adenocarcinomas were found to have only HGD at esophagectomy. Despite these impressive findings, the generalizability of these results to other centers is unknown, and at present, this screening strategy cannot be widely recommended.

Another approach is to ablate BE. Several techniques have been proposed, including medical therapy with proton-pump inhibitors, laser therapy, and photodynamic therapy. Gore et al.[111] treated 23 BE patients with 1 to 2 years of omeprazole, 40 mg/day. Barrett's epithelium regressed with a significant decrease in length and the appearance of islands of squamous epithelium. In a similar study, although no change in length of the BE segment was noted, squamous epithelial islands were demonstrated.[112] Wang et al.[113] randomized patients to omeprazole, 20 mg/day, or to photodynamic therapy and omeprazole. At 6 months, no regression of BE was observed in the omeprazole-treated group, whereas the length of BE decreased by more than 4 cm in 7 of 24 of the patients who underwent photodynamic therapy. The efficacy of photodynamic therapy is enhanced by a centering balloon allowing uniform and circumferential esophageal mucosal injury.[114] Salo et al.[115] have ablated BE in 4 patients with a neodynium-YAG laser after antireflux surgery. Ablation techniques are promising but remain experimental. Theoretical and practical concerns persist regarding the adequacy of BE ablation (full depth?), cost, and patient acceptance.

NONSPECIFIC ESOPHAGEAL INJURY

Radiation Esophagitis

Esophageal irradiation may result in esophagitis and stricture. Increased prostaglandin synthesis has been noted in exposed esophageal tissue, which implies that there may be a role for prostaglandin inhibitors in the prevention of radiation sequelae. In a small placebo-controlled trial of 28 patients, naproxen, 375 mg twice daily, offered no advantage over placebo.[116] Although no benefit of prostaglandin inhibition was observed, this may have been due to a type II error.

Radiation-induced strictures may be more difficult to dilate than peptic strictures. In a review of 103 patients, Swaroop et al.[117] achieved a 98% technical success rate and were able to dilate the esophagus of 78 patients to greater than 12.8 mm in a single session. One third of the patients noted persistent dysphagia. There were 9 minor and 3 major complications (2 perforations, 1 fistula). The median duration of dysphagia relief was only 16 weeks.

Corrosive Esophagitis

Although corrosive esophageal injury in adults is uncommon in this country, this is not true in other parts of the world. Broor et al.[118] reviewed 123 patients with strictures, 59 of which were due to corrosive injury. Although 94% of the corrosive strictures could be adequately dilated, corrosive strictures were six to seven times more likely to recur than peptic strictures. Corrosive strictures were also more likely to perforate during dilation (0.8% vs. 0.26%). Prevention of stricture formation after corrosive injury has to date been minimally successful. Epidermal growth factor and interferon-γ can prevent stricture formation following corrosive esophageal injury in rats.[119]

Infectious Esophagitis

Esophageal infections are seen primarily in immunocompromised patients. *Candida,* cytomegalovirus (CMV), and herpes simplex virus (HSV) are the major pathogens and are typically identified via endoscopy with biopsy or brushing. Multiple histopathologic techniques can then be applied, including conventional and centrifuged culture, standard histology, immunohistology, and DNA hybridization. Either conventional or centrifuged culture appears to have the highest diagnostic yield for the detection of CMV.[120] A new cytology balloon for blind esophageal brushing has been shown to have a similar yield to endoscopy with biopsy and brushing for the diagnosis of infectious esophagitis in patients with acquired immunodeficiency syndrome (AIDS).[121]

The most common esophageal infectious pathogen is *Candida.* Given the prevalence of esophageal candidiasis in patients with AIDS, most clinicians empirically treat such patients with a course of antifungal therapy. Wilcox[122] reports that this results in a 90% 1-week and 100% 2-week symptom response rate. If symptoms persist after a 1- to 2-week course of therapy, EGD is indicated. After successful treatment of esophageal candidiasis, infection frequently recurs or relapses. Parente et al.[123] randomized 106 AIDS patients after successful treatment of their first episode of esophageal candidiasis to placebo or prophylaxis with ketoconazole, 200 mg/day, or fluconazole, 50 mg/day. The 12-month cumulative probability of relapse was 38% in the prophylaxis group as compared with 84% in the placebo group. Fluconazole proved more efficacious than ketoconazole. Despite these findings, *Candida* prophylaxis in this group of patients cannot yet be recommended until the following issues have been examined: side effects, drug interactions, cost, and emergence of drug-resistant *Candida* strains.

Esophageal ulcers may directly result from infection with the human immunodeficiency virus (HIV). This theory is supported by ultrastructural evidence from electron microscopy.[124] Frager et al.[125] presented a series of ten AIDS patients with large solitary ulcers without evidence of HSV or CMV infection. In six patients

HIV was detected in the ulcer base but not in the surrounding mucosa. The ulcers of nine patients healed with steroid therapy.

ESOPHAGEAL TRAUMA/FOREIGN BODY

Esophageal Trauma

Management of suspected traumatic esophageal penetration depends on the clinical circumstances. If immediate surgical exploration is not indicated, the diagnosis can be made by esophagography or EGD. In a recent series,[126] water-soluble contrast esophagography achieved 100% sensitivity and 100% specificity. Esophagogastroduodenoscopy proved to be less specific in a series of 13 cases reviewed by Horwitz et al.[127] Although the sensitivity of EGD was 100%, the specificity was 83%, with 2 false-positives leading to unnecessary surgical exploration.

Esophagectomy is superior to primary repair in patients with esophageal perforation complicated by mediastinal sepsis and whose diagnosis is delayed (>24 hours). Salo et al.[128] noted a 68% mortality rate with primary repair as compared with a 13% mortality rate with esophagectomy ($P = .001$).

Esophageal Foreign Bodies

The aim of therapy in esophageal obstruction by a foreign body is its expedient removal before and without incurring a complication. The mainstay of therapy is endoscopic removal. Endoscopy, either rigid or flexible, was successful in 96% of 111 adult cases.[129] There were 2 perforations resulting in 1 death. Complications occur more frequently with rigid endoscopy. In a review of 193 adult and pediatric cases of foreign body extraction,[130] 59 adults underwent flexible EGD with 1 complication and 1 failure, whereas rigid esophagoscopy resulted in a 10% complication rate.

Glucagon has been proposed as a noninvasive alternative to EGD in the management of esophageal food impaction. In one series glucagon was successful in only 3 of 25 attempts.[129] Robbins and Shortsleeve[131] achieved a 69% success rate by using 1 mg of intravenous glucagon in addition to water (1 cup) and an effervescent agent (1 cup E-Z Gas II) taken orally. Although no complications were observed, one can not conclude that this technique is completely safe because of the small sample size (n = 43). Additionally, the use of barium to document foreign body impaction will thwart subsequent endoscopic attempts to remove the foreign body in patients who fail glucagon treatment. Flexible EGD remains the procedure of choice for foreign body extraction, and diagnostic contrast radiography should be avoided.

ESOPHAGEAL VARICES

Upper gastrointestinal bleeding caused by rupture of esophageal varices is a common and life-threatening complication of portal hypertension. Both medical and surgical therapies aimed at eliminating or decompressing esophageal varices are associated with significant morbidity. Investigators have thus sought to stratify patients according to bleeding risk. Burkhart et al.[132] used cine phase-contrast magnetic resonance flow measurements to identify patients at risk for esophageal variceal hemorrhage (EVH). In 32 patients with esophageal varices, stratification by portal venous flow greater or less than 15 mL/min-kg resulted in a 89% sensitivity and 90% specificity for the prediction of subsequent EVH (Fig 4).

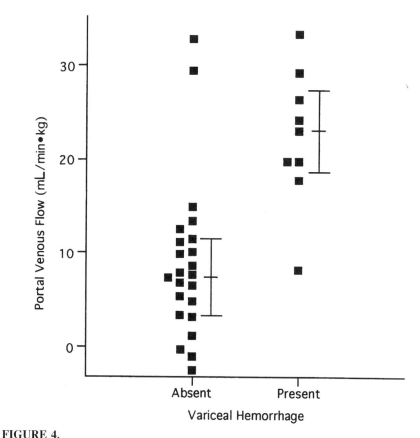

FIGURE 4.
Scatterplot of portal venous flow vs. the presence of variceal hemorrhage within 2 years before the magnetic resonance study. High flow was significantly associated with variceal bleeding on univariate ($P = .001$) and multivariate ($P = .006$) analysis. Three *horizontal bars* indicate 75th percentile *(top bar)*, and 25th percentile *(bottom bar)*. (From Burkhart DJ, Johnson CD, Ehman RL, et al: *Radiology* 188:643–648, 1993. Used by permission.)

Risk factors for recurrent EVH after endoscopic sclerotherapy have also been identified. Lin et al.[133] used CT to detect paraesophageal collaterals. Those patients harboring collaterals, as compared with those without, were at increased risk for variceal recurrence (57% vs. 16%, $P < .05$) and EVH (29% vs. 3%, $P < .05$) at a 20-month follow-up. Kokawa et al.[134] prospectively followed 197 patients with EVH who had undergone endoscopic sclerotherapy. Independent predictors for recurrent EVH included incomplete eradication of esophageal varices, the presence of hepatocellular carcinoma, and Child-Pugh class.

Treatment: Endoscopic Sclerotherapy

Sodium tetradecyl sulfate (STS) and ethanolamine are the most common sclerosants used for endoscopic sclerotherapy. A randomized comparison of the two revealed equivalent success in control of bleeding as well as no difference in the rates of subsequent esophageal ulceration, stricture formation, or perforation.[135] Sodium tetradecyl sulfate obliterated esophageal varices more rapidly than ethanolamine did (mean, 3.3 vs. 4.5 sessions, $P < .05$).

Nitrates have been shown to decrease variceal pressure[136] and have been used in conjunction with vasopressin in the setting of acute EVH. In a recent randomized clinical trial,[137] isosorbide-5-mononitrate was superior to placebo during the course of esophageal sclerotherapy because of less frequent rebleeding (11% vs. 38%, $P = .01$) and death (2 vs. 9, $P = NS$). The role of propranolol in patients undergoing esophageal sclerotherapy is less clear. In one randomized trial,[138] propranolol reduced bleeding from gastric varices and portal gastropathy. Furthermore, there was a trend toward a decreased rate of variceal recurrence and bleeding. In contrast, Acharya et al.[139] found no difference in bleeding or mortality in patients receiving propranolol during esophageal sclerotherapy. Propranolol has also been compared directly with esophageal sclerotherapy for patients after initial EVH. In a randomized trial, Teres and coworkers[140] noted a significantly ($P = .02$) reduced rate of rebleeding with esophageal sclerotherapy (64%) as compared with propranolol (45%). However, no survival benefit was demonstrated, and esophageal sclerotherapy was associated with a higher complication rate (primarily because of ulcer and stricture formation).

Treatment: Alternatives to Endoscopic Sclerotherapy

Endoscopic band ligation (EBL) offers a significant advantage over endoscopic sclerotherapy because of decreased rebleeding, more rapid obliteration of esophageal varices, and a reduced rate of ulcer and stricture formation. Laine et al.[141] randomized 77 patients to endoscopic sclerotherapy or EBL. Although EBL conferred no survival benefit, there was a trend to decreased rebleeding (26%) vs. endoscopic sclerotherapy (44%). Complications were much less frequent with EBL (0% stricture and 2.6% ulcer rates) than with endoscopic sclerotherapy (33% stricture and 15% ulcer rates). Finally, fewer ligation treatments were required to achieve variceal obliteration with EBL (4.2 vs. 7.2). Similar results were obtained by Gimson et al.[142] in another randomized trial. Endoscopic band ligation was superior to endoscopic sclerotherapy in reducing rebleeding (30% vs. 53%, $P < .05$) and the number of ligation sessions needed to achieve variceal obliteration (mean, 3.4 vs. 4.9, $P = .006$). Surprisingly, complication rates were similar in the two groups.

Although postsclerotherapy ulceration and stricture formation have been attributed to a direct sclerosant effect, Berner and coworkers[143] hypothesize that these complications result from sclerotherapy-induced GER. Esophageal dysmotility and GER were more common in endoscopic sclerotherapy patients (five of eight and five of five, respectively) than in EBL patients (one of seven for both dysmotility and GER). Adjunctive therapy to endoscopic sclerotherapy may reduce complication rates. Juhl et al.[144] reported that subcutaneous and paravariceal injection of recombinant EGF prevents esophageal ulcer and stricture formation in pigs.

Alternatives to endoscopic sclerotherapy for the management of EVH include octreotide therapy and placement of a transjugular intrahepatic portosystemic shunt (TIPS). Octreotide has similar efficacy to endoscopic sclerotherapy in the acute setting. In a trial[145] of 98 patients randomized to emergency endoscopic sclerotherapy or octreotide (50-μg/hr bolus followed by 50-μg/hr continuous infusion), there were no differences in initial control of bleeding, rebleeding, blood transfusion requirements, and mortality at 48 hours. Octreotide also compares favorably to the combination of terlipressin (a vasopressin analogue) and transdermal nitroglycerin. In a randomized trial,[146] octreotide proved to be more effective than combination therapy in the initial control of bleeding (78% vs. 59%, $P = .06$). The 48-hour mortality rate was 6% in the octreotide group vs. 12% in the terlipressin group ($P = $ NS).

A TIPS procedure produces excellent results in tertiary centers with a high volume of EVH patients. These results have not been duplicated outside of this setting, and the technique cannot be advocated for widespread use. Rossle et al.[147] have achieved a 93% technical success rate on their first 100 patients, with mean reduction in portal venous pressure of 57%. They have reported a 15% major complication rate, primarily as a result of bleeding and stent migration, with a procedure-related mortality of 1% and a 30-day mortality of 3%. At a 1-year mean follow-up, they noted a 10% shunt occlusion rate and a 21% shunt stenosis rate. Hepatic encephalopathy developed in 25% of the patients. Two other studies have noted less favorable results: 11% and 45% 30-day (or in-hospital) mortality as well as 30% and 57% major complication rates, respectively.[148, 149]

Although intra-abdominal shunting procedures for control of portal hypertension in patients after EVH have fallen into disfavor, surgical nonshunting options exist. Mariette et al.[150] have reported promising results with the Suigara procedure, which does not alter hepatic blood flow. The procedure consists of esophagogastric devascularization, splenectomy, and esophageal transection. In a study of 39 patients, there were no postoperative deaths, and 95% and 76% of the patients were free of variceal bleeding at 1 and 5 years, respectively, with similar (95% and 70%) 1- and 5-year survival rates. There was a 46% complication rate, including anastomotic stricture formation (28%) and portal venous thrombosis (18%), but no cases of hepatic encephalopathy or liver failure were seen.

ESOPHAGEAL CANCER

Esophageal cancer is one of the most common fatal cancers worldwide. Despite advances in detection, the prognosis of esophageal cancer remains poor. Over the past 20 years, the incidence of adenocarcinoma of the esophagus has risen sharply in Western countries. Barrett's esophagus has been associated with this epidemic of adenocarcinoma, but the cause remains unclear. Unfortunately, no breakthroughs in our understanding of this phenomenon occurred in the year of our review.

PALLIATION OF MALIGNANT DYSPHAGIA

Modalities available for palliation of malignant dysphagia include the following: surgery, serial dilation, chemotherapy, radiotherapy, laser ablation, ethanol-induced tumor necrosis (ETN), photodynamic therapy, brachytherapy, and stenting. Although effective, laser ablation is costly, incurs a 10% serious complication rate (primarily perforation and tracheoesophageal fistula [TEF]), and requires frequent sessions to maintain esophageal luminal patency. Sander and Poesl[151] achieved a 96% technical success rate with a 10% serious complication rate and 1% mortality rate. On average, 2.3 sessions were required to achieve luminal patency, and restenosis occurred at a mean of 1 month. Carter et al.[152] similarly noted that 92% of their patients returned to a semi-solid diet or better, but the procedure-related mortality was 4% with a 9% incidence of perforation or TEF.

Ethanol-induced tumor necrosis is a simple, inexpensive, yet effective palliative measure with minimal complications. Nwokolo et al.[153] achieved excellent results with 32 patients: the mean dysphagia grade was reduced from 3 to 1 in a median of one treatment session. Moreover, they incurred no complications. It should be noted that dilation to 12 mm before ETN therapy was required in 14 patients and dysphagia recurred at a median interval of about 1 month. Moreira et al.[154] also reported no complications in 9 cases. Chung et al.[155] have reported similar success with ETN, but noted 3 complications in 36 patients: 2 instances of TEF and 1 episode of mediastinitis. Given the ease, minimal cost, and low incidence of complications as compared with other modalities, ETN may emerge as a first-line therapy for the palliation of malignant strictures.

The use of plastic stents has been limited because of complications during placement as well as long-term complications of migration and obstruction. Expandable metal stents are easier to place and are subject to fewer short-term complications. Knyrim et al.[156] randomized 42 patients to plastic stent vs. metal Wallstents. Although the technical and functional success rates were comparable in both groups, 3 instances of perforation and 1 case of aspiration led to 3 procedure-related deaths in the plastic stent group as opposed to no immediate complications in the metal stent group. Recurrence of dysphagia was comparable in the two groups, with 5 plastic stent migrations offset by 5 metal stents obstructed by tumor ingrowth or overgrowth. Despite the high cost of metal stents, they proved more cost-effective.

SUMMARY

The study of esophageal disorders continues to be fruitful. This chapter has chronicled advances in the past year in our understanding of topics ranging from esophageal physiology to mucosal defense mechanisms. We have reviewed new therapies for esophageal varices and malignant dysphagia as well as promising new techniques such as botulinum toxin injection, laparoscopic fundoplication, and esophageal banding. We hope that this survey will complement current strategies for the clinical management of esophageal disorders.

REFERENCES

1. Castiglione F, Emde C, Armstrong D, et al: Nocturnal oeseophageal motor activity is dependent on sleep stage. *Gut* 34:1653–1659, 1993.
2. Mayrand S, Diamant NE: Measurement of human esophageal tone in vivo. *Gastroenterology* 105:1411–1420, 1993.
3. Anand N, Paterson WG: Role of nitric oxide in esophageal peristalsis. *Am J Physiol* 266:G123–G131, 1994.
4. Akbarali HI, Goyal RK: Effect of sodium nitroprusside on calcium currents in opossum esophageal circular muscle cells. *Am J Physiol* 266:G1036–G1042, 1994.
5. Saha JK, Hirano I, Goyal RK: Biphasic effect of SNP on opossum esophageal longitudinal muscle: Involvement of cGMP and eicosanoids. *Am J Physiol* 265:G403–G407, 1993.
6. Behar J, Guenard V, Walsh JH, et al: Vasoactive intestinal polypeptide and acetylcholine: Inhibitory and excitatory neurotransmitters in the cat esophagus. *Am J Physiol* 257:G380–G385, 1989.
7. Sohn UD, Chiu TT, Bitar KN, et al: Calcium requirements for acetylcholine-induced contraction of cat esophageal circular muscle cells. *Am J Physiol* 266:G330–G338, 1994.
8. Sohn UD, Harnett KM, De Petris G, et al: Distinct muscarinic receptors, G proteins and phospholipases in esophageal and lower esophageal sphincter circular muscle. *J Pharmacol Exp Ther* 267:1205–1214, 1993.
9. Huber O, Bertrand C, Bunnett W, et al: Tachykinins contract the circular muscle of the human esophageal body in vitro via NK2 receptors. *Gastroenterology* 105:981–987, 1993.
10. Huber O, Bertrand C, Bunnett N, et al: Tachykinins mediate contraction of the human lower esophageal sphincter in vitro via activation of NK2 receptors. *Eur J Pharmacol* 239:103–109, 1993.

11. Sandler AD, Schlegel JF, DeSautel MG, et al: Neuroregulation of a chemosensitive afferent system in the canine distal esophagus. *J Surg Res* 55:364–371, 1993.

12. Biancani P, Harnett KM, Sohn UD, et al: Differential signal transduction pathways in cat lower esophageal sphincter tone and response to ACh. *Am J Physiol* 266:G767–G774, 1994.

13. Pasricha NJ, Ravich WJ, Kalloo AN: Effects of intrasphincteric botulinum toxin on the lower esophageal sphincter in piglets. *Gastroenterology* 105:1045–1049, 1993.

14. Preiksaitis HG, Tremblay L, Diamant NE: Nitric oxide mediates inhibitory nerve effects in human esophagus and lower esophageal sphincter. *Dig Dis Sci* 39:770–775, 1994.

15. Jury J, Ahmedzadeh N, Daniel EE: A mediator derived from arginine mediates inhibitory junction potentials and relaxation in lower esophageal sphincter: An independent role for VIP. *Can J Physiol Pharmacol* 70:1182–1189, 1992.

16. Mao YK, Wang YF, Daniel EE: Distribution and characterization of vasoactive intestinal polypeptide binding in canine lower esophageal sphincter. *Gastroenterology* 105:1370–1377, 1993.

17. Mittal RK, Sivri B, Schirmer BD, et al: Effect of crural myotomy on the incidence and mechanism of gastroesophageal reflux in cats. *Gastroenterology* 105:740–747, 1993.

18. Klein WA, Parkman HP, Dempsey DT, et al: Sphincterlike thoracoabdominal high pressure zone after esophagectomy. *Gastroenterology* 105:1362–1369, 1993.

19. Goldblum JR, Whyte RI, Orringer MB, et al: Achalasia: A morphologic study of 42 resected specimens. *Am J Surg Pathol* 18:327–337, 1994.

20. Tung HN, Shirazi S, Schulze-Delrieu K, et al: Morphologic changes of myenteric neurons in the partially obstructed opossum esophagus. *J Submicrosc Cytol Pathol* 25:357–363, 1993.

21. Zhang ZG, Diamant NE: Repetitive contractions of the upper esophageal body and sphincter in achalasia. *Dysphagia* 9:12–19, 1994.

22. Kim CH, Cameron AJ, Hsu JJ, et al: Achalasia: Prospective evaluation of relationship between lower esophageal sphincter pressure, esophageal transit, and esophageal diameter and symptoms in response to pneumatic dilation. *Mayo Clin Proc* 68:1067–1073, 1993.

23. Sharma R, Achkar E: Predictors of pneumatic dilatation in the treatment of achalasia (abstract). *Gastroenterology* 106:177, 1994.

24. Nair LA, Reynolds JC, Parkman HP, et al: Complications during pneumatic dilation for achalasia or diffuse esophageal spasm. *Dig Dis Sci* 38:1893–1904, 1993.

25. Schwartz HM, Cahow CE, Traube M: Outcome after perforation sustained during pneumatic dilatation for achalasia. *Dig Dis Sci* 38:1409–1413, 1993.

26. Ellis FH: Oesophagomyotomy for achalasia: A 22-year experience. *Br J Surg* 80:882–885, 1993.

27. Pellegrini CA, Leichter R, Patti M, et al: Thoracoscopic esophageal myotomy in the treatment of achalasia. *Ann Thorac Surg* 56:680–682, 1993.

28. Jaakola A, Reinikainen P, Ovaska J, et al: Barrett's esophagus after cardiomyotomy for esophageal achalasia. *Am J Gastroenterol* 89:165–169, 1994.

29. Shoenut JP, Wieler JA, Micflikier AB: The extent and pattern of gastroesophageal reflux in patients with scleroderma esophagus: The effect of low-dose omeprazole. *Aliment Pharmacol Ther* 7:509–513, 1993.

30. Bhalla M, Silver RM, Shephard JO, et al: Chest CT in patients with scleroderma: Prevalence of asymptomatic esophageal dilation and mediastinal lymphadenopathy. *AJR Am J Radiol* 161:269–272, 1993.

31. Miller LS, Liu JB, Klenn PJ, et al: Endoluminal ultrasonography of the distal esophagus in systemic sclerosis. *Gastroenterology* 105:31–39, 1993.

32. Basilisco G, Barbera R, Molgora M, et al: Acid clearance and oesophageal sensitivity in patients with progressive systemic sclerosis. *Gut* 34:1487–1491, 1993.

33. Dantas RO, Meneghelli UG, Olivera RB, et al: Esophageal dysfunction does not always worsen in systemic sclerosis. *J Clin Gastroenterol* 17:281–285, 1993.

34. Gignoux CG, Bost R, Hostein J, et al: Role of upper esophageal reflex and belch reflex dysfunctions in noncardiac chest pain. *Dig Dis Sci* 38:1909–1914, 1993.

35. Williams D, Thompson DG, Heggie L, et al: Responses of human esophagus to experimental intraluminal distension. *Am J Physiol* 265:G196–G203, 1993.

36. Singh S, Richter JE, Bradley LA, et al: The symptom index, differential usefulness in suspected acid-related complaints of heartburn and chest pain. *Dig Dis Sci* 38:1402–1408, 1993.

37. Zierer ST, Sanowski RA, Young MF, et al: Can a single dose of omeprazole be used to identify gastroesophageal reflux and acid-related chest pain (abstract)? *Am J Gastroenterol* 88:1501, 1993.

38. Sifrim D, Janssens J, Vantrappen G: Failing deglutitive inhibition in primary esophageal motility disorders. *Gastroenterology* 106:875–882, 1994.

39. Behar J, Biancani P: Pathogenesis of simultaneous esophageal contractions in patients with motility disorders. *Gastroenterology* 105:111–118, 1993.

40. Janssens J, Annese V, Vantrappen G: Bursts of non-deglutitive simultaneous contractions may be a normal oesophageal motility pattern. *Gut* 34:1021–1024, 1993.

41. Johnston PW, Johnston BT, Collins BJ, et al: Audit of the role of oesophageal manometry in clinical practice. *Gut* 34:1158–1161, 1993.

42. Li M, Brasseur JG, Dodds WJ: Analyses of normal and abnormal esophageal transport using computer simulations. *Am J Physiol* 266:G525–G543, 1994.

43. Clouse RE, Staiano A: Topography of normal and high-amplitude esophageal peristalsis. *Am J Physiol* 265:G1098–G1107, 1993.

44. Williams D, Thompson DG, Marples M, et al: Diminished oesophageal traction forces with swallowing in gastro-oesophageal reflux disease and in functional dysphagia *Gut* 35:165–171, 1994.

45. Farkkila MA, Ertama L, Katila H, et al: Globus pharyngis, commonly associated with esophageal motility disorders. *Am J Gastroenterol* 89:503–508, 1994.

46. Ott DJ, Ledbetter MS, Koufman JA, et al: Globus pharyngeus: Radiographic evaluation and 24-hour pH monitoring of the pharynx and esophagus in 22 patients. *Radiology* 191:95–97, 1994.

47. Jerome-Zapadka M, Clarke MR, Sekas G: Recurrent upper esophageal webs in association with heterotopic gastric mucosa: Case report and literature review. *Am J Gastroenterol* 89:421–424, 1994.

48. Nakajima H, Munakata A, Saski Y, et al: pH profile of esophagus in patients with inlet patch of heterotopic gastric mucosa after tetragastrin stimulation: An endoscopic approach. *Dig Dis Sci* 38:1915–1919, 1993.

49. Kasapidis P, Xenos E, Mantides A, et al: Differences in manometry and 24-h ambulatory pH-metry between patients with and without endoscopic or histologic esophagitis in gastroesophageal reflux disease. *Am J Gastroenterol* 88:1893–1899, 1993.

50. Singh P, Taylor RH, Colin-Jones DG: Esophageal motor dysfunction and acid exposure in reflux esophagitis are more severe if Barrett's metaplasia is present. *Am J Gastroenterol* 89:349–357, 1994.

51. Williams D, Thompson DG, Heggie L, et al: Esophageal clearance function following treatment of esophagitis. *Gastroenterology* 106:108–116, 1994.

52. Deprez P, Flasse R: Healing of severe esophagitis improves esophageal motor dysfunction (abstract). *Gastroenterology* 106:70, 1994.

53. Howard JM, Reynolds RPE, Frei JV, et al: Macroscopic healing of esophagitis does not improve esophageal motility. *Dig Dis Sci* 39:648–654, 1994.

54. Coben RM, Weintraub A, DiMarino AJ, et al: Gastroesophageal reflux during gastrostomy feeding. *Gastroenterology* 106:13–18, 1994.

55. Wendl B, Pfeiffer A, Pehl C, et al: Effect of decaffeination of coffee or tea on gastro-oesophageal reflux. *Aliment Pharmacol Ther* 8:283–287, 1994.

56. Masclee AAM, Jansen JBMJ, Rovati LC, et al: Effect of cholestyramine and cholecystokinin re-

ceptor antagonist CR1505 (loxiglumide) on lower esophageal sphincter pressure in man. *Dig Dis Sci* 38:1889–1892, 1993.

57. Masclee AAM, Schrijver I, Ledeboer M, et al: Cholecystokinin provokes gastroesophageal reflux in patients with reflux disease (abstract). *Gastroenterology* 106:130, 1994.

58. Mittal RK, Stewart WR, Ramahi M, et al: The effects of psychological stress on the esophagogastric junction pressure and swallow induced relaxation. *Gastroenterology* 106:1477–1484, 1994.

59. Katz LC, Just R, Castell DO: Body position affects recumbent postprandial reflux. *J Clin Gastroenterol* 18:280–283, 1994.

60. Orr WC, Allen ML, Robinson M: The pattern of nocturnal and diurnal esophageal acid exposure in the pathogenesis of erosive mucosal damage. *Am J Gastroenterol* 89:509–512, 1994.

61. Saraswat MD, Dhiman RK, Mishra A, et al: Correlation of 24-hr esophageal pH patterns with clinical features and endoscopy in gastroesophageal reflux disease. *Dig Dis Sci* 39:199–205, 1994.

62. Collen MJ, Johnson DA, Sheridan MJ: Basal acid output and gastric acid hypersecretion in gastroesophageal reflux disease; correlation with ranitidine therapy. *Dig Dis Sci 39:410–417, 1994.*

63. Stein HJ, Feussner H, Kauer W, et al: Alkaline reflux: Assessment by ambulatory esophageal aspiration and pH monitoring. *Am J Surg* 167:163–168, 1994.

64. Tobey NA, Reddy SP, Keku TO, et al: Mechanisms of HCl-induced lowering of intracellular pH in rabbit esophageal cells. *Gastroenterology* 105:1035–1044, 1993.

65. Snow JC, Goldstein JL, Schmidt LN, et al: Rabbit esophageal cells show regulatory volume decrease: Ionic basis of effect of pH. *Gastroenterology* 105:102–110, 1993.

66. Hills BA: Oesophageal surfactant: Evidence for a possible mucosal barrier on oesophageal epithelium. *Aust N Z J Med* 24:41–46, 1994.

67. Hopwood D, Milne G, Jankowski J, et al: Secretory and adsorptive activity of oesophageal epithelium: Evidence of circulating mucosubstances. *Histopathology* 26:40–49, 1994.

68. Namiot Z, Sarosiek J, Rourk M, et al: Human esophageal secretion: Mucosal response to luminal acid and pepsin. *Gastroenterology* 106:973–981, 1994.

69. Sarosiek J, Yu Z, Namiot Z, et al: Impact of acid and pepsin on human esophageal prostaglandins. *Am J Gastroenterol* 89:588–594, 1994.

70. Sarosiek J, Hetzel DP, Yu Z, et al: Evidence on secretion of epidermal growth factor by the esophageal mucosa in humans. *Am J Gastroenterol* 88:1081–1087, 1993.

71. Brown CM, Snowdon CF, Slee B, et al: Measurement of bicarbonate output from the intact human oesophagus. *Gut* 34:872–880, 1993.

72. Namiot Z, Rourk RM, Piascik R, et al: Interrelationship between esophageal challenge with mechanical and chemical stimuli and salivary protective mechanisms. *Am J Gastroenterol* 89:581–587, 1994.

73. Rourk RM, Namiot Z, Sarosiek J, et al: Impairment of salivary growth factor secretory response to esophageal mechanical and chemical stimulation in patients with reflux esophagitis. *Am J Gastroenterol* 89:237–244, 1994.

74. Edmunds MC, Namiot Z, Sarosiek J, et al: Esophageal epidermal growth factor impairment persists despite healing of endoscopic changes in patients with reflux esophagitis (abstract). *Gastroenterology* 106:73, 1994.

75. DeVault KR, Georgeson S, Castell DO: Salivary stimulation mimics esophageal exposure to refluxed duodenal contents. *Am J Gastroenterol* 88:1040–1043, 1993.

76. Iftikhar SY, Ledingham S, Steele RJC, et al: Bile reflux in columnar-lined Barrett's esophagus. *Ann R Coll Surg Engl* 75:411–416, 1993.

77. Thompson JK, Koehler RE, Richter JE: Detection of gastroesophageal reflux: Value of barium studies compared with 24-hr pH monitoring. *AJR Am J Radiol* 162:621–626, 1994.

78. Ing AJ, Ngu MC, Breslin ABX: Pathogenesis of chronic cough associated with gastroesophageal reflux. *Am J Respir Care Med* 149:160–167, 1994.

79. Irwin RS, French CL, Curley FJ, et al: Chronic cough due to gastroesophageal reflux: Clinical, diagnostic, and pathogenetic aspects. *Chest* 104:1511–1517, 1993.

80. Bauman NM, Sandler AD, Schmidt C, et al: Reflex laryngospasm induced by stimulation of distal esophageal afferents. *Laryngoscope* 104:209–214, 1994.

81. Cox JGC, Winter RK, Maslin SC, et al: Balloon or bougie for dilatation of benign esophgeal stricture. *Dig Dis Sci* 39:776–781, 1994.

82. Marks RD, Richter JE, Rizzo J, et al: Omeprazole versus H_2-receptor antagonists in treating patients with peptic stricture and esophagitis. *Gastroenterology* 106:907–915, 1994.

83. Swarbrick ET, Gough AL, Christian J, et al: Prevention of recurrence of oesophageal stricture: A comparative study of lansoprazole and high dose ranitidine (abstract). *Gastroenterology* 106:189, 1994.

84. Ducrotte P, Guillemont F, Elouaer-Blanc L, et al: Comparison of omeprazole and famotidine on esophageal pH in patients with moderate to severe esophagitis: A cross-over study. *Am J Gastroenterol* 89:717–721, 1994.

85. Bate CM, Booth SN, Crowe JP, et al: Does 40 mg omeprazole daily offer additional benefit over 20 mg daily in patients requiring more than 4 weeks of treatment for symptomatic reflux oesophagitis? *Aliment Pharmacol Ther* 7:501–507, 1993.

86. Kuster E, Ros E, Toledo-Pimentel V, et al: Predictive factors of the long term outcome in gastro-oesophageal reflux disease: Six year follow up of 107 patients. *Gut* 35:8–14, 1994.

87. Urschel JD: Complications of antireflux surgery. *Am J Surg* 165:68–70, 1993.

88. Dunnington GL, DeMeester TR, and the Veterans Affairs gastroesophageal reflux disease study group: Outcome effect of adherence to operative principles of Nissen fundoplication by multiple surgeons. *Am J Surg* 166:654–657, 1993.

89. Bremner RM, DeMeester TR, Crookes PF, et al: The effect of symptoms and nonspecific motility abnormalities on outcomes of surgical therapy for gastroesophageal reflux disease. *J Thorac Cardiovasc Surg* 107:1244–1250, 1994.

90. Grande L, Toledo-Pimentel V, Manterola C, et al: Value of Nissen fundoplication in patients with gastro-oesophageal reflux judged by long-term symptom control. *Br J Surg* 81:548–550, 1994.

91. Luostarinen M, Isolauri J, Laitinen J, et al: Fate of Nissen fundoplication after 20 years: A clinical, endoscopic, and functional analysis. *Gut* 34:1015–1020, 1993.

92. Weerts JM, Dallemagne B, Hamoir E, et al: Laparoscopic Nissen fundoplication: Detailed analysis of 132 patients. *Surg Laparosc Endosc* 3:359–364, 1993.

93. Cadiere GB, Houben JJ, Bruyns J, et al: Laparoscopic Nissen fundoplication: Technique and preliminary results. *Br J Surg* 81:400–403, 1994.

94. Bittner HB, Meyers WC, Brazer SR, et al: Laparoscopic Nissen fundoplication: Operative results and short-term follow-up. *Am J Surg* 167:193–200, 1994.

95. Swanstrom L, Wayne R: Spectrum of gastrointestinal symptoms after laparoscopic fundoplication. *Am J Surg* 167:538–541, 1994.

96. Aye RW, Hill LD, Kraemer SJM, et al: Early results with the laparoscopic Hill repair. *Am J Surg* 167:542–546, 1994.

97. Collard JM, Verstraete L, Otte JB, et al: Clinical, radiological and functional results of remedial antireflux operations. *Int Surg* 78:298–306, 1993.

98. Li H, Walsh TN, O'Dowd G, et al: Mechanisms of columnar metaplasia and squamous regeneration in experimental Barrett's esophagus. *Surgery* 115:176–182, 1994.

99. Cameron AJ: Epidemiologic studies and the development of Barrett's esophagus. *Endoscopy* 25(suppl):635–636, 1993.

100. Zeroogian JM, Spechler SJ, Antonioli DA, et al: The high prevalence of short-segment Barrett's esophagus (abstract). *Gastroenterology* 106:216, 1994.

101. Reid BJ, Sanchez CA, Blount PL, et al: Barrett's esophagus: Cell cycle abnormalities in advancing stages of neoplastic progression. *Gastroenterology* 105:119–129, 1993.

102. Bount PL, Galipeau PC, Sanchez CA, et al: 17p allelic losses in diploid cells of patients with Barrett's esophagus who develop aneuploidy. *Cancer Res* 54:2292–2295, 1994.

103. Younes M, Lebovitz RM, Lechago LV, et al: p53 protein accumulation in Barrett's metaplasia, dysplasia, and carcinoma: A follow up study. *Gastroenterology* 105:1637–1642, 1993.

104. Jones DR, Davidson AG, Summers CL, et al: Potential application of p53 as an intermediate biomarker in Barrett's esophagus. *Ann Thorac Surg* 57:598–603, 1994.

105. Casson AG, Manolopoulos B, Troster M, et al: Clinical implications of p53 gene mutation in the progression of Barrett's epithelium to invasive cancer. *Am J Surg* 167:52–57, 1994.

106. Menke-Pluymers MBE, Hop WCJ, Dees J, et al: Risk factors for the development of an adenocarcinoma in columnar-lined (Barrett) esophagus. *Cancer* 72:1155–1158, 1993.

107. Falk GW, Catalano MF, Sivak MV, et al: Endosonography in the evaluation of patients with Barrett's esophagus and high-grade dysplasia. *Gastrointest Endosc* 40:207–212, 1994.

108. Rice TW, Falk GW, Achkar E, et al: Surgical management of high-grade dysplasia in Barrett's esophagus. *Am J Gastroenterol* 88:1832–1836, 1993.

109. Cameron AJ, Carpenter HC, Laukka MA, et al: Barrett's esophagus: Pathologic findings following resection for high grade dysplasia (abstract). *Am J Gastroenterol* 88:1483, 1993.

110. Levine DS, Haggitt RC, Blount PL, et al: An endoscopic biopsy protocol can differentiate high-grade dysplasia from early adenocarcinoma in Barrett's esophagus. *Gastroenterology* 105:40–50, 1993.

111. Gore S, Healy CJ, Sutton HR, et al: Regression of columnar lined (Barrett's) oesophagus with continuous omeprazole therapy. *Aliment Ther Pharmacol* 7:623–628, 1993.

112. Iqbal TH, Neumann CS, Gearty JC, et al: Omeprazole for 12–24 months in the treatment of patients with Barrett's esophagus (abstract). *Gastroenterology* 106:99, 1994.

113. Wang KK, Gutta K, Laukka MA: A prospective randomized trial of low dose photodynamic therapy in the treatment of Barrett's esophagus (abstract). *Gastroenterology* 106:208, 1994.

114. Overholt BF, Denovo RC, Panjehpour M, et al: A centering balloon for photodynamic therapy tested in a canine model. *Gastrointest Endosc* 39:782–787, 1993.

115. Salo JA, Hietala EM, Nemlander A, et al: Reversal of Barrett's esophagus by endoscopic laser ablation and antireflux surgery (abstract). *Gastroenterology* 106:171, 1994.

116. Soffer EE, Mitros F, Doornbos JF, et al: Morphology and pathology of radiation-induced esophagitis: Double-blind study of naproxen vs. placebo for prevention of radiation injury. *Dig Dis Sci* 39:655–660, 1994.

117. Swaroop VS, Desai DC, Mohandas KM, et al: Dilation of esophageal strictures induced by radiation therapy for cancer of the esophagus. *Gastrointest Endosc* 40:311–315, 1994.

118. Broor SL, Raju GS, Bose PP, et al: Long term results of endoscopic dilatation for corrosive oeseophageal strictures. *Gut* 34:1498–1501, 1993.

119. Berthet B, DiCostanzo J, Arnaud C, et al: Influence of epidermal growth factor and interferon-gamma on healing of oesophageal corrosive burns in rats. *Br J Surg* 81:395–398, 1994.

120. Hackman RC, Wolford JL, Gleaves CA, et al: Recognition and rapid diagnosis of upper gastrointestinal cytomegalovirus infection in marrow transplant recipients. *Transplantation* 57:231–237, 1994.

121. Brandt LJ, Coman E, Schwartz E, et al: Use of a new cytology balloon for diagnosis of symptomatic esophageal disease in acquired immunodeficiency syndrome. *Gastrointest Endosc* 39:559–561, 1993.

122. Wilcox CM: Short report: Time course of clinical response with fluconazole for *Candida* oesophagitis in patients with AIDS. *Aliment Pharmacol Ther* 8:347–350, 1994.

123. Parente F, Ardizzone S, Cernuschi M, et al: Prevention of symptomatic recurrences of esophageal

candidiasis in AIDS patients after the first episode: A prospective study. *Am J Gastroenterol* 89:416–420, 1994.

124. Chawla SK, Ramani K, Chawla K, et al: Giant esophageal ulcers of AIDS: Ultrastructural study. *Am J Gastroenterol* 89:411–415, 1994.

125. Frager D, Kotler DP, Baer J: Idiopathic esophageal ulceration in the acquired immunodeficiency syndrome: Radiologic reappraisal in 10 patients. *Abdom Imaging* 19:2–5, 1994.

126. Hatzitheofilou C, Strahlendorf C, Hakoyiannis S, et al: Penetrating external injuries to the oeseophagus and pharynx. *Br J Surg* 80:1147–1149, 1993.

127. Horwitz B, Krevsky B, Buckman RF, et al: Endoscopic evaluation of penetrating esophageal injuries. *Am J Gastroenterol* 88:1249–1253, 1993.

128. Salo JA, Isolauri JO, Heikkila LJ, et al: Management of delayed esophageal perforation with mediastinal sepsis: Esophagectomy or primary repair. *J Thorac Cardiovasc Surg* 106:1088–1091, 1993.

129. Blair SR, Graeber GM, Cruzzavala JL, et al: Current management of esophageal impactions. *Chest* 104:1205–1209, 1993.

130. Berggreen PJ, Harrison ME, Sanowski RA, et al: Techniques and complications of esophageal foreign body extraction in children and adults. *Gastrointest Endosc* 39:626–630, 1993.

131. Robbins MI, Shortsleeve MJ: Treatment of acute esophageal food impaction with glucagon, an effervescent agent, and water. *AJR Am J Radiol* 162:325–328, 1994.

132. Burkart DJ, Johnson CD, Ehman RL, et al: Evaluation of portal venous hypertension with cine phase-contrast MR flow measuremnts: High association of hyperdynamic portal flow with variceal hemorrhage. *Radiology* 188:643–648, 1993.

133. Lin CY, Lin PW, Tsai HM, et al: Influence of paraesophageal venous collaterals on efficacy of endoscopic sclerotherapy for esophageal varices. *Hepatology* 19:602–608, 1994.

134. Kokawa H, Shijo H, Kubara K, et al: Long-term risk factors for bleeding after first course of endoscopic injection sclerotherapy: A univariate and multivariate analysis. *Am J Gastroenterol* 88:1206–1211, 1993.

135. Chan ACW, Chung SCS, Sung JY, et al: A double-blind randomized controlled trial comparing sodium tetradecyl sulfate and ethanolamine oleate in the sclerotherapy of bleeding oesophageal varices. *Endoscopy* 25:513–517, 1993.

136. Saraya A, Sarin SK: Effects of intravenous nitroglycerin and metocloperamide on intravariceal pressure: A double-blind, randomized study. *Am J Gastroenterol* 88:1850–1853, 1993.

137. Bertoni G, Sassatelli R, Fornaciari G, et al: Oral isosorbide-5-mononitrate reduces the rebleeding rate during course of injection sclerotherapy for esophageal varices. *Scand J Gastroenterol* 29:363–370, 1994.

138. Avgerinos A, Rekoumis G, Klonis C, et al: Propranolol in the prevention of recurrent upper gastrointestinal bleeding in patients with cirrhosis undergoing endoscopic sclerotherapy: A randomized trial. *J Hepatol* 19:301–311, 1993.

139. Acharya SK, Dasarathy S, Saksena S, et al: A prospective randomized trial to evaluate propranolol in patients undergoing long-term endoscopic sclerotherapy. *J Hepatol* 19:291–300, 1993.

140. Teres J, Bosch J, Bordas JM, et al: Propranolol versus sclerotherapy in preventing variceal rebleeding: A randomized controlled trial. *Gastroenterology* 105:1508–1514, 1993.

141. Laine L, El-Newihi HM, Migikovsky B, et al: Endoscopic ligation compared with sclerotherapy for the the treatment of bleeding esophageal varices. *Ann Intern Med* 119:1–7, 1993.

142. Gimson AES, Ramage JK, Panos MZ, et al: Randomised trial of variceal banding ligation versus injection sclerotherapy for bleeding oesophageal varices. *Lancet* 342:391–394, 1993.

143. Berner JS, Gaing AA, Sharma R, et al: Sequelae after eseophageal variceal ligation and sclerotherapy: A prospective randomized study. *Am J Gastroenterol* 89:852–858, 1994.

144. Juhl KO, Jensen LS, Steiniche T, et al: Recombinant human epidermal growth factor prevents

sclerotherapy-induced esophageal ulcer and stricture formations in pigs. *Dig Dis Sci* 39:393–401, 1994.

145. Sung JJY, Chung SCS, Lai CW, et al: Octreotide infusion or emergency sclerotherapy for variceal haemorrhage. *Lancet* 342:637–641, 1993.

146. Silvain C, Carpentier S, Sautereau D, et al: Terlipressin plus transdermal nitroglycerin vs. octreotide in the control of acute bleeding from esophageal varices: A multicenter randomized trial. *Hepatology* 18:61–65, 1993.

147. Rossle M, Haag K, Ochs A, et al: The transjugular intrahepatic portosystemic stent-shunt procedure for variceal bleeding. *N Engl J Med* 330:165–1671, 1994.

148. Duggan A, Waugh RC, Perkins KW, et al: Transjugular intrahepatic portosystemic stent-shunt (TIPSS) for variceal haemorrhage: Initial results in 28 patients. *Aust N Z J Med* 24:136–140, 1994.

149. Hebbard GS, Fitt G, Thomson KR, et al: Transjugular intrahepatic portal-systemic shunts (TIPS)—initial experience and clinical outcome. *Aust N Z J Med* 24:141–148, 1994.

150. Mariette D, Smadja C, Borgonovo G, et al: The Sugiara procedure: A prospective experience. *Surgery* 115:282–289, 1994.

151. Sander RR, Poesl H: Cancer of the oesophageal–palliation-laser treatment and combined procedures. *Endoscopy* 25(suppl):679–682, 1993.

152. Carter R, Smith JS, Anderson JR, et al: Palliation of malignant dysphagia using the Nd:YAG laser. *World J Surg* 17:608–614, 1993.

153. Nwokolo CU, Payne-James JJ, Silk DBA, et al: Palliation of malignant dysphagia by ethanol tumour necrosis. *Gut* 35:299–303, 1994.

154. Moreira LS, Coelho RCL, Sadala RU, et al: The use of ethanol injection under endoscopic control to palliate dysphagia caused by esophagogastric cancer. *Endoscopy* 26:311–314, 1994.

155. Chung SCS, Leong HT, Choi CYC, et al: Palliation of malignant oesophageal obstruction by endoscopic alcohol injection. *Endoscopy* 26:275–277, 1994.

156. Knyrim K, Wagner HJ, Bethge N, et al: A controlled trial of an expansile metal stent for palliation of esophageal obstruction due to inoperable cancer. *N Engl J Med* 329:1302–1307, 1993.

CHAPTER 2

The Stomach*

Felix W. Leung, M.D.

Acting Director, Division of Gastroenterology, UCLA—San Fernando Valley Program; Sepulveda Veterans Administration Medical Center and Olive View Medical Center; Professor of Medicine, UCLA School of Medicine, Los Angeles, California

This chapter on the stomach will focus mainly on developments in the area of peptic ulcer disease during the past year and review studies on peptic ulcers; the epidemiology, treatment, and mechanism of the mucosa-damaging action of *Helicobacter pylori;* and reports on portal hypertensive gastropathy, ulcer bleeding, and dyspepsia. The chapter will close with an overview of the recent advances in our understanding of the mechanisms of mucosal injury and defense.

PEPTIC ULCERS

Predictors of Ulcer Occurrence, Giant Ulcers, Delayed Ulcer Healing, and Ulcer Relapse

Factors associated with giant duodenal ulcers were assessed[1] (Table 1). The mean basal acid output for 17 patients with giant duodenal ulcers (>2 cm) was 8 mEq/hr (range, 0.0 to 28 mEq/hr), and for the 167 patients with duodenal ulcers in the standard range (0.5 to 1.5 cm), it was 9 mEq/hr (range, 0.0 to 49 mEq/hr). The

---

*Supported by Veterans Administration Medical Research Funds.

TABLE 1.

Predictors of Ulcer Occurrence, Giant Ulcers, Delayed Ulcer Healing, and Ulcer Relapse

Risk Factors	Reference
Giant ulcer	
NSAID* use	1, 2
Delay in ulcer healing	
Decreased blood flow at ulcer margin, large ulcer, stigmata of recent hemorrhage, concurrent medical illness, frequent NSAID use, duodenal deformity	3
Prior ulcer history, large ulcer (>10 mm), smoking	4
Smoking, male sex, family history of ulcers	5
Ulcer relapse	
Duodenal erosions, smoking, psychological stress, heavy physical labor	6

*NSAID = nonsteroidal anti-inflammatory drug.

differences were not statistically significant. There was a significant difference in the percentages of ulcer complications in the patients with giant duodenal ulcers and those with duodenal ulcers in the standard range, 65% vs. 25% ($P = 0.001$), and in the percentage of patients using nonsteroidal anti-inflammatory drugs (NSAIDs) daily during the month preceding the upper gastrointestinal endoscopy, 53% vs. 8% ($P = 0.00001$). The results suggest that giant duodenal ulcers and the associated significant increase in complications are not attributable to increased basal acid output but are associated with increased NSAID use.

The relationship between a history of benign upper gastrointestinal ulcer disease, serologic evidence of achlorhydria (pepsinogen A, <17 µg/L), and a history of NSAID use was assessed in 857 consecutive outpatients without a prior history of gastrectomy in a rheumatology clinic (n = 430) and several internal medicine clinics (n = 427).[2] Interview data were validated against reviews of medical records, and blood for a determination of the serum pepsinogen A level was obtained. Of 857 patients interviewed, 36 (4.2%; confidence interval [CI], 2.9 to 5.5) had a pepsinogen A level lower than 17 µg/L. A history of benign upper gastrointestinal ulcer was confirmed in 3 (8%) of these 36 patients. The ulcers were benign during a follow-up period of 2.4 to 7 years. They were known to have pernicious anemia before (2 patients) or simultaneously (1 patient) with the diagnosis of a upper gastrointestinal ulcer and were using NSAIDs at that time. The data suggest that NSAID-induced benign ulcers can develop in the presence of pernicious anemia and achlorhydria.

In 97 consecutive patients with duodenal ulcer bleeding, an index of mucosal blood flow (index of oxygen saturation [ISO_2]) was assessed at the ulcer margin and the adjacent mucosa by endoscopic reflectance spectrophotometry.[3] The difference in the index of oxygen saturation (ΔISO_2 = ulcer margin ISO_2 − adjacent mucosa ISO_2) was determined. A higher ISO_2 (positive ΔISO_2) at the ulcer margin indicates an increase in blood flow at the ulcer margin. A lower ISO_2 (negative ΔISO_2) at the ulcer margin indicates that blood flow at the ulcer margin is reduced when compared with that in the adjacent mucosa. Endoscopic examinations were repeated until the ulcers had healed (n = 86). Relative to the adjacent mucosa, 78% of the ulcer margins had increased blood flow (positive ΔISO_2) and 22% had decreased blood flow (negative ΔISO_2). Stepwise multilinear regression analysis selected ΔISO_2, ulcer size, and stigmata of recent hemorrhage as predictors of delayed healing. Multivariate logistic regression analysis selected concurrent medical illness, duodenal deformity, frequent use of NSAIDs, and stigmata of recent hemorrhage as factors significantly associated with delayed (longer than 5 weeks) ulcer healing. The results support the hypothesis that prognostic factors are identifiable at the time of ulcer diagnosis, even in patients who are bleeding.

One prospective, multicenter, double-observer–blinded, randomized trial[4] assessed the risk factors for delayed healing of duodenal ulcers. Five hundred ninety-four patients with active duodenal ulcers were randomly assigned to receive famotidine, 40 mg, or ranitidine, 300 mg, at bedtime. Endoscopy was performed at entry and at 2, 4, and 8 weeks after therapy or until complete ulcer healing. After 4 weeks of treatment, by a "per protocol" analysis, three risk factors for nonhealing were statistically significant: prior ulcer history (63% healed as compared with 78% with no history, $P = .001$; odds ratio for nonhealing, 2.1; Cl, 1.4 to 3.1); ulcer size (62% of the ulcers 10 mm or larger healed at 4 weeks as compared with 76% of the smaller ulcers, $P = 0.001$; odds ratio, 1.9; Cl, 1.3 to 2.8); and smoking (62% of the smokers healed as compared with 78% of the nonsmokers; odds ratio, 2.1; Cl, 1.4 to 3.1). The presence of multiple risk factors resulted in additive risk: for patients with none, one, two, or three of the risk factors, the healing rate at 4 weeks was 87%, 77%, 63%, and 47%, respectively. Multiple risk factors also affected healing rates at 8 weeks. On the other hand, bleeding, alcohol use, and prior NSAID use did not influence ulcer healing. The data suggest that smoking, a prior ulcer history, and ulcer size of 10 mm or larger exert independent risks for nonhealing of duodenal ulcers.

A controlled, double-blind study in gastric ulcer maintenance therapy with nizatidine was performed in 241 patients.[5] Multivariate analysis showed that smoking habits (odds ratio, 2.35), male sex (odds ratio, 2.30), and ulcer family history (odds ratio, 2.7) are the major risk factors for relapse. Cigarette smoking was the most important factor.

In a prospective study of the risk factors for duodenal ulcer relapse during maintenance (150 mg daily) ranitidine therapy, 1,899 patients with chronic ulcer disease were evaluated.[6] Endoscopic examination was undertaken to confirm ulcer healing after 1 and 2 years and if symptoms relapsed. By the end of the first and second years, 247 and 432 patients had experienced at least one relapse, respectively. Univariate analysis indicated that all seven prospectively defined risk factors were associated with an increased 2-year relapse rate; of these, duodenal erosions distant from the healed ulcer (odds ratio, 2.23; Cl, 1.6 to 3.2; $P < .0001$), past or present smoking (odds ratio, 1.46; Cl, 1.1 to 1.9; $P = .0050$), psychological stress (odds ratio, 1.38; Cl, 1.1 to 1.7; $P = .0085$), heavy physical labor (odds ratio, 1.45; Cl, 1.1 to 2.0; $P = .0219$), and absence of NSAID intake (odds ratio, 1.54; Cl, 1.0 to 2.3; $P = .0464$) were independent risk factors on stepwise logistic regression analysis, whereas persistent symptoms at healing (odds ratio, 1.3; CI, 1.03 to 1.62; $P = .0310$) and frequent prior relapses (odds ratio, 1.45; CI, 1.0 to 2.0; $P = .0454$) were not. Multiple relapses in 107 patients (odds ratio, 5.6%; CI, 4.6% to 6.7%) were associated with duodenal erosions, smoking, stress, and heavy physical labor. Two-year relapse rates increased from 16% (CI, 11% to 20%) in the presence of no or one risk factor to 41% (CI, 26% to 56%) in the presence of four or five risk factors.

None of the studies reviewed in this section took into account the *H. pylori* status of the subjects. Studies that assessed the role of *H. pylori* in ulcer healing and relapse will be reviewed later.

Treatment of Peptic Ulcers

Free Radical Scavengers

One prospective randomized, double-blind study examined the influence of free radical scavengers on the healing and recurrence of refractory duodenal ulceration.[7] Allopurinol, an inhibitor of xanthine oxidase, the enzyme that forms superoxide radicals, and dimethyl sulfoxide (DMSO), a hydroxyl radical scavenger, were studied. Three hundred sixty-three consecutive patients with duodenal ulcers that did not heal despite 3 months of treatment with cimetidine and who were cigarette smokers and social drinkers were randomized to receive 800 mg cimetidine twice a day with 5 mL of vehicle for allopurinol (0.1M NaOH) or with either 50 mg allopurinol or 500 mg DMSO, each four times a day orally. In 315 patients who were evaluable for efficacy analysis, the healing rate at 8 weeks was 60% for cimetidine, 100% for cimetidine with DMSO, and 100% for cimetidine with allopurinol. The healing efficacy of cimetidine was therefore significantly ($P < .01$) enhanced by DMSO and allopurinol. The patients whose ulcers healed were provided maintenance treatment for 1 year. They received 800 mg cimetidine alone at bedtime or with either DMSO or allopurinol. In 218 patients who were evaluable for efficacy analysis, the cumulative relapse rate at 1 year was 29% for cimetidine, 8% for cimetidine with DMSO, and 7% for cimetidine with allopurinol. Dimethyl sulfoxide with cimetidine and allopurinol with cimetidine were superior to cimetidine alone ($P < .01$) in preventing ulcer relapse. The results indicate that antisecretory treatment combined with free radical inhibitor or scavenger treatment is associated with healing and a reduction in recurrence of duodenal ulceration.

Maintenance Therapy Reduces the Recurrence of Ulcers and Complications

A controlled, double-blind study with nizatidine in gastric ulcer maintenance treatment was performed. The study, which involved 241 patients, takes into account the following data: age, sex, family history of ulcers, smoking habits, alcohol consumption, previous ulcer treatment, number of ulcers, ulcer size and location, and current drug therapy (nizatidine or placebo). Multivariate analysis showed that placebo treatment (odds ratio, 2.45) is one of the major predictor of relapse. The data suggest that nizatidine treatment is significantly better than placebo in maintaining gastric ulcer remission.[5]

The effect of a 5-year maintenance program with ranitidine on the natural history of duodenal ulcer disease both during treatment and after drug withdrawal was assessed.[8] In one group of patients (n = 40), ranitidine (150 mg/day) was given continuously for 5 years. In another group of patients (n = 40), seasonal, 8-week prophylactic treatment with ranitidine (300 mg/day) in the spring and the fall was administered. Endoscopic examination was performed every year and whenever ulcer symptoms recurred. After the 5-year study, drug therapy was discontinued in both groups, and the patients underwent endoscopic examination after 3, 6, 12, and 18 months. The probability of duodenal ulcer recurrence was significantly lower in patients continuously receiving ranitidine ($P < 0.001$), and ulcer complications were significantly fewer in the group of patients receiving continuous treatment ($P < .03$). In the 18 months of follow-up after drug discontinuation, only 15% (4/26) of the patients receiving continuous treatment relapsed, whereas ulcer recurrence was diagnosed in 81% (26/32) of the patients receiving seasonal treatment ($P < .001$). The data suggest that low-dose continuous treatment with ranitidine modifies the recurrence of duodenal ulcer disease.

The effectiveness and safety of long-term maintenance therapy with histamine H_2-receptor blockers in preventing recurrent duodenal ulcer hemorrhage were evaluated in a double-blind study in patients with endoscopically documented hemorrhage from duodenal ulcers.[9] The patients were randomly assigned to maintenance therapy with ranitidine (150 mg at night) or placebo and were followed for up to 3 years. Endoscopy was performed at baseline (to document that the ulcers had healed), at exit from the study, and when a patient had persistent ulcer symptoms unrelieved by antacids or had gastrointestinal bleeding. Symptomatic relapses without bleeding were treated with ranitidine; if the ulcer healed within 8 weeks, the patient resumed taking the assigned study medication. The two groups were similar at entry, which usually occurred about 3 months after the index hemorrhage. After a mean follow-up of 61 weeks, 3 of the 32 patients treated with ranitidine had recurrent hemorrhage as compared with 12 of the 33 given placebo ($P < .05$). Half the episodes of recurrent bleeding were asymptomatic. One patient in the ranitidine group withdrew from the study because of asymptomatic thrombocytopenia during the first month. The data suggest that for patients whose duodenal ulcers heal after severe hemorrhage, long-term maintenance therapy with ranitidine is safe and reduces the risk of recurrent bleeding.

It must be pointed out that if the observations reviewed later regarding the beneficial effects of treatment of *H. pylori* infection on ulcer disease are reproducible, the results of studies using antisecretory therapy alone may become less important.

Prostaglandin in the Treatment of Nonsteroidal Anti-Inflammatory Drug–Induced Ulcerations

In a study to evaluate the long-term effect of misoprostol (600 to 800 μg/day) in the prevention of gastric ulcers and gastroduodenal erosions, 83 arthritis patients receiving chronic NSAID therapy were assessed.[10] Gastric ulcers developed in 4 (13%) of the 32 patients given misoprostol as compared with 11 (29%) of the 38 who received placebo (*P* < .05, life-table analysis). Of the 11 patients with an initial gastric ulcer, a further gastric ulcer developed in 6 as compared with 9 of 58 patients without an initial ulcer (*P* < .05). The data suggest that misoprostol decreases the cumulative development of NSAID-induced gastric ulcers.

To determine whether a prostaglandin analogue is effective treatment for NSAID-induced lesions, a 9-week double-blind trial compared placebo with enprostil, 35 μg twice daily and three times daily.[11] The use of antacids was not allowed. Three centers entered 145 patients with chronic inflammatory arthritis and osteoarthritis (mean age, 63 years) who required continuous fixed-dose NSAID therapy within the therapeutic dosage range. The minimum entrance criterion was the presence of either four gastric erosions or one gastric ulcer. Two pretreatment endoscopies within a 2-week interval were performed to establish the presence of stable baseline gastric lesions. Endoscopy was repeated at week 6 and week 9 during treatment. All groups were similar with regard to age distribution, sex, weight, height, tobacco usage, and alcohol consumption. The ulcer healing rates were 14%, 57%, and 68% at 6 weeks and 19%, 68%, and 74% at 9 weeks for the groups receiving placebo, enprostil twice daily, and enprostil three times daily, respectively (*P* < .01). No dose effect of enprostil was observed. Complete mucosal healing of all erosions and ulcers at 9 weeks occurred in 59% of the enprostil-treated patients and 10% of placebo-treated patients. Gastric erosions and gastric ulcers developed in 16% of the patients given placebo and 4% of the enprostil-treated patients. Eighteen percent of the enprostil-treated patients withdrew early from the study because of adverse experiences such as diarrhea and abdominal pain. The data suggest that gastric ulcers and erosions rarely heal spontaneously. Enprostil, 35 μg taken either twice daily or three times daily, heals NSAID-induced gastric ulcers and erosions and protects the mucosa from further NSAID-induced gastric injury, but there is a high incidence of diarrhea.

HELICOBACTER PYLORI

Epidemiology

A prospective 3-year cohort study in Canada examined the seroprevalence, conversion, and reversion of *H. pylori* infection as determined by immunoglobulin G antibodies.[12] The serum specimens were initially collected for a study of the prevalence and incidence of *Coxiella burnetii* infection in 900,000 inhabitants of Nova

Scotia. A computer-generated list of 4,500 persons were contacted by mail. Approximately 600 agreed to participate and provide three blood samples in 3 consecutive years. Some of the blood samples were heat-inactivated in the beginning and had to be discarded. For the *H. pylori* study the cohort consisted of 316 of these subjects aged 18 to 72 years. At least two suitable blood samples were available for each subject. The seroprevalence of *H. pylori* increased from 21% in the third decade to 50% in the eighth decade. The crude annual seroconversion rate was 1%, and the "spontaneous" seroconversion rate was 1.6%. Stepwise logistic regression with *H. pylori* infection as the dependent variable showed that only age was statistically associated with *H. pylori* infection ($P < .01$). Although a small cohort effect in this Canadian population could not be ruled out, the data suggested that there was a continuous risk throughout life that was highest in childhood and gradually decreased with age.

One study in the United Kingdom attempted to isolate *H. pylori* from stool specimens donated by 36 adults who had dyspepsia.[13] Fresh fecal samples were obtained and, after centrifugation to harvest bacteria, cultured onto *H. pylori*–sensitive growth media. Pure colonies of *H. pylori* were isolated from the feces of 12 of 25 subjects with dyspepsia proven to be *H. pylori*–positive at endoscopy and/or the ^{14}C urea breath test. Identification of the bacterium as *H. pylori* was confirmed phenotypically and genotypically (by polymerase chain reaction). The results indicate that transmission of *H. pylori* infection by the fecal-oral route is feasible. Whether this finding can be reproduced by other investigators and can be useful diagnostically remains to be confirmed.

One nested case-control study[14] determined whether pre-existing *H. pylori* infection increases the risk for duodenal or gastric ulceration. The subjects were born in 1900 to 1919 and identified by a 1942 Selective Service draft registration file. Those who died before the study, those with a prior history of gastrectomy or ulcer disease, and those who declined to participate were excluded. A cohort of 5,443 Japanese-American men who underwent a physical examination and phlebotomy from 1967 to 1970 were evaluated. An additional exclusion criterion was inadequately stored serum. One hundred fifty patients with gastric ulcers and 65 patients with duodenal ulcers were identified. The diagnosis was based on surgical or biopsy specimens, radiologic examination, or endoscopic or surgical reports. Each was matched with 1 control from the study cohort based on age at examination and date of serum collection. Subjects were excluded from the control group if they had a prior history of ulcer or cardiovascular disease or other cancer because their serum samples were needed for other tests. The presence of serum IgG antibody to *H. pylori* in the stored serum specimens from patients and from matched controls were tested by using an enzyme-linked immunosorbent assay. For gastric ulcers, 93% of the 150 patients and 78% of the matched controls had a positive antibody level for *H. pylori*–specific IgG, yielding an odds ratio of 3.2 (95% CI, 1.6 to 6.5). Ninety-two percent of the 65 patients with duodenal ulcers and 78% of the matched controls had a positive test result, yielding an odds ratio of 4.0 (CI, 1.1 to 14.2). A statistically significant increase was noted in the risk for gastric and duodenal ulcer as the level of antibody to *H. pylori* increased. Even when the diagnosis was made 10 or more years after the serum sample had been obtained, there was still a statistically significant association with *H. pylori* infection for both types of ulcer. The data suggest that pre-existing *H. pylori* infection increases the risk for the subsequent development of either duodenal or gastric ulcer disease.

Treatment of *Helicobacter pylori* Infection

In a prospective, single-blind, single-center study, 70 patients (3 dropped out) with active, *H. pylori*–positive (by histology and/or culture) gastric ulcers were randomly treated with either omeprazole, 20 mg twice daily, and amoxicillin, 1 g twice daily (group I; n = 35), or with omeprazole, 40 mg twice daily, and amoxicillin, 1 g twice daily for 2 weeks, followed by full-dose ranitidine for another 4 weeks (group II; n = 35).[15] Assessment of *H. pylori* status by means of the urease test, specific culture, and histologic and endoscopic examination was conducted before treatment and after 6 weeks. The overall proportion of *H. pylori* eradication was 88% (group 1, 91%; group 2, 85%, with no significant difference between groups). The ulcer healing rate was 79% after 6 weeks, 93% after 10 weeks, and 100% after 6 months. Complete pain relief occurred after a median of 2 days in group 1 and 1.5 days in group 2. Six patients (9%) had side effects that led to discontinuation of amoxicillin treatment in 3 of them (4.5%). The results suggest that the combination of omeprazole and amoxicillin is a highly effective and well-tolerated therapy regimen to eradicate *H. pylori* from the gastric mucosa of patients with gastric ulcer disease.

One study compared the efficacy of two omeprazole and amoxicillin doses in *H. pylori* eradication, ulcer healing, pain relief, and safety in the treatment of duodenal ulcer disease.[16] Ninety patients with active *H. pylori*–positive (by culture and/or histology) duodenal ulcer disease were randomly treated with either omeprazole, 20 mg twice daily, and amoxicillin, 1 g twice daily (group 1, n = 30); omeprazole, 40 mg twice daily, and amoxicillin, 1 g twice daily (group 2, n = 30); or omeprazole, 40 mg twice daily, and amoxicillin, 1 g three times daily (group 3, n = 30) for 2 weeks, followed by ranitidine at bedtime for another 4 weeks. Overall, *H. pylori* was eradicated in 83% and the ulcers healed in 92%, without statistically significant differences between the study groups. Complete pain relief occurred after a median of 1 day in all groups. Six patients had side effects during the therapy phase. Therapy was discontinued in 1 female patient. The data suggest that in the doses used, omeprazole with amoxicillin is a highly effective and well-tolerated therapy regimen to eradicate *H. pylori* in duodenal ulcer disease.

The efficacy and acceptability of low-dose, short-duration triple therapy in eradicating *H. pylori* from patients with duodenal ulcers was assessed in a prospective study of 105 patients with *H. pylori*–associated duodenal ulcer.[17] Patients were treated with H_2 antagonists (if required), followed by 2 weeks of triple therapy

consisting of colloidal bismuth subcitrate (Denol), one tablet four times daily between meals, tetracycline hydrochloride, 250 mg four times daily, and metronidazole, 400 mg twice daily. Four weeks and again 12 months after treatment, the
patients were assessed by gastroscopy and antral biopsy for ulceration and *H. py-*
lori as measured by the rapid urease test. Four patients withdrew because of drug
side effects. Of 101 patients completing treatment, *H. pylori* was eradicated in 91
(90%, or 87% of the total). Eight of the 10 patients in whom initial treatment failed
received one or more additional courses of triple therapy, with *H. pylori* being eradicated in 5. Mild nausea occurred in 6% and possible *Candida* infection in 3%. The
data suggest that this particular regimen of triple therapy was effective, safe, and
acceptable.

Eradication of *Helicobacter pylori* Without Antisecretory Therapy Heals Ulcers

Anti–*H. pylori* triple treatment of tripotassium dicitrato bismuthate (120 mg) and
amoxicillin (500 mg), each four times daily given for 7 days, and metronidazole,
400 mg five times a day given on days 5 to 7, was evaluated in one study.[18] A
change in the ^{14}C-urea breath test was used to document eradication of *H. pylori.*
Of 45 patients, 44 were available for follow-up. In 2 patients the ulcers initially
healed with clearance of *H. pylori* but recurred 3 weeks later. Both had
metronidazole-resistant *H. pylori*. Overall, 41 of 43 (95%; Cl, 81% to 99%) duodenal ulcers were healed at 1 month. *Helicobacter pylori* was eradicated in 28 of
44 (64%) patients (median follow-up, 10.2 months). In the 16 patients with persistent *H. pylori,* 1 duodenal ulcer had not healed at the 1-month follow-up, 2 had
recurrent ulcers. Within 3 weeks of finishing treatment, 5 had recurrent dyspepsia
but no recurrent ulcers on repeat endoscopy. This study suggests that 1 week of
anti–*H. pylori* triple treatment is effective in healing duodenal ulcers.

One hundred fifty-three patients with *H. pylori* infection and duodenal ulcers
were randomized to receive either a 1-week course of bismuth subcitate, tetracycline, and metronidazole (n = 76) or omeprazole for 4 weeks with the same three-
drug regimen for the first week (n = 77).[19] Endoscopy and antral biopsy specimens were obtained at entry and 4 weeks after treatment. One hundred thirty-two
patients were analyzed, 65 and 67, respectively. Duodenal ulcers healed in 60 (92%;
Cl, 86% to 100%) patients taking bismuth, tetracycline, and metronidazole as compared with 63 (95%; Cl, 88% to 100%) taking omeprazole in addition to the three
other drugs. *Helicobacter pylori* was eradicated in 61 (94%; Cl, 88% to 100%)
who received only three drugs as compared with 66 (98%; Cl, 96% to 100%) who
received omeprazole as well. Symptoms were reduced more effectively during the
first week in patients who received omeprazole ($P = .003$). The data suggest that a
1-week regimen of bismuth, tetracycline, and metronidazole for patients with *H.*
pylori and duodenal ulcers eradicates the organism and heals the ulcers in most

patients. Concurrent administration of omeprazole reduces ulcer pain more rapidly but has no effect on ulcer healing or eradication of *H. pylori.*

Low Reinfection Rate of *Helicobacter pylori* After Eradication

Of the patients whose *H. pylori* infections were successfully eradicated by triple therapy and omeprazole at 8 weeks, 90% remained *H. pylori*–negative at 1 year.[20] Of 68 patients who were reassessed after 12 months, 66 were still clear of *H. pylori,* but in 4, small superficial ulcers were present. Two patients were positive for *H. pylori,* 1 with and 1 without ulceration, for an *H. pylori* recurrence rate of 3% and an ulcer recurrence rate of 7%.[17] In one Australian study,[21] patients with endoscopically proven duodenal ulcers who had been treated with triple therapy resulting in documented eradication of *H. pylori* and cure of the ulcer for at least 4 years were recalled and had their *H. pylori* status determined by the ^{14}C-urea breath test. Those found positive for *H. pylori* underwent endoscopic confirmation of the infection. Of the 94 patients restudied with a follow-up range of 48 to 96 months or a total of 550 patient-years, only 2 (2%) were again *H. pylori*–positive. This gives an effective reinfection rate of 0.4% per patient year. Of 35 patients previously rendered *H. pylori*–negative, 32 (92%) remained *H. pylori*–negative after 7.1 years (mean).[22] These results suggest that following eradication of *H. pylori,* reinfection is an unusual phenomenon.

Eradication of *Helicobacter pylori* Enhances the Healing of Refractory Ulcers

One randomized crossover study[23] determined the distribution of *H. pylori* in the antral and duodenal mucosa of patients with duodenal ulcers refractory to 12 weeks of treatment with cimetidine. The study assessed the effect of adding antimicrobial agents to cimetidine on the healing of such refractory ulcers. Treatments included continued 800 mg of cimetidine at night for 4 weeks as compared with cimetidine plus 500 mg of amoxicillin three times a day for the first 2 weeks and 250 mg of metronidazole three times a day for the second 2 weeks. *Helicobacter pylori* status in the gastric antral and duodenal mucosa was evaluated by histology and bacterial culture before and at the end of each treatment period. Forty-eight patients were studied. At entry all patients had *H. pylori* identified in the antrum. In the duodenum, active chronic duodenitis was present in 66%, duodenal gastric metaplasia in 33%, and *H. pylori* in 50%, similar proportions of those in patients with nonrefractory duodenal ulcers. Healing occurred in 70% (30 of 43) of the patients during treatment with cimetidine and antimicrobials but in only 21% (6 of 28) during treatment with cimetidine alone ($P = .0003$). In patients who received antimicrobials, neither clearance (absence of *H. pylori* immediately after therapy) of *H. pylori* from the antrum (58% of the patients) or duodenum (71% of the colonized patients) nor eradication (absence of *H. pylori* 4 weeks after stopping antibiotic therapy) of *H. pylori* (33%) was significantly correlated with ulcer healing. When compared with historical data, the results of this study indicate that the distribution of *H. pylori* in refractory duodenal ulcers is similar to that of nonrefractory ulcers. The combination of amoxicillin and metronidazole with cimetidine, although unconventional, enhances healing of refractory duodenal ulcers.

Causal Role for *Helicobacter pylori* in the Pathogenesis of Ulcer Disease

To determine whether eradication of *H. pylori* infection reduces the rate of recurrence of gastric ulcers without maintenance therapy with H_2-receptor antagonists,[24] 30 patients with active gastric ulcers who were infected with *H. pylori* were first treated with omeprazole until scarring occurred. Patients then received plaunotol (a drug extracted from the plau-noi tree of Thailand) for 4 weeks and amoxicillin and metronidazole for 7 days. Eradication of *H. pylori* occurred in 26 (87%) of 30 patients. Histologic inflammatory changes improved, and there was no ulcer recurrence during a 12-month follow-up period in these patients. Of the 4 patients with persistent *H. pylori* infection, ulcers recurred in 3 (75%).

The ulcer recurrence rate of *H. pylori*–positive duodenal ulcers 1 year after eradication of the bacteria by triple therapy was assessed.[20] Patients with *H. pylori*–positive duodenal ulcers were randomized to receive either triple therapy for 1 week and omeprazole for 4 weeks (triple + omeprazole) (n = 78) or omeprazole alone for 4 weeks (n = 77). The patients were contacted every 3 months for symptom enquiry. At 1 year, all asymptomatic patients were offered gastroscopy. At 8 weeks when endoscopy was performed to document healing, 16 patients in the omeprazole group and four in the triple + omeprazole group had an ulcer. The patients underwent endoscopy when symptoms of epigastric pain or dyspepsia developed. During the 1-year period, symptomatic ulcers developed in 12 patients in the omeprazole group and no patient in the triple + omeprazole group. At follow-up endoscopy at 1 year, another 10 ulcers were detected in the omeprazole group and two in the triple + omeprazole group. In assessable patients, ulcers were detected in 39 of 61 (64%) in the omeprazole group and in 6 of 65 (9%) in the triple + omeprazole group after 1 year ($P < .001$). Of the patients whose *H. pylori* infections were successfully eradicated by triple + omeprazole at 8 weeks, 90% remained *H. pylori*–negative at 1 year. Triple therapy for 1 week eradicates *H. pylori* infection and significantly reduces duodenal ulcer relapses.

The long-term benefits of *H. pylori* eradication treatment in *H. pylori*–associated duodenal ulcers was reported in one study.[22] Sixty-three of 78 patients (81%) with duodenal ulcers from a trial of *H. pylori* eradication in 1985 and 1986 were reviewed clinically and had upper gastrointestinal endoscopy with gastric antral biopsy. Of 35 patients previously rendered *H. pylori*–negative, 32 (91%) remained *H. pylori*–negative after 7.1 years (mean). All patients initially *H. pylori*–positive remained infected unless *H. pylori* eradication treatment was given. Duodenal ulceration was found in 20% (5 of 25) of the patients remaining *H. pylori*–positive as compared with 3% (1 of 38) of the *H. pylori*–negative patients (*P* < .05). The reduction in duodenal ulcer relapse obtained from *H. pylori* eradication in *H. pylori*–associated duodenal ulceration extends to at least 7 years after treatment and is probably due to freedom from *H. pylori* infection. However, duodenal ulcers may recur in patients rendered *H. pylori*–negative because of factors other than reinfection with *H. pylori*.

The effect of treating *H. pylori* infection on the recurrence of peptic ulcer bleeding was evaluated in one study.[25] Sixty-six of 70 consecutive *H. pylori*–positive (by histology and/or culture) patients with conservatively and endoscopically managed peptic ulcer bleeding (duodenal ulcer, n = 39; gastric ulcer, n = 25; gastroduodenal ulcers, n = 2) were followed for a median period of 17 months (range 6 to 33 months). Patients were treated with seven different protocols, each of which included an attempt to eradicate *H. pylori* infection. Patients with (n = 42) and without (n = 24) bacterial eradication had similar demographic and clinical characteristics. Eradication of *H. pylori* was associated with a statistically significant reduction in ulcer recurrence (2% vs. 63%; *P* < .001) and bleeding relapse (0% vs. 38%; *P* = .01). The data suggest that *H. pylori* eradication markedly changes the natural history in patients with complicated duodenal and gastric ulcer disease. The conclusion, although potentially important, needs to be confirmed by double-blind, randomized, controlled trials.

Gastric Cancer and *Helicobacter pylori*

One case report described a patient with a nodular gastric mucosa–associated lymphoid tissue (MALT) lymphoma larger than 10 cm that caused hematemesis and weight loss. Antibiotic therapy for *H. pylori* resulted in full clinical recovery and resolution of the mass lesion and morphologic features of lymphoma on routine histologic examination. However, monotypic immunostaining of plasma cells persisted in a separate and grossly normal-appearing region of the stomach. The authors suggest that antibiotic therapy may be of benefit in patients with MALT lymphoma, mass lesions, and significant signs and symptoms, but a periodic search for residual lymphoma is needed.[26]

To evaluate the relation between gastric malignant MALT lymphoma and *H. pylori*, 162 surgical specimens of MALT lymphoma were retrospectively reviewed to determine the tumor type and inflammatory patterns.[27] In 121 cases, biopsy specimens obtained before surgery were available and stained with hematoxylin-eosin, periodic acid–Schiff, Giemsa, and Warthin-Starry stains. Residual lymphoid follicles were found less often in high-grade malignant than in low-grade malignant MALT lymphomas. Chronic active gastritis was shown within the mucosa at some distance from the tumors in 143 of 146 specimens. In all the cases for which biopsy specimens could be evaluated, colonization of the mucosa by *H. pylori* had occurred. Lymphoid follicles and lymphoid aggregates were detected in 83% of the antral and 85% of the body mucosa specimens. Although the authors suggest that these data support the hypothesis that *H. pylori* plays a role in the development of MALT lymphomas causality cannot be established from these findings of association alone.

Whether *H. pylori* infection is also a risk factor for primary gastric non-Hodgkin's lymphoma was assessed in one study.[28] This nested case-control study involved two large cohorts (N = 230,593). Serum had been collected from cohort members and stored, and all subjects were followed for cancer. Thirty-three cases of gastric non-Hodgkin's lymphoma occurred a median of 14 years after serum collection. Patients with gastric lymphoma were significantly more likely than matched controls to have evidence of previous *H. pylori* infection (matched odds ratio, 6.3; Cl, 2 to 20). No association was found between nongastric non-Hodgkin's lymphoma and previous *H. pylori* infection. The results suggest that non-Hodgkin's lymphoma affecting the stomach, but not other sites, is associated with previous *H. pylori* infection. A causative role for the organism is plausible but remains unproved.

Mechanism of the Mucosa-Damaging Action of *Helicobacter pylori*

Adhesion of *H. pylori* to human gastric surface mucous cells in vitro is characterized by a close membrane-to-membrane association between *H. pylori* and the target cells.[29] This phenomenon suggests a specific receptor-ligand interaction (Table 2).

Pathogenic strains of *H. pylori* cause progressive vacuolation and death of epithelial cells. To identify the nature of the vacuoles, the distribution of markers of various membrane traffic compartments was studied. The results indicate that the vacuoles specifically originate from late endosomal compartments.[30]

Intravital microscopy was used to continuously monitor leukocyte adherence and emigration and albumin leakage in rat mesenteric venules during perfusion with a water extract of *H. pylori*.[31] Leukocyte adherence and emigration and microvascular albumin leakage were increased. Perivenular mast cell degranulation and the formation of platelet-leukocyte aggregates within postcapillary venules were also elicited. The early phase (within 10 minutes) of albumin leakage was attenuated by pretreatment with a mast cell stabilizer. The late (30 minutes) phase of albumin leakage was reduced by monoclonal antibodies directed against either CD11b/CD18 or intercellular adhesion molecule type 1 (ICAM-1). A monoclonal antibody against P-selectin also inhibited the platelet-leukocyte aggregation and reduced the later

TABLE 2.

Mechanism of Mucosal Damaging Action of *Helicobacter Pylori*

Mechanism	Reference
Adhesion to mucous cells by receptor-ligand interaction	29
Vacuolation based on components derived from late endosomal compartments	30
Vascular albumin leakage dependent on mast cell, CD11b/CD18, ICAM,* and P-selectin	31
Reactive oxygen metabolites in antral tissue and neutrophils	32, 33
Increase in pepsinogen I	34
Reduced inhibition of G-cell secretion of gastrin by decreased antral release of somatostatin	35
Mast cell–dependent histamine release	36
Increased mucosal interleukin-6 and interleukin-8	37

*ICAM = intercellular adhesion molecule.

phase of albumin leak. One study measured the production of reactive oxygen metabolites by *H. pylori* in human antral mucosal biopsy specimens.[32] Two related chemiluminescence techniques were used to compare *H. pylori*–positive (n = 105) and *H. pylori*–negative patients (n = 64) with a similar spectrum of macroscopic disease. Both techniques showed that excess mucosal reactive oxygen metabolite production is associated with *H. pylori* gastric antral infection. When a suspension of *H. pylori* was added to isolated human neutrophils, luminol-dependent chemiluminescence, a measure of toxic oxidants from neutrophils, exhibited a 12-fold increase.[33]

One report[34] addressed the short- and long-term effects of eradication of *H. pylori* on serum pepsinogen I, gastrin, and insulin concentrations. Insulin was included because postprandial hyperinsulinemia had been reported in patients with duodenal ulcers and the investigators in this study wanted to determine the effect of *H. pylori* therapy on basal insulin levels as well. Fifty-three patients with proven duodenal ulceration and *H. pylori* infection received a 2-week course of colloidal bismuth subcitrate, amoxicillin, and metronidazole, and endoscopy was performed at 1.5, 3, 6, and 12 months after entry. *Helicobacter pylori* status was assessed by a urease test and histology. Among 43 patients in whom *H. pylori* was eradicated throughout the follow-up year, the mean basal pepsinogen I level was 108 ng/mL before treatment but decreased significantly to 85, 77, 80, and 75 ng/mL at 1.5, 3, 6, and 12 months, respectively, post-treatment. The basal gastrin level was 100 pg/mL before treatment and fell significantly to 72, 64, 65, and 59 pg/mL, respectively, post-treatment. Of the 4 patients in whom the *H. pylori* was not eradicated, there was no significant change in the median basal pepsinogen I and gastrin concentrations. Among the 6 patients in whom the *H. pylori* was again detectable within the follow-up year, the fallen serum concentration of pepsinogen I and gastrin returned to the pretreatment level. There was no significant change in basal insulin concentration after triple therapy in either the successfully eradicated or failed group. The data indicate that there is a close correlation between *H. pylori* and higher serum concentrations of pepsinogen I and gastrin in patients with duodenal ulcers.

One study addressed the reason for the hypergastrinemia associated with *H. pylori* infection.[35] The antral concentrations of α-amidated gastrin (bioactive) and total progastrin products were significantly higher in *H. pylori*–infected patients than in those not infected. The antral somatostatin concentration was significantly decreased in infected patients. The results suggest that the increased gastrin secretion from antral G cells in *H. pylori*–infected patients may be a result of reduced inhibition by somatostatin.

Fifty-five elderly patients with chronic antral gastritis (CAG) were studied to assess the relationship between *H. pylori* status and CAG subtypes.[38] Twenty-eight patients (51%) were *H. pylori*–positive and 27 (49%) were *H. pylori*–negative. *Helicobacter pylori* positivity had a significantly greater association with features of severe active CAG (chronic inflammation and polymorphonucleocyte activity) than did *H. pylori* negativity. Use of NSAIDs correlated with a predominantly *H. pylori*–negative gastritis that was relatively asymptomatic. The association between dyspeptic symptoms in elderly people and an *H. pylori*–positive gastritis was suggested in this report.

To assess the interaction between *H. pylori,* bile acids, mast cells and histamine release the following study was performed. Bile acids alone induce in vitro histamine release from rat serosal and mucosal mast cells. No significant histamine release was obtained when incubating any *H. pylori* preparations (culture, formalin-killed bacteria, crude cell wall preparation) alone with mast cells. Histamine release induced by bile acids was significantly enhanced without any significant increase in lactate dehydrogenase activity when whole washed or formalin-killed bacterial cells or crude cell walls were incubated with mast cells in the presence of cholic (0.3mM), deoxycholic (0.3mM), or lithocholic (0.3mM) acids; chenodeoxycholyglycine (0.3mM); and deoxycholyltaurine (3mM).[36] The results suggest a link between human *H. pylori* infection, bile acids, and histamine release and possible involvement of gastric mucosal mast cells in the pathogenesis of *H. pylori*–associated gastritis.

One study found enhanced mucosal interleukin-6 and interleukin-8 (mediators of infection) in *H. pylori*–positive dyspeptic patients.[37] Tissue homogenates of mucosal biopsy specimens from *H. pylori*–positive and *H. pylori*–negative patients were prepared. Twenty-nine of 43 patients (67%) were histologically positive for *H. pylori;* all had chronic gastritis. The mucosal levels of interleukin-6 and interleukin-8 were significantly higher in *H. pylori*–positive patients than in the *H. pylori*–negative patients ($P < .001$). A significantly higher percentage of samples with increased interleukin-8 was found in patients colonized by *H. pylori* with active superficial chronic gastritis (86%) as compared with quiescent superficial gastritis (13%) ($P < 0.01$), and the median and range were, respectively, 400 (0 to 1000) and 0 (0 to 200) pg/mg protein ($P < .001$). In patients with active superficial gastritis, a significant correlation between interleukin-6 and interleukin-8 was found ($P = 0.01$). Although the authors conclude that these results suggest a possible pathogenetic role for interleukin-6 and interleukin-8 in *H. pylori*–associated gastritis, a causal relationship cannot be established by these correlation data alone.

PORTAL HYPERTENSIVE GASTROPATHY

Factors Associated With Gastropathy

One hundred eighteen patients with portal hypertension (102 with cirrhosis, 16 with noncirrhotic portal fibrosis) were evaluated.[40] Congestive gastropathy (or what other authors define as portal hypertensive gastropathy) was present in 71 (60%) patients with portal hypertension, 41 (58%) of whom had mild (discreet areas of erythema with or without a mosaic pattern) and 30 (42%) had severe (cherry-red spots) portal hypertensive gastropathy. Portal hypertensive gastropathy was observed with equal frequency in patients with cirrhosis (63%) and noncirrhotic portal fibrosis (44%). The incidence of portal hypertensive gastropathy was higher in patients with severe liver disease, in those with a past history of hematemesis in those with esophageal varices, and in those with gastric varices. Severe portal hypertensive gastropathy was commonly observed in patients with large esophageal varices and in those with gastric varices. There was significant dilation of gastric mucosal vessels in patients with portal hypertension, but in this regard there was no significant difference between patients with and without portal hypertensive gastropathy.

Somatostatin Attenuates Increased Gastric Perfusion

Gastric perfusion has been found to be increased in cirrhotic patients with portal hypertensive gastropathy. This phenomenon may contribute to gastric bleeding in these patients. Drugs reducing gastric mucosal perfusion may be beneficial in the treatment of bleeding portal hypertensive gastropathy. In one study,[41] gastric mucosal perfusion was assessed by means of laser-Doppler flowmetry and reflectance spectrophotometry in 36 cirrhotic patients with portal hypertensive gastropathy in basal conditions and after double-blind administration of placebo or somatostatin. Intravenous bolus injection of 250 μg somatostatin induced a rapid, marked decrease ($-32\% \pm 8\%$, $P < .05$) in gastric perfusion (laser-Doppler flowmetry) that lasted for only 6 minutes. Changes in the hemoglobin content of the gastric mucosa paralleled those of the laser-Doppler signal. The oxygen content of the gastric mucosa was mildly reduced ($-7\% \pm 1\%$, $P < .05$). When the bolus injection was followed by a continuous infusion of somatostatin, the reduction in gastric perfusion (laser-Doppler flowmetry) was maintained, although the magnitude of the reduction ($-17\% \pm 7\%$) was significantly smaller than that observed immediately after the bolus ($P < .05$); the hemoglobin content of the gastric mucosa was also significantly reduced ($-8\% \pm 1\%$), but no changes were observed in the oxygen content. Placebo administration had no effect on any of these parameters. The data suggest that the increased gastric perfusion in cirrhotic patients with portal hypertensive gastropathy can be effectively decreased by somatostatin administration.

ULCER BLEEDING

Predictors of Bleeding

Eighty-four consecutive cases of peptic ulcer hemorrhage from 1986 to 1988 in patients already hospitalized for other diseases were reviewed.[42] Forty-one followed major surgery, whereas 43 were associated with other severe conditions. The bleeding site was duodenal in two thirds. The patients' mean age was 67 ± 15 years. Fifty percent had recently received NSAIDs, one third were taking anticoagulants, and 10% were receiving corticosteroids. In 39 (46%), bleeding was shown to be persistent or recurrent. Five (6%) underwent endoscopic and 18 (21%) underwent surgical therapy. Twenty-nine (34%) died. Active bleeding and endoscopic stigmata were statistically significant risk factors for further bleeding. The latter was shown to be significantly related to mortality. The results suggest that NSAIDs and anticoagulants, in association with stress and aging, are very frequently involved in peptic ulcer bleeding in hospitalized patients.

Injection Therapy in the Management of Bleeding Peptic Ulcers

Fifty-two patients with bleeding ulcers that continuously bled after water irrigation were randomized to receive endoscopic injection therapy with either 1:10,000 epinephrine in water (group 1) or distilled water (group 2). Twenty-five of 27 patients in group 1 vs. 22 of 25 patients in group 2 achieved initial hemostasis after endoscopic injection therapy ($P < .05$). Rebleeding developed in 3 patients in each group after initial hemostasis. No significant difference in the amounts of solution required for successful hemostasis was noted between the two groups. The authors suggest that a local tamponade effect with distilled water is as effective and safe as diluted epinephrine solution for endoscopic injection therapy.[43]

A prospective, randomized trial was performed to assess whether second-look endoscopy could improve the efficacy of injection therapy for bleeding ulcers.[44] One hundred four patients with active arterial bleeding or a nonbleeding visible vessel were enrolled. All received an injection of 1:10,000 adrenaline. They were randomized to receive a second elective endoscopy within the first 24 hours with repeated injection if a visible vessel was still identified (n = 52) or no repeat endoscopy (n = 52). The groups were well matched for clinical and endoscopic data. A tendency toward better results was noted in the group that received second-look endoscopy in regard to further bleeding, need for emergency surgery, transfusion requirements, length of hospital stay, and mortality rate. The authors did not recommend the routine use of second-look endoscopy.

One hundred seven consecutive patients with significant stigmata of ulcer hemorrhage were randomized to endoscopic injection of 3 to 10 mL of 1:100,000 adrenaline (55 patients, group 1) or to a combination of adrenaline and 5% ethanolamine (52 patients, group 2).[45] The groups were well matched with regard to risk factors. There were no significant differences in rebleeding, surgical operations, median blood transfusion requirements, and hospital stay. The authors concluded that the addition of a sclerosant did not confer an advantage over injection with epinephrine alone.

DYSPEPSIA

Gastric Emptying of Solids

Gastric emptying of a solid meal and of ten indigestible radiopaque solids was measured with scintigraphic and radiologic techniques in 50 healthy volunteers (controls), 41 patients with insulin-dependent diabetes mellitus, and 50 patients with functional dyspepsia[46] (Table 3). Gastroparesis to digestible solids was found in 51% of the diabetic patients and 74% of the patients with dyspepsia. Whereas all healthy volunteers emptied all ten indigestible solids in less than 4 hours, only 51% and 32% of diabetics and dyspeptics, respectively, achieved this emptying time (P < .01).

Gastroduodenal Reflex and Intragastric Distribution of Food

The relationship between functional dyspepsia, hypersensitivity to gastric distension, and gut reflex dysfunction was assessed.[47] In 10 patients with dyspepsia

TABLE 3.
Dyspepsia

Abnormalities Demonstrated in Patients With Dyspepsia	Reference
Decreased solid emptying	46
Defective gastric relaxatory response to duodenal distension	47
Increased and premature distribution of food to the distal end of the stomach	48
Increased self-reported abuse	49

and 12 healthy controls, perception and gut reflex response (measured as isobaric volume changes by gastric and duodenal barostats) to gastric distension, duodenal distension, and somatic stimulation were measured. Patients with dyspepsia had gastric hypersensitivity to distension (discomfort threshold at 6.4 ± 0.4 mm Hg vs. 8.3 ± 0.6 mm Hg in controls; $P < .05$). Duodenal and somatic sensitivity was normal. Patients with dyspepsia recognized their clinical symptoms in all gastric but in only $58\% \pm 12\%$ of the duodenal distension trials. Patients with dyspepsia showed defective gastric relaxatory responses to duodenal distension (68 ± 30 mL gastric expansion vs. 239 ± 12 mL in controls; $P < 0.05$). The results suggest that patients with dyspepsia are selectively hypersensitive to gastric distension. This sensory dysfunction is associated with impaired reflex reactivity of the stomach.

One study examined the hypothesis that food maldistribution in the stomach may cause symptoms in dyspeptic patients.[48] Eleven patients with functional dyspepsia characterized by chronic severe postprandial bloating without organic abnormality and 12 healthy volunteers ingested a standard meal labeled with technetium 99m. In controls, food remaining predominantly in the proximal half of the stomach after ingestion and was then redistributed to the distal half. In the patients, however, initial activity in the proximal half after ingestion (48%; Cl, 40% to 65%) was significantly lower ($P < 0.05$) than in controls (60%; Cl, 39% to 73%) and was distributed more fully to the distal half of the stomach with a peak distal activity (56%; Cl, 34% to 58%) that was consistently higher than in controls (36%; Cl, 33% to 42%) ($P < .05$). The results suggest that in these dyspeptic patients, intragastric distribution of food is abnormal.

Ten consecutive patients with functional dyspepsia and prepyloric erosions were studied twice on separate days, once without drug administration and once after the intake of one tablet of glyceryl trinitrate, 2.6 mg, 2 hours before the ingestion of 500 mL of meat soup. Without glyceryl trinitrate, postprandial antral area distension and symptoms scores were positively correlated ($r = 0.64$, $P = .05$). After the administration of glyceryl trinitrate, antral area distension both in the fasting state and 10 minutes postprandially was reduced ($P = .02$ and $P = .01$, respectively), whereas the amplitude and the motility index of antral contractions were unaffected. Abdominal discomfort was not significantly reduced by glyceryl trinitrate ($P = .13$). The data raise questions about the causal relationship between symptoms and antral distension in patients with functional dyspepsia.[50]

Role of Endoscopic Evaluation

One study compared two strategies for the management of dyspepsia—treatment based on the results of prompt endoscopy (group 1) and empiric H_2-blocker treatment with diagnostic endoscopy only in cases of therapeutic failure or symptomatic relapse within 1 year (group 2).[51] Eligible patients had symptoms severe enough to justify empiric H_2-blocker therapy. Symptoms, drug consumption, and sick-leave

days were assessed through monthly diaries. Patients with nonorganic dyspepsia diagnosed by endoscopy did not receive ulcer drugs. Of 414 patients randomized, 373 completed 1-year follow-up. Organic disease was found at endoscopy in 68 (33%) of 208 group 1 patients (ulcers in 45). Endoscopy was done in 136 (66%) of 206 group 2 patients. Case selection for endoscopy was not improved by the empiric treatment strategy. The prevalence of organic disease was no higher among patients who underwent endoscopy after a poor response to H_2 blockers than among those who received prompt endoscopy. Forty percent of the expected ulcer cases remained undiagnosed in the group receiving empiric treatment. After 1 year there were no differences in symptoms or quality-of-life measures. The empiric treatment strategy in dyspepsia was associated with higher costs, mainly due to a higher number of sick-leave days and the cost of ulcer drug use. The data suggest that prompt endoscopy is a cost-effective strategy in dyspeptic patients with symptoms severe enough to justify empiric H_2-blocker treatment.

Role of Self-Reported Abuse

The link between abuse (self-reported sexual, physical, emotional, and verbal abuse in childhood and adulthood) and irritable bowel syndrome was assessed in one survey study.[49] Residents of Olmsted County, Minnesota, ranging in age from 30 to 49 were randomly selected; 1,248 subjects were contacted by mail. Of the 919 responders (74%), the age-adjusted prevalence of any abuse was 41% in women and 11% in men, for an age- and sex-adjusted prevalence of 26%. Symptoms of irritable bowel syndrome, dyspepsia, and frequent heartburn were reported by 14%, 23%, and 12%, respectively. There was a significant association between irritable bowel syndrome and sexual abuse, emotional or verbal abuse, and abuse in childhood and adulthood. Similarly, dyspepsia and heartburn were both significantly associated with abuse. In the population, 31% had visited a physician for gastrointestinal symptoms; the odds of visiting a physician were highest in those reporting abuse in adulthood and childhood. The data suggest that self-reported abuse is common in middle-aged subjects; those who report abuse are more likely to have symptoms consistent with irritable bowel syndrome, dyspepsia, or heartburn and to visit a physician for bowel symptoms. This type of association, however, does not establish causality among the parameters studied.

Role of Treatment of *Helicobacter pylori*

The soundness of therapeutic trials to establish whether *H. pylori* plays a role in functional dyspepsia was critically evaluated.[39] A broad-based MEDLINE search to identify all treatment trials published between 1984 and 1993 was performed. All functional dyspepsia trials were systemically analyzed for potential design

strengths and weaknesses. Eight reported that anti–*H. pylori* therapy was efficacious and eight failed to detect a statistically significant benefit. In all studies one or more serious methodologic weakness was identified, including nonrandomized, non–placebo-controlled designs, lack of maintenance of blindness, application of inadequate outcome measures, failure to eradicate infection and follow patients after therapy, and inadequate study power. The findings suggest that there is a need for well-designed trials in *H. pylori*–positive dyspepsia.

MECHANISMS OF MUCOSAL INJURY AND DEFENSE

The redundancy of the gastroduodenal defense mechanism is illustrated by the many studies of different pathways of mucosal injury and protection. A synopsis of recent studies is presented (Table 4).

Aspirin, Thromboxane B₂, and Prostaglandin

A randomized, placebo-controlled study was designed to determine whether a dose of aspirin exists that might inhibit thromboxane-dependent platelet function without causing gastric mucosal injury.[52] Five male and 11 female healthy volun-

TABLE 4.
Mechanisms of Mucosal Injury and Defense

Mechanism	Reference
Low-dose aspirin (3 or 10 mg/day) reduces serum thromboxane B_2 without significant inhibition of gastric prostaglandin	52
Increased epidermal growth factor is associated with increased cellular proliferation during NSAID* ingestion	53
Endogenous vasopressin prevents restraint water immersion stress–induced gastric ulcers via the V_1 receptor	54
Vasopressin V_1 receptor contributes to gastric lesions induced by ethanol, reserpine, cold-restraint stress, hemorrhagic shock, and indomethacin	55
High-dose capsaicin treatment reduces gastric CGRP and increases the size of acetic acid–induced gastric ulcer	56
Low-dose capsaicin pretreatment increases prostaglandin and decreases acidified bile salt–induced gastric mucosal injury	57
CGRP released from gastric enteric neurons mediates gastric mucosal resistance to ulceration	58
Ulcer healing is associated with increased laminin receptor expression	59
Misoprostol enhances ulcer healing by increasing mucosal regeneration	60
Ammonia impairs ulcer healing by suppressing cell cycling of regenerative epithelium and fibroblasts in the ulcer margin	61

*NSAID = nonsteroidal anti-inflammatory drug; CGRP = calcitonin gene–related peptide.

teers received placebo or aspirin, 324, 1,300, or 2,600 mg/day for 2 days in the first part of the study. Significant ($\sim$50%) inhibition of gastric juice prostaglandin output was observed with daily aspirin doses of 324 to 2,600 mg. A significant increase in gastric juice hemoglobin output occurred only with 2,600 mg/day. In the second part, volunteers received placebo or aspirin, 3, 10, 30, or 81 mg/day for 8 days. Significant inhibition ($\sim$50%) of gastric prostaglandin E_2 output was noted at a daily aspirin dose of 30 mg. Lower aspirin doses did not reduce prostaglandin E_2 output significantly, although these doses did significantly reduce serum thromboxane B_2 in a dose-related manner. These data suggest that aspirin can significantly reduce serum thromboxane B_2 at doses of 3 or 10 mg/day, which are significantly below the threshold dose for significant gastric prostaglandin inhibition and acute stomach mucosal injury.

Epidermal Growth Factor

Patients with arthritis underwent endoscopy with collection of saliva and gastric juice for epidermal growth factor measurement before and 2 weeks after continuous NSAID ingestion. During this period patients also received either the prostaglandin analogue misoprostol or placebo in addition to their NSAID. In the misoprostol group (n = 5), there was no observed mucosal damage and no change in either salivary or gastric juice epidermal growth factor. In the placebo group (n = 10), erosions developed in 3 patients. Salivary epidermal growth factor did not change (3.02 $\pm$ 0.54 vs. 2.80 $\pm$ 0.41 ng/mL), but gastric juice epidermal growth factor increased from 0.42 $\pm$ 0.12 to 0.69 $\pm$ 0.14 ng/mL ($P <$ .05). The data suggest that the increased epidermal growth factor could contribute to the increased cellular proliferation observed during NSAID ingestion and may represent an important mechanism underlying gastric mucosal adaptation.[53]

Vasopressin

To elucidate the role of vasopressin in the development of stress-induced gastric ulcers, mucosal lesions after restraint and water immersion were examined in Brattleboro strain rats with hereditary hypothalamic diabetes insipidus (vasopressin deficient) and in Long-Evans rats used as controls.[54] Restrained animals were immersed in water for 2 hours, and the size of lesion was expressed as a percentage of the lesion area to the total glandular mucosal area, which was defined as the ulcer index. In vasopressin-deficient rats, the ulcer index was significantly higher than in control rats. Intracerebroventricular administration of vasopressin reduced the ulcer index in vasopressin-deficient rats, and intracerebroventricular administration of the V_1 antagonist [d(CH$_2$)$_5$Tyr(Me)]AVP elevated the ulcer index in control rats. These results indicate that endogenous vasopressin plays a role in preventing the formation of gastric ulcers induced by stress via a central V_1 receptor. In another study, [Mca_1, $TyrMe_2$, Arg_8]vasopressin, a vasopressin pressor (V_1) receptor antagonist, reduced the gastric mucosal injury induced by ethanol, indomethacin, reserpine, cold-restraint stress, and hemorrhagic shock in a dose-dependent manner. Endogenous vasopressin deficiency, as in Brattleboro homozygous rats, had a similar effect. [Lys_8]vasopressin injected exogenously aggravated all types of lesions in normal rats. Circulating vasopressin levels were increased by ethanol, reserpine, cold-restraint stress, and hemorrhagic shock, but not by indomethacin. The intramucosal vasopressin content was found to be elevated in all models. Specific vasopressin binding sites were shown on the blood vessels of the gastric mucosa. The data suggest that vasopressin plays a significant role in the generation of these lesions.[55] The results of these two studies are perplexingly contradictory. The role of endogenous vasopressin in the formation of gastric mucosal lesions remains to be characterized.

Sensory Nerves

The effects of ablation of sensory neurons on acetic acid–induced chronic gastric ulcers in rats were investigated at morphologic and biochemical levels by computerized imaging analysis of the ulcerated area, histologic examination, and neuropeptide determination.[56] Afferent nerve ablation, as a result of treating the rats with a neurotoxic dose of capsaicin (50 + 50 mg/kg subcutaneously over a 2-day period), produced a significant increase in the ulcer area at 1 and 2 weeks after acetic acid injection. The delay in ulcer healing was associated with a marked and persistent decrease in tissue calcitonin gene–related peptide (CGRP)-like immunoreactivity. These findings suggest that capsaicin-sensitive afferent fibers may play a role in the healing of chronic experimental gastric ulcers in rats.

In another study, before injury with topical 5 mmol/L acidified taurocholate (pH 1.2), rat stomachs were pretreated with either vehicle or capsaicin (160 mmol/L), both with and without prior administration of either lidocaine (1%) or indomethacin (5 mg/kg subcutaneously). Pretreatment with a neurostimulatory dose of topical capsaicin significantly ($P < .05$) decreased bile acid–induced net luminal ion fluxes and luminal DNA accumulation (a marker of gastric mucosal cell exfoliation), an effect blocked by both lidocaine and indomethacin. Both local neuronal blockade and cyclooxygenase inhibition block the protective effect of capsaicin, findings corroborated by gross and histologic injury analysis. This study suggests that sensory neurons may mediate gastric mucosal protection from bile acid injury by increasing the synthesis of endogenous prostaglandins.[57]

The role of CGRP in gastric mucosal resistance to ulceration was assessed.[58] Intra-arterial capsaicin (concentration range, 10^{-7} to 10^{-5} mol/L) stimulated a prompt and sustained release of immunoreactive CGRP in the vascular perfusate,

84% of which coeluted with rat $CGRP_{1-37}$ by gel filtration. Intragastric capsaicin (range, 10^{-5} to 10^{-4} mol/L) failed to release CGRP into the vascular perfusate. In separate experiments, intragastric capsaicin (10^{-6} mol/L) or intravenous $CGRP_{1-37}$ (10 µg/kg/hr) reduced the number and area of mucosal lesions caused by hydrochloric acid (HCl) and indomethacin as compared with vehicle treatment. Rats depleted of endogenous CGRP were more susceptible to gastric ulceration than were normal rats. Intragastric capsaicin failed to protect the mucosa of CGRP-depleted rats, whereas exogenous intravenous CGRP was effective. The data suggest that CGRP released from gastric enteric neurons mediates gastric mucosal resistance to ulceration by noxious agents.

Laminin Receptor

Laminin, an extracellular adhesive protein, is presumed to be able to facilitate the migration of epithelial cells to the site of mucosal damage. A study was performed to confirm that laminin receptors play a role in mucosal repair. In rats with acetic acid–induced gastric ulcers, binding assays revealed that ulcer healing was accompanied by an increase in mucosal expression of laminin receptor. A 2.7-fold increase in receptor expression occurred by the 4th day following ulcer development and reached a maximum of an 8.6-fold increase by the 14th day when the ulcer was essentially healed. Drug treatment that evokes enhanced mucosal cell laminin receptor expression promotes re-epithelialization and hence hastens ulcer healing.[59]

Mucosal Regeneration

In a study of mucosal regeneration in experimental ulcer healing, gastric ulcers were induced by the application of acetic acid. Rats were treated with 200 mg/kg aspirin, 100 µg/kg misoprostol, a combination of both treatments, or methylcellulose vehicle for up to 2 weeks starting 2 days after ulcer induction. Aspirin delayed ulcer healing when compared with controls, whereas misoprostol significantly reversed this effect. Quantitative histologic studies revealed that misoprostol cotreatment significantly increased mucosal regeneration when compared with aspirin treatment alone.[60]

Ammonia

Another study assessed the direct effect of ammonia on the healing of experimental ulcers. In the rats with acetic acid–induced gastric ulcers, the 0.02% ammonia treatment group showed a significant increase in the ulcer index (long diameter $\times$ short diameter; square millimeters) in the fourth and eighth weeks. This group also showed suppressed cell cycling of the regenerative epithelium and fibroblasts in the ulcer margin, which suggests direct toxicity of ammonia. The data indicate that healing of acetic acid–induced ulcers was delayed by continuous administration of 0.02% ammonia.[61]

Mucosal Blood Flow

In a model of canine vascularized chambered gastric mucosa, topical application of 5mM sodium taurocholate at pH 1.2 to the mucosa results in luminal hydrogen ion loss and surface epithelial cell injury (luminal accumulation of DNA). However, gross mucosal injury does not occur because of a protective increase in gastric mucosal blood flow. To test the hypothesis that mucosal acid-base status influences mucosal blood flow and surface cell injury, studies employing the aforementioned model and intra-arterial sodium chloride, bicarbonate, or HCl were performed. When compared with the sodium chloride group, the bicarbonate group had no increase in gastric mucosal blood flow after exposure to 5mM sodium taurocholate at pH 1.2. Simultaneously, however, surface epithelial cell loss was reduced by 48%, 604 $\pm$ 72 with sodium chloride vs. 314 $\pm$ 59 μg/30 minutes DNA with bicarbonate, $P < 0.025$. Infusion of intra-arterial HCl generated a large increase in gastric mucosal blood flow without an increase in surface epithelial cell injury as compared with intra-arterial sodium chloride. The data suggest that mucosal acid-base status is an important modulator of mucosal blood flow. The change in mucosal blood flow protects the gastric mucosa during bile acid–induced injury.[62]

To assess the mechanism of mucosal adaptation to the ulcerogenic action of aspirin, the following study was performed. After repeated administration of aspirin, the mucosal damage progressively declined and was accompanied by a significant augmentation in gastric blood flow. A reduction in blood neutrophil count, mucosal neutrophil infiltration, and leukotriene B_4 release was observed. The results suggest that adaptation of the rat stomach to repeated aspirin exposure appears to be mediated by a significant increase in gastric blood flow and a reduction in neutrophil activation and leukotriene B_4 release.[63]

Mucus and Surfactant Phospholipids

The effect of omeprazole on gastric mucosal injury induced by hemorrhagic shock in rats was investigated.[64] Omeprazole and ranitidine did not affect mean arterial blood pressure under both basal conditions and induction of hemorrhagic shock. Both significantly inhibited gastric acid output from anesthetized, pylorus-ligated rats. Omeprazole but not ranitidine increased gastric mucus secretion and caused a significant reduction in hemorrhagic shock–induced damage to gastric mucosa. The increase in mucus secretion by omeprazole may be important in its protective action against hemorrhagic shock–induced mucosal injury.

Aging and Mucosal Prostaglandin

One study determined the effect of aging on gastric mucosal eicosanoid formation and aspirin-induced injury in Fischer 344 rats.[65] Rats of three different age groups (3, 12, and 21 months) were killed after an overnight fast, and gastric mucosal formation of prostaglandins and leukotrienes was determined. Gastric mucosal prostaglandin formation decreased with aging, whereas no significant changes in mucosal leukotriene formation were noted in any age groups. Rats of various ages were killed 3 hours after receiving aspirin (100 mg/kg intragastrically) or vehicle (for controls). Gastric mucosal eicosanoid formation and gross mucosal injury were assessed. No gastric mucosal lesions were present in any rats treated with the vehicle alone. In contrast, aspirin caused significant mucosal injury in all age groups, but significantly more mucosal lesions were noted in the older rats. These observations indicate that gastric mucosal prostaglandin synthesis decreases with aging in rats and that aged animals are more susceptible to aspirin-induced acute gastric mucosal injury.

Nonulcerogenic Anti-Inflammatory Agents

Cyclooxygenase (COX) exists in two forms. COX-1 is in most tissues (constitutive) and is involved in the physiologic production of prostaglandins. COX-2 is cytokine-inducible (inducible) and is expressed in inflammatory cells. Carrageenan administration to the subcutaneous rat air pouch induces a rapid inflammatory response characterized by high levels of prostaglandins and leukotrienes in the fluid exudate. The time course of the induction of COX-2 mRNA and protein coincided with the production of prostaglandins in the pouch tissue and cellular infiltrate. Carrageenan-induced COX-2 immunoreactivity was localized to macrophages obtained from the fluid exudate as well as to the inner surface layer of cells within the pouch lining. Dexamethasone inhibited both COX-2 expression and prostaglandin synthesis in the fluid exudate but failed to inhibit prostaglandin synthesis in the stomach. Furthermore, NS-398, a selective COX-2 inhibitor, and indomethacin, a nonselective COX-1/COX-2 inhibitor, blocked proinflammatory prostaglandin synthesis in the air pouch. In contrast, only indomethacin blocked gastric prostaglandin and, additionally, produced gastric lesions. These results suggest that inhibitors of COX-2 are potent anti-inflammatory agents that do not produce the typical side effects (e.g., gastric ulcers) associated with the nonselective COX-1–directed anti-inflammatory drugs.[66]

Nonsteroidal anti-inflammatory drugs inhibit mucosal prostaglandin synthesis and promote neutrophil adhesion to endothelium as part of their ulcerogenic property. Nitric oxide is a potent inhibitor of neutrophil function. The combination of a nitric oxide donor and an NSAID in a single compound is postulated to provide the anti-inflammatory effect of the NSAID devoid of the proinflammatory and ulcerogenic side effect. One study examined the effect of addition of a nitroxybutyl moiety to diclofenac on its ulcerogenic properties. The diclofenac derivative nitrofenac (after the addition of a nitroxybutyl moiety) was compared with diclofenac.[67] The addition of a nitroxybutyl moiety to diclofenac markedly reduces the ulcerogenic properties of this compound without interfering with its ability to inhibit COX activity or reduce acute inflammation. In another study, the short-term ulcerogenic and anti-inflammatory properties of nitroxybutyl derivatives were compared with those of the parent NSAIDs.[68] The derivatives of flurbiprofen and ketoprofen caused significantly less short-term gastric mucosal injury at all doses tested despite producing comparable suppression of prostaglandin synthesis. The NSAID derivatives also showed comparable anti-inflammatory activity to the native compounds. The flurbiprofen derivative inhibited collagen-induced platelet aggregation significantly more than the native NSAID did. Plasma nitrate/nitrite levels increased significantly after administration of the flurbiprofen derivative, consistent with the release of nitrogen oxide. The data suggest that the addition of a nitroxybutyl moiety to two NSAIDs markedly reduces the ability of these agents to induce short-term gastric injury but does not interfere with their ability to suppress inflammatory processes, inhibit prostaglandin synthesis, or inhibit platelet aggregation.

Angiotensin

One study tested the hypothesis that vasodilator prostaglandins attenuate in angiotensin II–induced gastric vasoconstriction.[69] Angiotensin II produced statistically significant, dose-related increases in the vascular resistance of a mechanically perfused ex vivo canine stomach segment. Indomethacin and meclofenamic acid (both COX inhibitors) blocked the vasodilator response to intra-arterial arachidonic acid and augmented the maximal increase in perfusion pressure during angiotensin II infusion. Angiotensin II produced dose-related increases in gastric venous but not arterial levels of 6-ketoprostaglandin $F_{1\alpha}$, the major metabolite of prostacyclin. These results are consistent with the hypothesis that release of vasodilatory prostaglandins attenuates the vasoconstrictor response to angiotensin II in the gastric microcirculation.

Another study tested whether the angiotensin converting the enzyme inhibitor captopril would prevent stress ulceration when given after the onset of canine hemorrhagic shock and whether any detrimental effects would result from enhancing splanchnic perfusion with captopril during hemorrhagic shock.[70] Captopril treatment was associated with a decrease in gastric mucosal injury and with a marked decrease in systemic acidosis. Captopril enhanced blood flow to the small intestine, pancreas, liver, and spleen during shock, but not flow to the stomach. The data suggest that captopril reduces the stress ulceration produced by canine hemorrhagic shock by alleviating systemic acidosis through enhanced perfusion of other viscera rather than by a specific enhancement of gastric perfusion.

Neuropeptides

Intracisternal but not intraperitoneal injection of rat pancreatic polypeptide (62.5, 250, and 1,000 ng per rat) into pylorus-ligated rats resulted in a dose-dependent stimulation of gastric acid and pepsin secretion. This effect of centrally administered pancreatic polypeptide was completely blocked by vagotomy and by pretreatment with atropine. Intracisternal but not intraperitoneal injection of pancreatic polypeptide (500 to 2,000 ng per rat) dose-dependently increased the severity of gastric lesions induced by intravenous 2-deoxy-D-glucose (a gastric ulcerogenic manipulation) or subcutaneous indomethacin. These results suggest that pancreatic polypeptide acts centrally in the brain to stimulate gastric acid and pepsin secretion through a vagal, muscarinic pathway and exerts an ulcerogenic action on the gastric mucosa.[71]

Adhesion Molecules

The adhesion of polymorphonuclear leukocytes (PMNs) to the vascular endothelium plays a role in the induction of gastric mucosal injury by ethanol, ischemia-reperfusion, NSAIDs, and aspirin. Polymorphonuclear leukocyte adhesion induced by NSAIDs, in particular, may be related to an increase in leukotrienes and/or a reduction in prostaglandin levels in the tissue. Adhesion of PMNs to the vascular endothelium is dependent on a range of molecules, including lymphocyte function–associated antigen type 1 (LFA-1; CD11a) on the leukocyte and ICAM-1 on the endothelial cell. The distribution and sequence of expression of leukocyte LFA-1 and endothelial ICAM-1 adhesion molecules in the mucosa after treatment with NSAIDs was investigated.[72] The number of ICAM-1–stained blood vessels in the mucosa increased significantly after 30 minutes of treatment with intragastric aspirin and indomethacin before any appreciable mucosal damage was evident. This increase was reversed by treatment with misoprostol in both aspirin- and indomethacin-treated animals. There was no significant increase in LFA-1–positive cells until after 60 minutes of NSAID treatment. The results suggest that the adhesion molecules LFA-1 and ICAM-1 are expressed in the normal gastric mucosa and that the number of ICAM-1–stained blood vessels increases rapidly after NSAID treatment. This increase in ICAM-1 expression may be associated with an inhibition of prostaglandin synthesis by NSAIDs. These results provide further support for the role of early vascular changes in NSAID gastropathy.

Tumor Necrosis Factor Alpha

Pentoxifylline is a methylxanthine derivative that exerts a number of hematologic, hemodynamic, and anti-inflammatory effects. Pentoxifylline reduces PMN adhesion in vitro in septic shock and ischemia-reperfusion models and inhibits the synthesis and release of tumor necrosis factor α (TNF-α) from macrophages. Pentoxifylline reduces indomethacin-induced mucosal damage and neutrophil margination in a dose-dependent manner without exerting any effect on gastric mucosal prostaglandin concentrations. The effect of pentoxifylline was not affected by pretreatment with a nitric oxide inhibitor. Pentoxifylline prevented the indomethacin-induced increase in TNF-α concentrations in a dose-dependent fashion.[73] Pentoxifylline attenuates indomethacin-induced gastric mucosal injury and neutrophil margination by modulating indomethacin-induced release of TNF-α.

Modulation of Angiogenesis as a New Approach to Ulcer Treatment

Human basic fibroblast growth factor (bFGF) is an endothelial mitogen that stimulates angiogenesis and the proliferation of other cells such as fibroblasts and smooth muscle cells. After this peptide was stabilized to acid and pepsin by site-specific mutagenesis, a study tested whether bFGF might accelerate the healing of experimental duodenal ulcers. This mutein peptide (bFGF-CS23) was administered orally in comparison with cimetidine to rats with duodenal ulcers induced by cysteamine. Oral bFGF-CS23 therapy maintained for 21 days at 100 ng/100 g twice daily resulted in (1) a significant acceleration of healing of duodenal ulcers, i.e., a reduction in mean ulcer area by 83% in the bFGF-CS23–treated rats as compared with only 61% after cimetidine therapy and 40% for untreated controls; (2) complete healing with no residual ulcer in 62% of the bFGF-CS23–treated rats as compared with only 7% of the untreated rats; and (3) a ninefold increase in angiogenesis in the ulcer bed as compared with untreated controls. A single dose of the bFGF-CS23 mutein had no effect on gastric output of HCl or pepsin, but daily treatment for 2 or 3 weeks resulted in enhanced acid and pepsin outputs. The data suggest that chronic duodenal ulcers can be healed rapidly by stimulating angiogenesis and other wound-healing processes in the ulcer bed without a reduction of gastric acid.[74]

SUMMARY

Several reports deal with predictors of ulcer occurrence, giant ulcers, delayed ulcer healing, and ulcer relapse. Free radical scavengers are effective in the treatment of duodenal ulcers. Antisecretory maintenance treatment prevents not only ulcer recurrence but also recurrence of complications of ulcer disease. Prostaglandins such as misoprostol and enprostil can be used in the treatment of NSAID-induced ulcerations, but diarrhea is an important side effect.

Recent reports have focused on the search for simpler regimens for the treatment of gastric *H. pylori* infection. Eradication of *H. pylori* without antisecretory therapy is sufficient to allow healing of duodenal ulcers. Once eradicated, the re-infection rate of *H. pylori* appears to be low. Eradication of *H. pylori* enhances the healing of refractory ulcers. Ulcer recurrence data continue to support a possible causal role for *H. pylori* in the pathogenesis of duodenal ulcer disease. *Helicobacter pylori* treatment also reduces the recurrence of ulcer complications. An association between gastric malignancy and *H. pylori* continues to receive attention. The mechanisms of the mucosa-damaging action of *H. pylori* involve receptor-ligand interaction, endosomal vacuoles, and intercellular adhesion molecules.

Factors associated with portal hypertensive gastropathy include large esophageal varices and gastric varices. Somatostatin transiently attenuates increased gastric perfusion in portal hypertensive gastropathy. Predictors of ulcer bleeding and injection therapy continue to occupy center stage in discussions on the management of bleeding peptic ulcers.

Studies on dyspepsia have revealed an increase in emptying time for indigestable solids in diabetic dyspeptics and an impairment in gastric reflex relaxation in response to duodenal distension have been described. Maldistribution of food in dyspeptics remains a controversial issue. Prompt endoscopy is a cost-effective strategy in dyspeptic patients with symptoms severe enough to justify empiric H_2-blocker treatment. The trials to evaluate the efficacy of *H. pylori* eradication in dyspeptics are inadequate. Self-reported abuse is an issue to be considered in subjects with functional dyspepsia.

Recent advances in our understanding of the mechanisms of mucosal injury and defense include the following. Aspirin can significantly reduce serum thromboxane B_2 at doses that are significantly below the threshold dose for significant gastric prostaglandin inhibition and acute stomach mucosal injury. Increased epidermal growth factor increases cellular proliferation during NSAID ingestion and may represent an important mechanism underlying gastric mucosal adaptation. Endogenous vasopressin plays a role in preventing the formation of gastric ulcers induced by stress via a central V_1 receptor and in the development of gastric mucosal lesions induced by ethanol. Capsaicin-sensitive CGRP-containing afferent fibers play a role in the healing of chronic experimental gastric ulcers in rats. They mediate gastric mucosal protection from bile acid injury by increasing the synthesis of endogenous prostaglandins. Calcitonin gene–related peptide released from gastric enteric neurons mediates gastric mucosal resistance to ulceration by noxious agents. Drug treatment that evokes enhanced mucosal cell laminin receptor expression promotes re-epithelialization and hence hastens ulcer healing. Misoprostol cotreatment significantly increases mucosal regeneration when compared with aspirin treatment alone. Healing of acetic acid–induced ulcers is delayed by the continuous administration of 0.02% ammonia. A change in mucosal blood flow protects the gastric mucosa during bile acid–induced injury. Adaptation of the rat stomach to repeated aspirin exposure appears to be mediated by a significant increase in gastric blood flow and a reduction in neutrophil activation and leukotriene B_4 release. Omeprazole causes a significant reduction in hemorrhagic shock–induced damage to gastric mucosa, inhibition of gastric acid output from anesthetized pylorus-ligated rats, and an increase in gastric mucus. Aged animals are more susceptible to aspirin-induced acute gastric mucosal injury. Inhibitors of COX-2 are potent anti-inflammatory agents that do not produce the typical side effects. The development of NSAIDs without gastroduodenal ulcerogenic effects is undergoing active investigation. Release of vasodilatory prostaglandins attenuates the vasoconstrictor response to angiotensin II in the gastric microcirculation. Captopril alleviates the stress ulceration produced by canine hemorrhagic shock by alleviating systemic acidosis through enhanced perfusion of other viscera rather than a specific enhancement of gastric perfusion. Pancreatic polypeptide is capable of acting centrally in the brain to stimulate gastric acid and pepsin secretion through a vagal, muscarinic pathway and in so doing exerts an ulcerogenic action on the gastric mucosa. The adhesion molecules LFA-1 and ICAM-1 are expressed in normal gastric mucosa, and the number of ICAM-1–stained blood vessels increases rapidly after NSAID treatment. Pentoxifylline prevents the indomethacin-induced increase in TNF-α. Modulation of angiogenesis as a new approach to ulcer treatment has also been reported.

Acknowledgment

I would like to thank A. Bruce Ivie for his assistance in the preparation of this manuscript.

REFERENCES

1. Collen MJ, Santoro MJ, Chen YK: Giant duodenal ulcer. Evaluation of basal acid output, nonsteroidal antiinflammatory drug use, and ulcer complications. *Dig Dis Sci* 39:1113–1116, 1994.
2. Janssen M, Dijkmans BA, Vandenbroucke JP, et al: Achlorhydria does not protect against benign upper gastrointestinal ulcers during NSAID use. *Dig Dis Sci* 39:362–365, 1994.
3. Leung FW, Wong DN, Lau J, et al: Endoscopic assessment of blood flow in duodenal ulcers. *Gastrointest Endosc* 40:334–341, 1994.
4. Reynolds JC, Schoen RE, Maislin G, et al: Risk factors for delayed healing of duodenal ulcers treated with famotidine and ranitidine. *Am J Gastroenterol* 89:571–580, 1994.
5. Battaglia G: Risk factors of relapse in gastric ulcer: A one-year, double-blind, comparative study of nizatidine versus placebo. *Ital J Gastroenterol* 26(suppl 1):19–22, 1994.
6. Armstrong D, Arnold R, Classen M, et al: RUDER—a prospective, two-year, multicenter study of risk factors for duodenal ulcer relapse during maintenance therapy with ranitidine. *Dig Dis Sci* 39:1425–1433, 1994.

7. Salim AS: Role of free radical scavengers in the management of refractory duodenal ulceration. A new approach. *J Surg Res* 56:45–52, 1994.

8. Susi D, Neri M, Ballone E, et al: Five-year maintenance treatment with ranitidine: Effects on the natural history of duodenal ulcers disease. *Am J Gastroenterol* 89:26–32, 1994.

9. Jensen DM, Cheng S, Kovacs TO, et al: A controlled study of ranitidine for the prevention of recurrent hemorrhage from duodenal ulcer. *N Engl J Med* 330:382–386, 1994.

10. Elliott SL, Yeomans ND, Buchanan RR, et al: Efficacy of 12 months' misoprostol as prophylaxis against NSAID-induced gastric ulcers. A placebo-controlled trial. *Scand J Rheumatol* 23:171–176, 1994.

11. Sontag SJ, Schnell TG, Budiman-Mak E, et al: Healing of NSAID-induced gastric ulcers with a synthetic prostaglandin analog (enprostil). *Am J Gastroenterol* 89:1014–1020, 1994.

12. Veldhuyzen van Zanten SJ, Pollak PT, Best LM, et al: Increasing prevalence of Helicobacter pylori infection with age: Continuous risk of infection in adults rather than cohort effect. *J Infect Dis* 169:434–437, 1994.

13. Kelly SM, Pitcher MC, Farmery SM, et al: Isolation of Helicobacter pylori from feces of patients with dyspepsia in the United Kingdom. *Gastroenterology* 107:1671–1674, 1994.

14. Nomura A, Stemmermann GN, Chyou PH, et al: Helicobacter pylori infection and the risk for duodenal and gastric ulceration. *Ann Intern Med* 120:977–981, 1994.

15. Labenz J, Ruhl GH, Bertrams J, et al: Medium- or high-dose omeprazole plus amoxicillin eradicates Helicobacter pylori in gastric ulcer disease. *Am J Gastroenterol* 89:726–730, 1994.

16. Labenz J, Ruhl GH, Bertrams J, et al: Medium- and high-dose omeprazole plus amoxicillin for eradication of Helicobacter pylori in duodenal ulcer disease. *Dig Dis Sci* 39:1483–1487, 1994.

17. Iser JH, Buttigieg RJ, Iseli A: Low dose, short duration therapy for the eradication of Helicobacter pylori in patients with duodenal ulcer. *Med J Aust* 160:192–196, 1994.

18. Logan RP, Gummett PA, Misiewicz JJ, et al: One week's anti–Helicobacter pylori treatment for duodenal ulcer. *Gut* 35:15–18, 1994.

19. Hosking SW, Ling TK, Chung SC, et al: Duodenal ulcer healing by eradication of Helicobacter pylori without anti-acid treatment: Randomised controlled trial. *Lancet* 343:508–510, 1994.

20. Sung JJ, Chung SC, Ling TK, et al: One-year follow-up of duodenal ulcers after 1-wk triple therapy for Helicobacter pylori. *Am J Gastroenterol* 89:199–202, 1994.

21. Borody TJ, Andrews P, Mancuso N, et al: Helicobacter pylori reinfection rate, in patients with cured duodenal ulcer. *Am J Gastroenterol* 89:529–532, 1994.

22. Forbes GM, Claser ME, Cullen DJ, et al: Duodenal ulcer treated with Helicobacter pylori eradication: Seven-year follow-up. *Lancet* 343:258–260, 1994.

23. Boyd HK, Zaterka S, Eisig JN, et al: Helicobacter pylori and refractory duodenal ulcers: Crossover comparison of continued cimetidine with cimetidine plus antimicrobials. *Am J Gastroenterol* 89:1505–1510, 1994.

24. Karita M, Morshed MG, Ouchi K, et al: Bismuth-free triple therapy for eradicating Helicobacter pylori and reducing the gastric ulcer recurrence rate. *Am J Gastroenterol* 89:1032–1035, 1994.

25. Labenz J, Borsch G: Role of Helicobacter pylori eradication in the prevention of peptic ulcer bleeding relapse. *Digestion* 55:19–23, 1994.

26. Weber DM, Dimopoulos MA, Anandu DP, et al: Regression of gastric lymphoma of mucosa-associated lymphoid tissue with antibiotic therapy for Helicobacter pylori. *Gastroenterology* 107:1835–1838, 1994.

27. Eidt S, Stolte M, Fischer R: Helicobacter pylori gastritis and primary gastric non-Hodgkin's lymphomas. *J Clin Pathol* 47:436–439, 1994.

28. Parsonnet J, Hansen S, Rodriguez L, et al: Helicobacter pylori infection and gastric lymphoma. *N Engl J Med* 330:1267–1271, 1994.

29. Nilius M, Bode G, Buchler M, et al: Adhesion of Helicobacter pylori and Escherichia coli to human and bovine surface mucus cells in vitro. *Eur J Clin Invest* 24:454–459, 1994.

30. Papini E, de Bernard M, Milia E, et al: Cellular vacuoles induced by Helicobacter pylori originate from late endosomal compartments. *Proc Natl Acad Sci U S A* 91:9720–9724, 1994.

31. Kurose I, Granger DN, Evans DJ Jr, et al: Helicobacter pylori–induced microvascular protein leakage in rats: Role of neutrophils, mast cells, and platelets. *Gastroenterology* 107:70–79, 1994.

32. Davies GR, Simmonds NJ, Stevens TR, et al: Helicobacter pylori stimulates antral mucosal reactive oxygen metabolite production in vivo. *Gut* 35:179–185, 1994.

33. Suzuki M, Miura S, Mori M, et al: Rebamipide, a novel antiulcer agent, attenuates Helicobacter pylori induced gastric mucosal cell injury associated with neutrophil derived oxidants. *Gut* 35:1375–1378, 1994.

34. Chen TS, Tsay SH, Chang FY, et al: Effect of eradication of Helicobacter pylori on serum pepsinogen I, gastrin, and insulin in duodenal ulcer patients: A 12-month follow-up study. *Am J Gastroenterol* 89:1511–1514, 1994.

35. Odum L, Petersen HD, Andersen IB, et al: Gastrin and somatostatin in Helicobacter pylori infected antral mucosa. *Gut* 35:615–618, 1994.

36. Masini E, Bechi P, Dei R, et al: Helicobacter pylori potentiates histamine release from rat serosal mast cells induced by bile acids. *Dig Dis Sci* 39:1493–1500, 1994.

37. Gionechetti P, Vaira D, Campieri M, et al: Enhanced mucosal interleukin-6 and -8 in Helicobacter pylori–positive dyspeptic patients. *Am J Gastroenterol* 89:883–887, 1994.

38. Gillanders IA, Scott PJ, Smith GD: Helicobacter pylori and chronic antral gastritis in elderly patients. *Age Ageing* 23:277–279, 1994.

39. Talley NJ: A critique of therapeutic trials in Helicobacter pylori–positive functional dyspepsia. *Gastroenterology* 106:1174–1183, 1994.

40. Parikh SS, Desai SB, Prabhu SR, et al: Congestive gastropathy: Factors influencing development, endoscopic features, Helicobacter pylori infection, and microvessel changes. *Am J Gastroenterol* 89:1036–1042, 1994.

41. Panes J, Pique JM, Bordas JM, et al: Effect of bolus injection and continuous infusion of somatostatin on gastric perfusion in cirrhotic patients with portal-hypertensive gastropathy. *Hepatology* 20:336–341, 1994.

42. Loperfido S, Monica F, Maifreni L, et al: Bleeding peptic ulcer occurring in hospitalized patients: Analysis of predictive and risk factors and comparison with out-of-hospital onset of hemorrhage. *Dig Dis Sci* 39:698–705, 1994.

43. Lai KH, Peng SN, Guo WS, et al: Endoscopic injection for the treatment of bleeding ulcers: Local tamponade or drug effect? *Endoscopy* 26:338–341, 1994.

44. Villanueva C, Balanzo J, Torras X, et al: Value of second-look endoscopy after injection therapy for bleeding peptic ulcer: A prospective and randomized trial. *Gastrointest Endosc* 40:34–39, 1994.

45. Choudari CP, Palmer KR: Endoscopic injection therapy for bleeding peptic ulcer; a comparison of adrenaline alone with adrenaline plus ethanolamine oleate. *Gut* 35:608–610, 1994.

46. Caballero-Plasencia AM, Muros-Navarro MC, Martin-Ruiz JL, et al: Gastroparesis of digestible and indigestible solids in patients with insulin-dependent diabetes mellitus or functional dyspepsia. *Dig Dis Sci* 39:1409–1415, 1994.

47. Coffin B, Azpiroz F, Guarner F, et al: Selective gastric hypersensitivity and reflex hyporeactivity in functional dyspepsia. *Gastroenterology* 107:1345–1351, 1994.

48. Troncon LE, Bennett RJ, Ahluwalia NK, et al: Abnoirmal intragastric distribution of food during gastric emptying in functional dyspepsia patients. *Gut* 35:327–332, 1994.

49. Talley NJ, Fett SL, Zinsmeister AR, et al: Gastrointestinal tract symptoms and self-reported abuse: A population-based study. *Gastroenterology* 107:1040–1049, 1994.

50. Hausken T, Berstad A: Effect of glyceryl trinitrate on antral motility and symptoms in patients with functional dyspepsia. *Scand J Gastroenterol* 29:23–28, 1994.

51. Bytzer P, Hansen JM, Schaffalitzky de Muckadell OB: Empirical H_2-blocker therapy or prompt endoscopy in management of dyspepsia. *Lancet* 343:811–816, 1994.

52. Lee M, Cryer B, Feldman M: Dose effects of aspirin on gastric prostaglandins and stomach mucosal injury. *Ann Intern Med* 120:184–189, 1994.

53. Kelly SM, Jenner JR, Dickinson RJ, et al: Increased gastric juice epidermal growth factor after non-steroidal anti-inflammatory drug ingestion. *Gut* 35:611–614, 1994.

54. Honda K, Fukuda S, Ishikawa SE, et al: Role of endogenous vasopressin in development of gastric ulcer induced by restraint and water immersion. *Am J Physiol* 266:R1448–R1453, 1994.

55. Laszlo F, Karacsony G, Pavo I, et al: Aggressive role of vasopressin in development of different gastric lesions in rats. *Eur J Pharmacol* 258:15–22, 1994.

56. Tramontana M, Renzi D, Calabro A, et al: Influence of capsaicin-sensitive afferent fibers on acetic acid–induced chronic gastric ulcers in rats. *Scand J Gastroenterol* 29:406–413, 1994.

57. Mercer DW, Ritchie WP Jr, Dempsey DT: Sensory neuron–mediated gastric mucosal protection is blocked by cyclooxygenase inhibition. *Surgery* 115:156–163, 1994.

58. Gray JL, Bunnett NW, Orloff SL, et al: A role for calcitonin gene–related peptide in protection against gastric ulceration. *Ann Surg* 219:58–64, 1994.

59. Slomiany BL, Piotrowski J, Czajkowski A, et al: Gastric mucosal laminin receptor expression with ulcer healing by ebrotidine. *Gen Pharmacol* 25:451–455, 1994.

60. Penney AG, Andrews FJ, O'Brien PE: Effects of misoprostol on delayed ulcer healing induced by aspirin. *Dig Dis Sci* 39:934–939, 1994.

61. Hata M, Yamazaki Y, Ueda T, et al: Influence of ammonia solution on gastric mucosa and acetic acid induced ulcer in rats. *Eur J Histochem* 38:41–52, 1994.

62. Sullivan TR Jr, Dempsey DT, Milner R, et al: Effect of local acid-base status on gastric mucosal blood flow and surface cell injury by bile acid. *J Surg Res* 56:112–116, 1994.

63. Konturek SJ, Brzozowski T, Stachura J, et al: Role of neutrophils and mucosal blood flow in gastric adaptation to aspirin. *Eur J Pharmacol* 253:107–114, 1994.

64. Blandizzi C, Gherardi G, Natale G, et al: Protective action of omeprazole against gastric mucosal injury induced by hemorrhagic shock in rats. *Dig Dis Sci* 39:2109–2117, 1994.

65. Lee M, Feldman M: Age-related reductions in gastric mucosal prostaglandin levels increase susceptibility to aspirin-induced injury in rats. *Gastroenterology* 107:1746–1750, 1994.

66. Masferrer JL, Zweifel BS, Manning PT, et al: Selective inhibition of inducible cyclooxygenase 2 in vivo is antiinflammatory and nonulcerogenic. *Proc Natl Acad Sci U S A* 91:3228–3232, 1994.

67. Wallace JL, Reuter B, Cicala C, et al: A diclofenac derivative without ulcerogenic properties. *Eur J Pharmacol* 257:249–255, 1994.

68. Wallace JL, Reuter B, Cicala C, et al: Novel nonsteroidal anti-inflammatory drug derivatives with markedly reduced ulcerogenic properties in the rat. *Gastroenterology* 107:173–179, 1994.

69. Wood JG, Yan ZY, Cheung LY: Role of prostaglandins in angiotensin II–induced gastric vasoconstriction. *Am J Physiol* 267:G173–G179, 1994.

70. Cullen JJ, Ephgrave KS, Broadhurst KA, et al: Captopril decreases stress ulceration without affecting gastric perfusion during canine hemorrhagic shock. *J Trauma* 37:43–49, 1994.

71. Okumura T, Pappas TN, Taylor IL: Stimulation of gastric secretion and enhanced gastric mucosal damage following central administration of pancreatic polypeptide (PP) in rats. *Dig Dis Sci* 39:2398–2406, 1994.

72. Andrews FJ, Malcontenti-Wilson C, O'Brien PE: Effect of nonsteroidal anti-inflammatory drugs on LFA-1 and ICAM-1 expression in gastric mucosa. *Am J Physiol* 266:G567–G664, 1994.

73. Santucci L, Fiorucci S, Giansanti M, et al: Pentoxifylline prevents indomethacin induced acute gastric mucosal damage in rats: Role of tumour necrosis factor alpha. *Gut* 35:909–915, 1994.

74. Szabo S, Folkman J, Vattay P, et al: Accelerated healing of duodenal ulcers by oral administration oif a mutein of basic fibroblast growth factor in rats. *Gastroenterology* 106:1106–1111, 1994.

CHAPTER 3

Small Bowel Review

G. E. Wild, M.D.

Cell and Molecular Biology Collaborative Network in Gastrointestinal Physiology, Department of Medicine, Division of Gastroenterology, McGill University, Montreal, Quebec, Canada

J. A. Thompson, M.D.

Cell and Molecular Biology Collaborative Network in Gastrointestinal Physiology, Medical College of St. Bartholomew's Hospital, London, England

A. B. R. Thomson, M.D.

Cell and Molecular Biology Collaborative Network in Gastrointestinal Physiology, Nutrition and Metabolism Research Group, Department of Medicine, Division of Gastroenterology, University of Alberta, Edmonton, Canada

AMINO ACIDS, PEPTIDES, AND FOOD ALLERGIES

Intestinal dipeptidyl peptidase IV (DPP IV) plays a role in the hydrolysis of prolyl peptides and in the assimilation of proline-rich proteins.[1] In rats fed a high-proline diet, there is increased angiotensin converting enzyme (ACE) activity and increased DPP IV activity, as well as increased mRNA abundance.[2] Feeding a high-proline (gelatin) diet increases brush border membrane (BBM) ACE levels, as well as DPP IV activity and its corresponding mRNA.[2] Dipeptidyl peptidase IV expression is controlled primarily at the transcriptional level.[3] Forskolin treatment of Caco-2 cells leads to a reduction in transport of this protein from the Golgi apparatus to the

BBM and a 50% reduction in the amount of active DPP IV present in the BBM.[4] Both transcriptional and post-translational events may be involved in the final control of expression of this differentiation-dependent BBM hydrolase.

Nucleotides are important in infant nutrition and play a role in development of the gastrointestinal tract. Nucleotides may also be beneficial to the function of enterocytes. Nucleotide content may be an important factor by which dietary intake influences gene expression in the intestinal epithelium.[5] An exogenous source of nucleotides from the diet may optimize the function of dividing tissue, particularly when growth is rapid and the diet is low in nucleotides.[6] Nucleotides may decrease protein leakage and the production of nitric oxide during intestinal ischemia.[7] Supplementing the diet with the nucleotide adenosine alters intestinal morphology, as well as alters intestinal blood flow by way of vasodilatation. Nucleotide supplements enhance normal enterocyte growth and maturation, as well as spare the need for exogenous glutamine in cell maintenance and development.[8] Synthetic pathways for purine and pyrimidines are influenced by the dietary intake of nucleotides, and these may be important in gut mucosal defense.[9]

Several anticancer and anti–acquired immunodeficiency syndrome (AIDS) drugs, including 5-fluorouracil (5-FU) and azidodeoxythymidine (AZT), are absorbed by the nucleoside transporter. Nucleoside transport in the small intestine appears to be an Na^+-dependent process, and a uridine transporter in the small intestine has been identified by using mRNA-injected *Xenopus laevis* oocytes.[10] This transport system is similar to that functioning in the BBM of the small intestine.

Caco-2 cells have been used to study the intestinal permeability of peptides, and the values obtained in cell culture correlate with those obtained from an in situ perfused ileum model.[11, 12] The cell culture transport of peptides may be increased in Caco-2 cells with the calcium channel blocker verapamil, and in this human enterocyte-like carcinoma cell line there may be a saturable, apically polarized peptide transport system.[13]

Exudation of plasma across the gut mucosa occurs in the setting of inflammatory bowel disease, and this plasma protein loss into the intestinal lumen may correlate with the severity of inflammation. The intestinal exudation of protein in response to challenges such as an allergen is markedly inhibited in the rat by administration of the nonsystemic glucocorticoid budesonide given by gavage 24 hours before challenge.[14]

The polyamines (spermine, spermidine, and putrescine) are important in the growth, differentiation, and multiplication of gastrointestinal cells. Polyamines are regulated by their biosynthesis from ornithine. Ornithine decarboxylase (ODC), the key rate-limiting enzyme in the formation of polyamines, is mainly located at the tip of the villous enterocytes, and feeding plays an important role in regulating the circadian rhythm of ODC activity. The increase in ODC activity in the duodenum at 1700 hours (when rats normally do not feed), but not at other time points, is abolished by subdiaphragmatic vagotomy, whereas vagotomy has no effect on the feeding pattern of rats.[15] This suggests that the increase in duodenal ODC activity in the late afternoon is due to a signal from the upper brain structure through the vagus and is not due to luminal nutrient factors. The polyamine transport system appears to be Na^+ dependent in some but not in all tissues. For example, there are two different Na^+-independent uptake systems in the rat intestine for spermine and spermidine, systems that are distinct from the electrical potential–dependent uptake system for monocationic compounds.[16] In an IEC-6 duodenal crypt cell line, the BBM but not the basolateral membrane transports polyamines.[17]

There are three chloride-dependent intestinal transporters for amino acids: the imino, the taurine, and the β-alanine carrier.[18] Taurine is a nonprotein amino acid whose uptake into HT-29 and Caco-2 cells is under the control of protein kinase C (PKC), with the underlying mechanism being one of regulation by phosphorylation of the transporter protein.[19] The phorbol ester phorbol myristate acetate (PMA) activates PKC in HT-29 and Caco-2 cells in culture and reduces the uptake of taurine.

Transport of amino acids across the intestinal enterocyte membrane results from the action of a number of Na^+-dependent and Na^+-independent transport systems arranged in series at the apical and basolateral cell membranes. In addition, simple passive diffusion may occur via the paracellular pathway or across the basolateral membrane. Dipeptides and tripeptides may be absorbed across the BBM via pH-dependent, H^+-coupled mechanisms localized at both the apical and basolateral membranes. Studies of dipeptide/tripeptide absorption are difficult to interpret because there is hydrolysis of some peptides by BBM hydrolases. This technical problem can be overcome by using substrates that are resistant to hydrolysis such as carnosine or glycylsarcosine (Gly-Sar). In Caco-2 cells there is coupling of the transintestinal transport of the dipeptide Gly-Sar to the transmembrane proton electrochemical gradient.

The dipeptide Gly-Sar is transported in Caco-2 cells in both absorptive (apical-to-basal) and secretory (basal-to-apical) directions, with transport and accumulation in both directions enhanced in the presence of a pH gradient.[20] A proton-dependent but Na^+-independent amino acid transporter has been identified at the apical membrane of human intestinal Caco-2 cells.[21, 22] Caco-2 cells also possess an apically localized Na^+-independent electrogenic hydrogen/imino acid transporter for L-proline.[23] Caco-2 cell monolayers have been used to study dipeptide/H^+ transport via a symport.[21, 22] In Caco-2 cells the basolateral dipeptide transporter is distinct from the BBM H^+/dipeptide cotransporter.[24] Voltage-clamping BBM vesicles (inside negative) with a K^+ gradient (in the presence of valinonycin) accelerate dipeptide uptake, which is consistent with the electrogenic nature of dipeptide/H^+ transport. Thus it is the electrochemical gradient for H^+ rather than that for Na^+ that plays a major role in dipeptide/tripeptide absorption across the apical membrane of the intestinal enterocyte.

An Na^+-dependent neutral L-α-amino acid transporter from rabbit small intestine has been purified and reconstituted.[25] The Na^+-independent neutral and basic amino acid transporter is intensely labeled in the small intestine within enteroendocrine cells and submucosal neurons, which suggests that this transporter may have multiple functions in the small intestine.[26] L-Lysine transport systems have been demonstrated in isolated oocytes.[27]

Injection of poly (A)$^+$ RNA (mRNA) isolated from rabbit intestinal mucosa into

X. laevis oocytes results in an increase in Na^+-independent uptake of L-leucine, cystine, and arginine.[28] There is an Na^+-independent system that can be inhibited by leucine with high affinity when Na^+ is present, but this affinity is reduced in its absence. In addition, there is an Na^+-independent system that is inhibited by leucine with high affinity only when Na^+ is present.[27]

Glutamine is the most abundant free amino acid in the body and has been shown to be the major respiratory fuel for the absorptive cells of animal and human intestine.[29] These metabolically active cells derive glutamine both from the diet (by uptake across the intestinal BBM) and from an endogenous source (by uptake across the basolateral membrane). Rats with chronic portal hypertension have lower uptake of glutamine into BBM vesicles, with a reduced value of the maximal transport rate (Vmax) of both the Na^+-dependent and the Na^+-independent transport processes and with similar changes in the Vmax for transport across the basolateral membrane.[30]

Although most dietary proteins are degraded by luminal enzymes in the gastrointestinal tract, β-lactoglobulin and α-lactalbumin are found in an intact antigenic form in the intestinal lumen. About 10% to 20% of β-lactoglobulin is absorbed in rabbit ileum, and passage of the intact protein is inhibited both by colchicine, a microtubule-depolymerizing agent, and by galactose.[31] Bovine serum albumin is transported across rat jejunum by a saturable energy-dependent process that uses the microtubular network and is regulated by the enteric nervous system, primarily through cholinergic nerves acting on muscarinic receptors.[32] Neural factors may influence the uptake of macromolecules from the gut lumen during intestinal anaphylaxis.[33] During postnatal development, pretranslational, translational, and posttranslational levels of control are important in regulation of the expression of BBM hydrolysis.

Epidermal growth factor (EGF) is a 53–amino acid polypeptide that has been implicated in the regulation of a wide variety of physiologic and pathophysiologic processes such as cellular growth, tissue repair, and neoplasia.[34] Epidermal growth factor upregulates amino acid transport activity in jejunal BBM vesicles from adult rats by a process that may involve an increase in de novo biosynthesis of transporter protein.[35] Epidermal growth factor decreases glucose transport, which indicates that the Na^+-dependent glucose cotransporter is regulated independently from and opposite to amino acid transporters. Epidermal growth factor increases nutrient absorption in association with mucosal hyperplasia, but the change in absorption is not attributable to this morphologic alteration.[36]

SMOOTH MUSCLE FUNCTION AND INTESTINAL MOTILITY

The muscularis externa of the small intestine and the stomach consists of the thin longitudinal muscle layer on the outside and a thick circular muscle layer on the inside of the wall. The enteric nerves in the small intestine innervate the two muscle layers in a reciprocal fashion and those in the stomach in a complementary manner.[37] The electrical activity recorded from the small intestinal smooth muscle consists of slow waves and spike potentials that determine the segmental pattern of contractile activity. During the fasting stage, there is a cyclic, propagated myoelectric pattern of activity that appears to serve as a "housekeeper" and periodically sweep the intestine clean until the next meal. This is called the migrating myoelectric complex (MMC). The MMC is characterized by periodic cycling of a pattern of regular and irregular spike activity dominated by a several minute–long band of excitation during which spike potentials are associated with the slow waves. This "activity front" begins in the stomach and in the upper part of the small intestine and migrates as far as the ileocecal junction at a rate of about 1 mm/sec. Phase III (activity front) of the MMC is an interdigestive housekeeper that is immediately preceded by increased secretion of gastric acid, pepsin, pancreatic enzymes, and bile. Impedance planimetry has been used to measure tone and compliance in the human duodenal wall in situ, and both compliance and tone change between the different phases of the MMC.[38] The patterns of jejunal contractions can sustain a propagated single spike burst; isolated or repetitive spike bursts characterize the postprandial state in healthy humans and are dependent on digestive flow.[39]

Myoelectric spike activity correlates with smooth muscle contractions as well as with changes in luminal pressure, and the MMC propels interdigestive nutrients distally. Phase I of the MMC consists of electrical and motor quiescence, phase II has irregular activity, and phase III consists of several minutes of maximal electrical and mechanical activity that may begin in either the stomach or small intestine and propagates distally. The intrinsic intramural nerves of the gastrointestinal tract control the initiation and propagation of the MMC. After feeding, there is persistent cycling at the fasted (MMC) rate in rat small intestine, and factors controlling myoelectric cycling during the fasted state may persist after feeding and allow continued net aboral propulsion of food.[40] Migrating myoelectric complexes are found less frequently in germ-free as compared with normal rats; luminal control by the resident microflora may be important for physiologic cycling and aboral propagation of the MMC but appears to be of no major consequence for the postprandial myoelectric response.[41] Alcohol has only minor effects on postprandial contractile activity but abolishes the circadian variation of the MMC that is normally seen in healthy subjects.[42] The fact that breath alcohol content is low at the time of onset of sleep suggests that the effects on the MMC may be mediated through central rather than local mechanisms. Small intestinal transit is prolonged during acute hyperglycemia.[43]

Nitric oxide is a physiologic messenger[44] involved in nonadrenergic noncholinergic (NANC) relaxation of the gastrointestinal tract. In the human jejunum, nitric oxide mediates inhibitory nerve input.[45] Nonadrenergic, noncholinergic relaxation evoked in the muscles of the small intestine is suppressed by nitric oxide synthetase (NOS) inhibitors. Nitric oxide–containing NANC neurons play an important role in regulating MMC and cyclic motor activity during the fasting state and their disruption by a meal.[37] In the developing small intestine, nitric oxide–containing neurons cluster near the myenteric plexus.[46] Inhibition of nitric oxide production leads to a reversible circulating leukocyte-independent increase in epithelial permeability.[47] Inhibition of NOS also activates mast cells in the mucosa and consequently increases epithelial permeability.[48] Exogenous nitric oxide–donating compounds can modulate electrolyte transport in the guinea pig intestine in vitro.[49]

Nitric oxide is a vasodilator derived from the endothelium from L-arginine by way of the calcium-dependent constitutive enzyme NOS. Nitric oxide plays a physiologic role in the regulation of gastrointestinal blood flow and is important in modulation of intestinal vascular integrity under conditions such as acute endotoxic channeling.[50] Inhibition of NOS abolishes or reduces relaxation from enteric nerve stimulation, and these effects may be overcome with L-arginine. There is tonic calcium-dependent nitric oxide output from perfused intestinal segments of canine intestine, and nitric oxide acts to directly inhibit muscle by inhibiting the release of an excitatory mediator. This output may be a primary inhibitory determinant of contractile activity.[51]

In the enteric nervous system, NOS is colocalized in a population of neurons in the myenteric plexus that contain vasoactive intestinal peptide (VIP). These neurons project onto the circular and longitudinal muscle layers and are involved in the control of muscle relaxation. Vasoactive intestinal peptide release is facilitated by and may be dependent on nitric oxide production.[52] During stretch-induced relaxation of the rat colon, nitric oxide is produced by muscle cells and in neurons, and relaxation represents the combined effects of VIP and nitric oxide on muscle cells and enhancement of VIP release by nitric oxide.[53]

Myenteric neurons can be divided into four types based on their electrophysiologic behavior. Patch-clamp methods may be applied to study the cellular neurophysiology of myenteric neurons in guinea pig small intestine, and such methods have revealed two populations of neurons.[54] The interstitial cells of Cajal in the intermuscular space between the circular and longitudinal muscle layers of the small intestine may serve as pacemaker cells. Interstitial cells of a different class have been found in the deep muscular plexus at the small intestine in specialized smooth muscle cells.[55]

Galanin, a gut-brain neuropeptide, stimulates rat jejunal contraction,[56] and in the canine gastrointestinal tract galanin is present in the neurons of the myenteric and submucous plexuses. In canine small intestine, galanin may act as an inhibitory neuromodulator.[57] Motilin plays a role in controlling MMCs, the cyclic bursts of contractile activity that occur in the fasting state. Motilin released from the enterochromaffin cells of the proximal portion of the small intestine appears to be involved in stimulating or recruiting the gastric contractions during phase II, and in humans the receptor for motilin has been localized on smooth muscle cells in the gastric antrum and in the upper part of the duodenum. Erythromycin, a motilin receptor agonist, is a potential gastrointestinal prokinetic agent.[58]

The phospholipase A_2 but not phospholipase C pathway is involved in the muscarinic receptor–induced calcium influx in ileal smooth muscle.[59] Acetylcholine and norepinephrine are enteric neurotransmitters, and serotonin (5-hydroxytryptamine [5-HT]) would appear to be an enteric neurotransmitter responsible for mediating a prolonged excitatory postsynaptic potential. Anti-idiotypic antibodies that recognize 5-HT receptors on myenteric neurons of guinea pig small intestine are present on myenteric and submucosal neurons.[60]

Serotonin is a potent stimulant of intestinal fluid and electrolyte secretion and is a mediator of diarrhea in patients with the carcinoid syndrome. The nomenclature and classification of 5-HT receptors, as well as their putative role in the gastrointestinal tract, have been reviewed.[61] At least four main types of receptors have been described in the intestine, and all four types appear to influence the gastrointestinal tract. There is a mucosal 5-HT$_2$ receptor located on guinea pig small intestinal crypt cells, and 5-HT stimulates concentration-dependent production of inositol-1,4,5-triphosphate (IP$_3$) in dispersed enterocytes.[62] In the canine jejunum, enteric neurons with 5-HT$_3$ receptors play a role as sensory neurons or interneurons in the ascending excitatory and the descending inhibitory pathways of the peristaltic reflex elicited by stroking the mucosa, and the ascending limb is composed of cholinergic interneurons and motor neurons.[63] There are a variety of antagonists to the 5-HT$_3$ receptor, such as ondansetron, that are effective in controlling cancer chemotherapy–induced emesis. A series of quinoline carboxylic acid derivatives are a new class of 5-HT$_3$ receptor antagonists, and it has been suggested that this group of agents may potentially be tested in the future as a form of therapy for patients with irritable bowel syndrome (IBS).[64]

Serotonin is one of the transmitters responsible for the mediation of slow excitatory postsynaptic potentials in type 2/AH neurons of the myenteric plexus. The receptor responsible for the 5-HT–induced rise in cyclic adenosine monophosphate (cAMP) in ganglia isolated from the guinea pig myenteric plexus is not a known subtype of 5-HT receptor.[65] Inhibition of the release of acetylcholine and the tachykinins is an important regulator of motor activity. The second neuromediator contributing to the inhibitory function of the enteric nervous system is 5-HT, which is known to be present in enteric nerves and is released on depolarization. Adenosine and 5-HT receptors on enteric nerve endings are coupled to the inhibition of tachykinin release via distinct mechanisms, putatively distinct G proteins.[66] The gastrointestinal tract is the main source of 5-HT in humans, and 5-HT is found predominantly within the enterchromaffin cells of the mucosa, as well as within the myenteric plexus. The different 5-HT receptors may be involved in stress-induced colonic motor activity in rats.[67] A selective 5-HT reuptake inhibitor, paroxetine, reduces MMC periodicity in healthy humans and has a prokinetic action in the human small intestine.[68] The clinical significance of these findings remains to be established.

The two opioid precursors proenkephalin and prodynorphin are synthesized in neurons of the myenteric plexus of the gut and are processed into a variety of active opioid peptides. There are three distinct opioid receptors present on muscle cells of the circular but not the longitudinal neuropathy.[80] Chronic intestinal pseudo-obstruction may be ameliorated by cisapride (a substituted benzamide) in a subgroup of patients, particularly patients with an idiopathic intestinal motility disorder not associated with abdominal vagal dysfunction.[81]

Patients with Chagas' disease (American trypanosomiasis) have a combination of rapid gastric emptying and delayed transit of liquids through the more distal segments of the small bowel.[82] Occurrence of the MMC is reduced in animals with chronic portal hypertension.[83] Interestingly, altered proximal small bowel motility may be observed in patients with cirrhosis and may contribute to the bacterial overgrowth syndrome seen in some of these individuals.[84] Prominent cluster activities may develop in the intestinal remnant in animals that have undergone distal bowel resection, and this motor disruption may contribute to the symptomatology as well as the clinical features of patients with short-bowel syndrome.[85] Surgery decreases the MMC period to the equivalent of the absolute refractory period, thereby eliminating phase II, which returns as the MMC period lengthens; cisapride given as 30 mg three times daily into the rectum of patients after intra-abdominal surgery induced some changes in motor activity but did not accelerate the recovery of normal bowel motility.[86]

BLOOD FLOW AND INTESTINAL ISCHEMIA

The search continues for the identification of naturally occurring mediators of intestinal ischemia-reperfusion injury, as well as for the elucidation of its pathophysiologic process. Oxygen-derived free radicals are involved in the intestinal mucosal damage during ischemia-reperfusion. Neutrophils are a major source of the free radical production that occurs during reperfusion after ischemia, and radicals formed in the xanthine oxidase reaction seem to function as a primer for the neutrophils.[87] Indeed, infiltrated neutrophils rather muscle layer of the intestine.[69] Peripheral cholecystokinin (CCK) receptors may be involved in modification of the small intestinal transit produced by infusion of lipid into the distal end of the small intestine.[70] This so-called ileal brake is mediated in part by endogenous opiate pathways and may also be related to the release of peptide YY.[71] Luminal bile salts inhibit terminal ileal motility by a process that is independent of peptide YY release.[72]

The antidiarrheal agent loperamide is devoid of central opiate-like effects. The antisecretory effect of loperamide is accompanied by motor changes when loperamide reaches the myenteric m-opiate receptors.[73] Loperamide blocks the exercise effect on the upper part of the gut and may prove effective in treating some intestinal symptoms induced by physical activity.[74] Loperamide oxide is converted to loperamide in the intestinal lumen, and although loperamide inhibits the rise in short-circuit current associated with sodium-linked glucose absorption, the rate at which loperamide appears is not sufficient to inhibit absorptive processes.[75] Opiates reduce propulsive peristalsis; reduce pancreatic, biliary, and electrolyte/fluid secretions; and increase intestinal fluid absorption and blood flow. Morphine accumulates in the intestinal tissue of rats and contributes to its antidiarrheal effect, but loperamide does not accumulate in the rat intestinal lumen.[76]

A detailed discussion of the question "is IBS a motility disorder?" has been published.[77, 78] Although the pathophysiology of IBS remains unclear, it is widely believed that IBS is commonly associated with disordered gastrointestinal motility. Abdominal symptoms in IBS may originate from organs other than the colon. In patients with "diarrhea-predominant" IBS, ambulatory small intestinal motility studies do not show any abnormality in MMCs.[79]

Intestinal pseudo-obstruction is a clinical syndrome characterized by symptoms and signs of intestinal obstruction despite the absence of mechanical blockade of the intestinal lumen. Intestinal pseudo-obstruction in patients with amyloidosis is caused by either myopathy or then xanthine oxidase may be the primary source of free radicals under these conditions.[88] The relationship between histologic damage and radical production is unclear.[87]

Immature intestine does not effectively regulate blood flow or oxygen uptake. This may be a factor that predisposes the developing intestine to tissue hypoxia. The intestinal microvasculature in the immature rat appears to lack vasodilatory mechanisms that are active in the adult rat, and this may make the developing intestine prone to mucosal damage during periods of decreased perfusion.[89] Ischemia and subsequent reperfusion affect the efficacy of intrinsic vascular regulation in the postnatal intestinal circulation, with the intestine from older but not younger subjects maintaining the intrinsic capacity to preserve tissue oxygenation in response to a hypotensive challenge.[90]

A variety of approaches have been used in experimental models to improve ischemia-reperfusion injury to the bowel, including treatment with free radical scavengers, xanthine oxidase inhibitors, and iron chelators; depletion of neutrophils; and the administration of platelet-activating factor (PAF) antagonists. Another avenue has been to attempt to protect the intestinal mucosa by the intraluminal instillation of protease inhibitors, nutritional supplements, or oxygen. Intraluminal infusion of 10% glucose minimizes mucosal damage and increases mucosal adenosine triphosphate (ATP) content, which thus suggests that intraluminal oxygenation improves the mucosal hyperpermeability induced by ischemia-reperfusion.[91] The clinical usefulness of these observations remains to be established.

The early clinical diagnosis of acute intestinal ischemia and infarction is difficult. During intestinal ischemia the resident microbial flora of the intestine multiply rapidly. Shortly after superior mesenteric artery ligation, the tips of the villi begin to slough and form a membrane of necrotic material and bacteria. D-lactate is a byproduct of bacterial metabolism that is neither produced nor metabolized by mamamlian cells. There are increased blood concentrations of lactate early after the production of intestinal ischemia in a rat model, and this may prove to be a useful marker in human ischemic disease.[92]

CELIAC DISEASE

Celiac disease (CD) is usually seen in childhood and in early adult life, but it is being diagnosed in increasing numbers of elderly patients. In a district general hospital in England, 19% of their adult patients with CD had the disease diagnosed when they were older than 60 years. Over half of these older patients had had a long history of unexplained symptoms or abnormalities on blood tests but in whom the diagnosis of CD had been missed.[93] Thus it is suggested that clinicians should be alert to the possibility of CD in the elderly, particularly in patients with nonspecific gastrointestinal complaints in the presence of unexplained anemia. In fact, CD may be underdiagnosed in adults in England, and IgA antiendomysial antibody (EmA) testing is useful when selecting suspected cases of CD for a confirmatory biopsy.

Untreated CD carries an increased risk of malignancy, and thus there are sound reasons why cases of unsuspected disease should be diagnosed and treated. IgA EmAs have a high degree of sensitivity and specificity for gluten-sensitive enteropathy, and after gluten withdrawal the elevated IgA-EmA titers decline to zero in patients with CD who comply with their gluten-free diet.[94] Antireticulin antibody (ARA) is less sensitive and less specific for the diagnosis of CD, but these parameters improve greatly when the conventional test is adapted to detect IgA ARA of the R1 type. Indeed, IgA Ra-ARA is reliable and valuable in assisting in the early recognition and treatment of occult CD.[95] Antigliadin antibody (AGA) detection by enzyme-linked immunosorbent assay (ELISA) is easier than detection by ARA or EmA. Recently, a new IgA-class AGA ELISA test has been developed that shows 100% sensitivity and specificity in detecting symptomatic adults with CD. A word of caution is in order: AGAs are frequently detected in adult Estonians, and positivity increases with age and "represents a normal response to dietary antigens in the elderly."[96] Thus positivity for AGA in this population does not predict silent undetected CD.

The term "potential CD" may be more appropriate in clinical practice than the term "latent CD." In patients referred for jejunal biopsy in whom histologic findings are normal, the α/δ T-cell receptor intraepithelial lymphocyte (IEL) count may be increased, the celiac-like intestinal antibody pattern may be positive, and the total IEL count may be increased. In these individuals, clinical tests of gluten sensitivity may be required to establish the prevalence of CD.[97]

The classic definition of CD is being challenged by the emerging evidence that latent or potential CD is not particularly rare. Patients with latent CD are those who eat a normal gluten-containing diet, who have apparently normal jejunal histology, but who at some other time before or since have had a gluten-sensitive enteropathy. Those with CD whose intestinal lesions are resolved on a gluten-free diet and whose jejunal biopsy samples are classified as "normal" for diagnostic purposes may still express subtle pathologic or immunologic abnormalities similar to those of untreated CD. These include increased numbers of IELs, increased γ/δ T-cell receptor expression by IELs, abnormal jejunal permeability, and high levels of IgM antigliadin antibody. The CD-like intestinal antibody pattern is seen in patients with dermatitis herpetiformis without enteropathy, and this as well as a high IEL count may be markers of latent gluten-sensitive enteropathy.[98]

A person sensitive to gluten almost invariably has at least two of the genes DQB1*0201 and DQA1*0501. In addition to gluten, unknown environmental factors may trigger the development of jejunal damage. In family members of patients with CD, the density of both α/β and γ/δ T-cell receptor–bearing cells is frequently higher than in controls, even when the villous structure is normal. The increase in the density of γ/δ T-cells is linked with the CD marker DQ gene. When 75 healthy family members of patients with CD were studied by small bowel biopsy, 11 (15%) had clinically silent CD. Many family members of patients with CD have signs of inflammation in morphologically normal jejunum, and these inflammatory changes together with CD marker DQ genes may point to latent CD.[99]

Chronic ingestion of small amounts of gluten (100 mg/day) in children with CD results in an increased IEL count, a decrease in the villous height/crypt depth ratio, but normal intestinal permeability. However, when higher amounts of gluten (500 mg/day) are ingested, there are more pronounced cytologic changes as well as an increase in intestinal permeability as assessed by analysis of the urinary ratio of cellobiose/mannitol.[100]

Transmission electron microscopic examination of the small intestine in children with CD in remission has shown that the layer of BBM glycocalyx is thin or absent whereas the glycocalyx in persons with treated CD is greater as compared with that of controls.[101] Interestingly, in the rectal mucosa in adults with CD, morphometry shows increased populations of plasma cells, lymphocytes, and mast cells, as well as increases in CD3- and γ/δ-positive lymphocytes within both the lamina propria and the epithelium.[102]

Celiac disease is caused by the prolamine of wheat, rye, barley, and possibly oats. The peptides resulting from digestion with the proteolytic enzymes trypsin and pepsin damage the enterocytes of the small intestine and induce the symptoms of CD. Mucosal pathology in CD is dependent on T-cell–mediated reactivity in genetically predisposed subjects. There are homologous sequences within peptides derived from the N-terminal sequence of α-gliadin, residues 1 to 68, that are toxic to celiac mucosal explants in organ culture. The peptide Frazer III-2-VIII is part of the γ/δ fraction and is markedly toxic to duodenal explants from patients with active CD.[103]

The molecular genetics of gluten sensitivity have been reviewed.[104] The total villous atrophy in CD is associated with increased IEL T-cell infiltration and polyclonal expansion of γ/δ-positive T-cell receptor–bearing IELs. This expansion persists several years after gluten withdrawal. The presence of IELs bearing the CD56 natural killer marker in active CD is associated with a better clinical tolerance to gluten challenge than in patients with CD whose biopsy specimens do not have this IEL marker. Celiac disease is associated with particular HLA alleles, and some CD4-positive T cells using the α/β T-cell receptor located in the lamina propria may initiate the disease process. A particular HLA-DQ heterodimer encoded by the DQA1*0501 and DQB1*0201 genes in a *cis* or *trans* configuration may confirm the primary disease susceptibility.[105]

When small intestinal biopsy samples from patients with CD who are eating a gluten-free diet are challenged ex vivo with gluten, CD4-positive T cells in the lamina propria are activated and express CD25 (interleukin-2 receptor λ chain).

These activated T cells recognize gluten when presented by the HLA-DQ(α1*0501,β1*0201) heterodimer. There may be preferential mucosal presentation of gluten-derived peptides by HLA-DQ(α1*0501,β1*0201) in CD, which may explain the HLA association.[106] However, differences in the concordance rates for CD between monozygotic twins and siblings who share HLA haplotypes suggest that genes outside the HLA loci also contribute to CD susceptibility. Current thoughts on the mechanisms of inheritance of CD favor a "two-locus" model consisting of one gene linked to the HLA complex and one non–HLA-linked gene associated with recessive inheritance.

A number of T-cell receptor genes have been excluded as playing a major role in susceptibility to CD.[107] The traditional view that enteropathy-associated T-cell lymphoma (EATCL) is a complication of CD is supported by new immunohistochemical evidence that both diseases have similar subsets of intestinal mucosal T cells. Because patients with CD may be asymptomatic, it is difficult to prove that a monoclonal lymphocytic intestinal infiltrate can develop in previously normal bowel. A case of EATCL has been described that was diagnosed by biopsy of a lymphomatous pleural mass in a patient in whom an initial diagnosis of CD had been made 12 months previously.[108]

Since the widespread use of upper gastrointestinal tract endoscopy, descriptions of the endoscopic appearance of the second part of the duodenum in patients with CD have been reported, including a reduction in the number or an absence of duodenal folds and scalloping of the valvulae conniventes. A prospective study of 100 patients referred for endoscopy and intestinal biopsy showed severe villus atrophy in 36 patients, 34 of whom had endoscopic markers suggestive of CD, including a reduction in the number or loss of Kerckring's folds in 27, a mosaic pattern in 14, scalloped folds in 12, and visbility of the underlying blood vessels in 5. A reduction in the number or loss of Kerckring's folds was the most sensitive (76%) and specific (98%) single endoscopic change suggesting the presence of CD.[109]

Bone mineral density is reduced in many patients with CD, and these persons may possibly be candidates for screening for osteopenia. Indeed, the incidence of unsuspected asymptomatic CD is nearly tenfold higher than expected in patients with clinical osteoporosis who are screened with IgA antibodies to gliadin.

On Doppler ultrasound flowmetry, the mean basal blood flow is 50% higher in the superior mesenteric artery in patients with untreated CD than in healthy controls, and postprandial mesenteric blood flow is increased and delayed in time[110] (Fig 1).

The D-xylose hydrogen breath test may be a useful and practical means for the post-treatment follow-up of patients with CD.[111] Carnitine is crucial for mitochondrial energy production, and the total serum carnitine concentration is lower in patients with CD than in patients with nonactive disease or in controls.[112] Serum carnitine concentrations do not correlate with the degree of the intestinal lesion. Oral supplementation with L-carnitine can correct the deficiency.

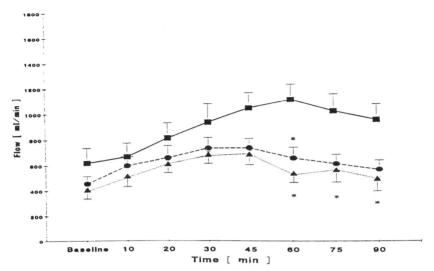

FIGURE 1.

Flow in the superior mesenteric artery in the basal condition and after a mixed test meal (Ensure Plus) in healthy controls *(triangles)*, patients with untreated celiac disease *(squares)*, and gluten-free diet–treated patients *(circles)*; mean ± SEM. Flow in untreated patients is significantly different from that in treated patients and healthy persons ($P < .002$). (From Alvarez D, Vazquez H, Bai JC, et al: *Dig Dis Sci* 38:1175–1182, 1993. Used by permission.)

GASTROINTESTINAL LYMPHOMA

Gastrointestinal lymphoma is a relatively uncommon tumor in most parts of the world; it accounts for 30% to 69% of all extranodal lymphomas but only 1% to 11% of gastrointestinal malignant neoplasms. However, in Saudi Arabia, malignant non-Hodgkin's lymphoma is relatively common, and multimodality treatment has been shown to be superior to therapy with either surgery alone or chemotherapy alone[113] (Fig 2). A prospective multicenter study from France also supported the concept that combined radical surgery and chemotherapy according to histologic grading is associated with prolonged remission in patients with primary digestive tract lymphomas.[114]

Immunoproliferative small intestinal disease (IPSID), also known as "Mediterranean" lymphoma or α heavy chain disease, is a disorder characterized by a diffuse and intense plasma cell infiltrate in the lamina propria of the small intestine that may give rise to a malignant lymphoma. Most cases have been reported from the underprivileged population of the Middle East and the Mediterranean basin, but cases of IPSID have also been described in Africa, Europe, Asia, as well as South, Central, and North America.[115]

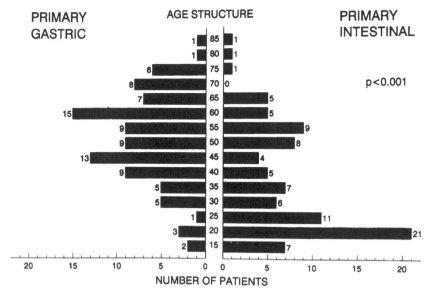

FIGURE 2.

Age distribution of adult patients with primary gastric and primary intestinal non-Hodgkins lymphoma. (From Amer MH, El-Akkad S: *Gastroenterology* 106:846–858, 1994. Used by permission.)

WHIPPLE'S DISEASE

The topic of Whipple's disease has been reviewed.[116] The gram-positive actinomycete *Tropheryema whippelii* has been isolated and characterized by application of the polymerase chain reaction.[117] The endoscopic findings of Whipple's disease include a combination of yellow-white plaques and an erythematous, erosive, or mildly friable mucosa. In spite of the endoscopic findings, intestinal epithelial cells themselves appear normal on light and electron microscopy, and major histocompatibility complex (MHC) class I expression is preserved.[118] Lactase and MHC class II expression are reduced or absent, and antibiotic treatment results in normalization of the intestine within 3 to 6 months.

There is evidence for both an associated humoral and cellular immune defect in patients with Whipple's disease, but no consistent abnormality has been shown. Reductions of complement receptor 3 α-chain–expressing monocytes and transient inhibitory serum factors have been described and may explain the impaired ability of patients with Whipple's disease to eliminate bacteria.[119] Extraintestinal lymphoma has been reported in a 45-year-old with Whipple's disease who died despite antibiotic treatment and nutrition support.[120]

Central nervous system (CNS) symptoms may rarely be the only initial manifestation in patients with Whipple's disease, and the CNS is the most common site of disease relapse after treatment with drugs that do not penetrate uninflamed meninges, such as tetracycline. This observation has led to the recommendation that antibiotics such as trimethoprim-sulfamethoxazole (TMP-SMX), which has more reliable CNS penetration, be used as first-line therapy.[121] However, a single case of CNS relapse during therapy with TMP-SMX has been reported, and response was obtained with cefixime.[122]

PERMEABILITY

The topic of intestinal permeability has been reviewed.[123] Failure of intestinal barrier function results in the spread of bacteria from the gut to systemic organs, and this has been termed *bacterial translocation.* Bacterial translocation is increased in animal models where nutrients are given by the parenteral route, whereas enteral feeding reverses this process. Bacterial translocation is increased if there is pre-existing protein energy malnutrition, and dietary fiber reduces the deleterious effect of endotoxin on translocation; glutamine is not effective in preventing elemental diet–induced bacterial translocation.[124]

Dexamethasone administration is associated with a significant increase in bacterial adherence to the mucosa, and bacterial–mucosal cell interactions may be responsible for alterations in intestinal permeability after dexamethasone administration.[125] In the rat, morphine-induced prolongation in bowel transit promotes bacterial translocation secondary to an overgrowth of enteric bacteria in the intestinal lumen.[126] There is probably an important clinical significance of this translocation.[127] Enteral diet supplementation with these amino acids may improve mucosal permeability.[128]

Increased intestinal permeability has been found in several diseases such as celiac sprue, rheumatoid arthritis, Crohn's disease, and nonsteroidal anti-inflammatory drug (NSAID)-induced enteritis. Intestinal permeability has been assessed clinically by using a variety of different probes, and generally it is recommended that two probes be used.[123] Mannitol permeability of the intestinal barrier is mediated by passive diffusion and by solvent drag.[129] Permeation of the intestine by ^{51}Cr-ethylendiaminetetraacetic acid (EDTA) is by passive diffusion, possibly by the paracellular route. Increased permeation after oral administration may occur with inflammation of the small or large bowel, and intestinal permeability to this probe is increased in patients with infectious diarrhea.[130]

In Caco-2 cell monolayers, intestinal paracellular permeability is regulated by the activity of enterocyte PKC, and the increase in cellular permeability induced by binding of carbachol to the muscarinic receptor is mediated by activation of PKC.[131] Exposure of T84 monolayers to phorbol ester downregulates PKC.[132] Contraction of microfilaments in the terminal web separates the tight junctions between adjacent enterocytes and increases the permeability of the mucosa. Actively transported nutrients may induce terminal web contraction as a result of activation of Na^+-dependent cotransport systems.[133]

Indomethacin increases intestinal permeability by mechanisms other than changes in prostanoid or PAF metabolism.[134] Mucosal permeability in the rat intestine is increased by ischemia-reperfusion injury, by hypoxia, and by high-dose indomethacin, but not by low-dose indomethacin, cold, or theophylline.[135] Nonsteroidal anti-inflammatory drugs increase intestinal permeability; early after NSAID exposure, there are microvascular changes in villi and inhibition of cyclooxygenase activity. In the second stage after NSAID exposure there is neutrophil infiltration.[136] Administration of synthetic prostaglandin E analogues immediately preceding exposure to NSAIDs prevents the expected increase in epithelial permeability, as well as prevents the macroscopic lesions in the small intestine and stomach.[134] Depletion of neutrophils in the rat by using antiserum largely prevents the expected increase in ^{51}Cr-EDTA clearance and intestinal morphologic changes in the rat.[137]

Intestinal permeability commonly increases in patients after elective and emergency major vascular surgery, and it has been proposed that this is due to reperfusion injury rather than the ischemic period of the intestine itself.[138] There is reversible impairment of small bowel transcellular transport after cardiopulmonary bypass, and gut permeability is increased.[139]

Prolonged cow's milk challenge in suckling rats increases gut permeability to intact proteins, and attempts to alter the microflora by oral bacteriotherapy using *Lactobacillus casei* GG counteracts this permeability disorder.[140] During rotavirus enteritis in suckling rats, administration of oral *L. casei* GG reduced uptake of horseradish peroxidase. This suggests that feeding cow's milk amplifies rotavirus infection–associated intestinal dysfunction whereas intestinal implantation of lactobacilli may counteract it.[141]

The lipid component of milk formula that appears to be responsible for increased intestinal permeability upon reperfusion of ischemic jejunal ileum in developing piglets is a long-chain fatty acid such as oleic acid.[142, 143] Luminal perfusion with oleate in concentrations similar to that found in premature infant formula produces a dose- and age-dependent mucosal injury in developing pig intestine. The lipid-induced changes in mucosal permeability appear to be a function of the fatty acid chain length and are not affected by the degree of saturation of the fatty acid.[142, 143] This lipid-induced injury also increases in proportion to the concentration of the fatty acid, and the oleic acid–induced injury can be abolished when the carboxylic group of the fatty acid is esterified with an ethyl group.[144] Bile salts are capable of producing mucosal damage, and part of this effect may be the result of increased leukotriene B_4 synthesis in Caco-2 cells.[145]

INVESTIGATIONAL TESTS

The ^{14}C-D-xylose breath test has been used to detect bacterial overgrowth in patients with gastrointestinal disorders, but when compared with small bowel aspirate and cultures, the sensitivity and specificity of the breath test were only 60% and 40%, respectively.[146] There may also be limitations to the use of measurement of H_2 excretion following lactulose ingestion for the assessment of bacterial over-growth.[147] The commonly used criteria of an increase in breath H_2 concentration of greater than 20 ppm over the fasting value was initially accepted, and it was proposed that persons with lower levels of H_2 excretion after the ingestion of 10 to 20 g of the nonabsorbable carbohydrate lactulose be termed "nonproducers" of H_2. The conventional criterion of a 20-ppm increase in breath H_2 had 100% specificity but failed to identify lactulose malabsorption in 47% and 24% of subjects at 4 and 8 hours of testing, respectively.[148] These authors suggested that true H_2 nonpro-ducers are rare and that a sum of breath H_2 at 5, 6, and 7 hours of greater than 15 ppm yielded better separation between H_2 producers and nonproducers.

The topic of radiology of the small intestine has been reviewed,[149] as has the topic of laparoscopic surgery.[150] The small bowel enema (enteroclysis) is both sen-sitive (93%) and specific (97%) in detecting small intestinal lesions, with the cor-rect specific diagnosis being made in approximately two thirds of examinations that were considered to be abnormal.[151] Leiomyomas and adenomatous polyps are the most common form of benign small intestinal tumors. These are rare. Conventional barium studies may not be adequate to demonstrate these lesions, whereas barium infusion techniques are useful.[152] Plain abdominal radiography and barium exami-nations represent the standard methods of abdominal imaging to detect small bowel obstruction. Abdominal computed tomography (CT) has been shown to be useful for diagnosing the causes of small bowel obstruction with an overall accuracy of 65%; 2 of 55 patients had false-positive and 13 had false-negative results for indi-viduals with low-grade obstruction.[153]

GASTROINTESTINAL HORMONES

When infant rodents are given insulin, there is premature intestinal maturation and activation of the expression of BBM disaccharidases, as well as microsomal and cytostolic enzymes. The BBM enzymatic response of immature enterocytes to insulin is mediated by binding of the hormone to its enterocyte receptor, and the response is transduced into the cell without the de novo synthesis of polyamines.[154]

The L cells of the intestinal mucosa contain an mRNA identical to that encoding proglucagon in the pancreatic A cells. The precursor molecule proglucagon is re-ferred to as enteroglucagon or GLI. Enteroglucagon is found in higher concentra-tions in the ileum, and the highest levels of change in plasma enteroglucagon oc-cur in resection models in which the ileum is conserved.[155]

Cholecystokinin is produced by I cells in the proximal portion of the intestine and is secreted into the circulation after the ingestion of food. Food components in the intestinal lumen have a direct effect on the apical surfaces of the gut endocrine cells to stimulate hormone secretion. When the effects of nutrients on CCK release from perfused cells were compared with changes in circulating plasma CCK levels in fed rats, orally administered protein was the only nutrient to stimulate CCK re-lease in rats.[156] Thus at least in the rat, protein stimulates CCK release postprandially via an indirect mechanism. Proteins appear to exert their stimulatory effect on CCK secretion via trypsin inhibition, and dietary trypsin inhibitors evoke increased pancreatic enzyme secretion via CCK secretion into the blood. The CCK-releasing peptide (monitor peptide) binds to the jejunal mucosal cells and has trypsin-like specificity.[157]

The pharmacodynamic effect of a long-acting analogue of somatostatin, octreotide (Sandostatin), has been reviewed.[158] Somatostatin receptors are present in high density in most intramural veins (but not arteries) of the intestines of patients with Crohn's disease or ulcerative colitis.[159] There is a family of receptors that bind somastatin in different tissues, and two such receptors have been cloned and sequenced. There is a distinct somatostatin receptor subtype in gastrointestinal tissues.[160] Somatostatin may be an effective antisecretory agent in patients with a variety of causes of secretory diarrhea, including children with intractable diarrhea of infancy.[161]

Depending on their size, functional neuroendocrine tumors can be diagnosed preoperatively by imaging procedures such as transabdominal ultrasonography, CT, angiography, or magnetic resonance imaging. Endoscopic ultrasound and somatostatin receptor scintigraphy are the most sensitive imaging methods for localization of these tumors.[162]

Oral administration of thyrotropin releasing hormone (TRH) in humans and in other animals is followed by an increase in plasma thyroid-stimulating hormone (TSH) concentrations. This indicates that sufficient TRH is absorbed intact from the intestine to elicit a physiologic response. Thyroid releasing hormone absorbed in vivo into rabbit BBM vesicles by a passive process,[163] although a paracellular route is also present for uptake of TRH across Caco-2 cell monolayers.[164, 165]

In both suckling and adult rats, intraluminal EGF stimulates intestinal epithelial cell proliferation.[166] In vitro, EGF exerts its mitogenic effects after binding to specific high-affinity receptors, which then activate an intrinsic receptor tyrosine kinase. Intraluminal EGF stimulates rapid tyrosine phosphorylation of the EGF receptor on the basolateral membrane of the enterocyte.[167]

An intricate interplay of cellular, hormonal, neural, and physical factors is responsible for the regulation of small bowel absorption. Circulating hormones have been implicated in meal-induced jejunal absorption, and peptide YY given in physiologic concentrations increases the small bowel absorption of water and electrolytes in canine small bowel in vivo.[168]

ENTERIC INFECTIONS AND HUMAN IMMUNODEFICIENCY VIRUS ENTEROPATHY

Giardiasis is the most common protozoal infection of the gastrointestinal tract. In a small proportion of patients, chronic infection with *Giardia lamblia* will develop, and treatment failures have been documented in both immunocompetent and immunodeficient patients. In a patient with hypogammaglobulinemia and chronic giardiasis, two *Giardia* isolates were obtained that differed in their characteristics of susceptibility to metronidazole and quinacrine, DNA fingerprinting, profiles of iodinated surface proteins, ^{35}S-methionine protein profiles, and isoenzyme patterns.[169]

Clostridium difficile is the agent responsible for antibiotic-associated diarrhea and pseudomembranous colitis.[170] This organism releases two protein exotoxins: toxin A, an enterotoxin, and toxin B, a cytotoxin. Toxin A is the principal agent responsible for fluid secretion and inflammation and may activate mucosal inflammatory cells as well as release inflammatory mediators. Ketotifen pretreatment of rats with *C. difficile* toxin A–induced enteritis reduces secretion and permeability, as well as epithelial cell inflammation and necrosis.[171] The usefulness of this agent in humans needs to be explored.

The canine hookworm *Ancylostoma caninum* may cause obscure abdominal pain and eosinophilic enteritis, with or without blood eosinophilia.[172] The diagnosis can be confirmed by an ELISA.

The gastrointestinal tract is a major target organ for disease associated with human immunodeficiency virus (HIV) infection.[173] In patients with AIDS, diarrhea and weight loss are common, even in community-based HIV-infected patients.[174] Approximately half of these patients have intestinal parasites, but there is no association between the presence of symptoms and stool parasites. Of 165 HIV-infected patients who were initially asymptomatic, intestinal symptoms subsequently developed in 72% over 36 months of actuarial follow-up. Patients with a greater degree of immunosuppression (as indicated by a lower CD4 count) were more prone to gastrointestinal symptoms. In Africa, HIV infection in children is associated with an 11-fold increased risk of death from diarrhea.[175]

Endoscopic as well as histopathologic abnormalities are common in HIV-infected adults, especially in patients with low CD4 counts.[176] In HIV-infected children with chronic gastrointestinal symptoms, there is shortening and irregularity of microvilli even in the absence of pathogens.[177]

Intestinal permeability as assessed by the ratio of lactulose/rhamnose is increased, and the absorption of xylose and 3-*O*-methyl-D-glucose is decreased in patients with HIV disease, especially in the presence of diarrhea.[178] Direct infection of HT-29 human cells with the AIDS virus reduced BBM enzyme activity, and infected cultures responded to calcium ionophore stimulation with an exaggerated increase in intracellular calcium.[179]

Cryptosporidium infection is a common cause of diarrhea in patients with AIDS. Microtubules are important in host cell invasion by *Cryptosporidium parvum*.[180] In addition to the sodium-glucose malabsorption arising from structural damage in *Cryptosporidium*-infected piglets, part of the diarrhea is attributed to local prostanoid production.[181] Severe morphologic abnormalities, including flattening of the villi, are associated with high-intensity infections.[182]

Microsporidia may be present in patients with HIV infection, but it is uncertain that this is necessarily a cause of chronic diarrhea.[183] Infection with the microsporidian *Enterocytozoon bieneusi* is commonly observed in HIV-positive patients.[184]

ONTOGENY AND AGING

The topic of ontogenic development of nutrient transport in rat intestine has been reviewed.[185] In rat embryonal and fetal intestine, GLUT-2 is present in the basolateral membrane of the enterocytes on day 18. The kinetics of expression of GLUT-5 is almost the same as for GLUT-2 except that GLUT-5 is localized to the BBM.[186] The activity and abundance of the sodium-dependent glucose transporter type 1 (SGLT-1) declines during the postnatal development of lambs, and this decline can be prevented by the intraluminal infusion of glucose. First detectable just below the crypt-villus junction, SGLT-1 mRNA rises to reach a peak level approximately 150 μm above this point; it then gradually declines toward the villus tip.[187] This pattern of mRNA accumulation along the villus is similar in all regions of the small intestine and in all age groups, but the decline in expression of mRNA does not coincide with the fall in either the activity or the amount of SGLT-1 protein. This suggests that expression of this sugar transporter is controlled at the post-transcriptional level, at least during the postnatal development of ovine intestine.

The development profile of BBM enzyme expression is modified by the effects of thyroxine and glucocorticosteroid "steroids," and this interaction may be synergistic.[188] Glucocorticosteroids are potent regulatory factors of sucrase activity in the developing rat's small intestine, but not in adult rats. In postnatal rats, administration of dexamethasone causes a precocious appearance of sucrase isomaltase (SI) mRNA as well as sucrase activity, and these changes are due to faster emergence of SI-bearing enterocytes from the intestinal crypts.[189] These authors suggest that there are three distinct phases of glucocorticoid action on the developing intestine: an early phase caused by activation of the gene, a later phase caused by changes in cell kinetics, and a final loss of responsiveness to steroids. Dexamethasone doubles the activity of intestinal glutaminase activity and its mRNA but has little effect on glutamine synthetase, which suggests that these enzymes, which are important for the oxidation of glutamine, are regulated by different mechanisms.[190] The enzyme Na^+/K^+-ATPase in the basolateral membrane plays a pivotal role in the small intestinal uptake of nutrients such as glucose and amino acids. The level of Na^+/K^+-ATPase activity changes during postnatal maturation, and these levels can be modulated by dietary manipulation, hormones, and drugs. Betamethasone increases the activity of Na^+/K^+-ATPase in the colon but not in the small intestine.[191]

Epidermal growth factor is present in milk, and this hormone may be involved in the regulation of postnatal development of the gastrointestinal tract. For example, in the rat, EGF may be involved in the postnatal maturation of intestinal sucrase activity.[192] Transamniotic fetal feeding (TAFF) represents the process of continuous infusion of nutrients or hormones into the amniotic fluid, which is then swallowed by the fetus and undergoes somatic utilization. Infusion of EGF into rabbit amniotic cavities results in an increased length of intestine, increased BBM lactase and maltase activities, and a trend to increase the intestinal uptake of glucose and proline.[193]

Prostaglandins may also play a role in the development of the intestine in early life: prostaglandin E_2 accelerates enzymatic and morphologic intestinal maturation.[194] The feeding of colostrum increases sucrase activity in piglets.[170] In addition to the known effects of corticosteroids, thyroxine, insulin, EGF, and prostaglandins modify enzymatic development in the postnatal intestine. Some dietary factors are involved in this maturational process as well. For example, orally administered polyamines induce structural and biochemical changes that are characteristic of mature intestine.[195] Spermine surgically placed in the lower part of the distal end of the small intestine of suckling rats induces BBM sucrase and decreases lactase activities in the proximal as well as the distal portions of the small intestine.[196]

Sodium-dependent bile acid uptake in rat ileum is abruptly expressed on day 17 of postnatal life, and taurocholate feeding results in precocious development of ileal bile acid transport and the induction of sucrase activity.[197] The topic of the effect of aging on intestinal lipid absorption has been reviewed.[198] A state of hypoproliferation occurs in epithelial cells of the small intestine of older as compared with younger rodents.[199] A crucial factor for the maintenance of adequate intestinal function is the ability of the intestine to adapt to a changing environment. The tricarboxylic acid cycle is suppressed with aging in jejunal epithelial cells.[200] The adaptation of intestinal nutrient absorption in response to changes in the dietary level of carbohydrate or protein is impaired in aged mice.[201] A high-protein diet fails to increase aminopeptidase activity in the jejunum of old rats, as is the case in younger animals, and this reduced adaptive capability of the jejunum may be partially compensated for by enhanced ileal function.[202] The site density of intestinal glucose transporters declines with age.[203] The reduction in villus height occurring in the jejunum of aged rats is balanced in the ileum by an increase in villus height, enhanced BBM hydrolytic enzyme activity, and a higher absorptive capacity.

DIABETES MELLITUS

Gastrointestinal symptoms are common in patients with diabetes mellitus and include common complaints such as postprandial pain, bloating, and altered bowel habits. In type I diabetic patients with cardiac autonomic neuropathy, hyperactivity in the interdigestive state is common and correlates with symptoms.[204] In association with insulin-induced hypoglycemia in rats, there is increased sugar uptake across both the BBM and basolateral membrane of mature villus cells near the villus tip, possibly as the result of an increased electrochemical gradient driving force for Na^+/sugar cotransport rather than as the result of any change in the number of transporters.[205] Increased expression of $SGLT_1$, $GLUT_2$, and $GLUT_5$ occurs in the small intestine of the diabetic rat.[206] The alterations in transporter expression may serve to increase nutrient transport in a perceived state of starvation. 3-Hydroxy-3-methylglutaryl coenzyme A (HMG CoA) reductase is the rate-limiting enzyme in cholesterol synthesis and is increased in the intestines of animals with experimental diabetes mellitus. This increased activity is associated with enhanced abundance of the HMG CoA reductase protein; although the intestinal levels of HMG CoA reductase mRNA is increased in diabetic intestine, the levels in the diabetic liver do not change.[207]

Insulin administered by mouth encounters the proteolytic activity of the gastrointestinal tract and also faces the relative impermeability of the intestinal epithelium to the transport of peptides. When insulin is introduced into the lumen of the rat duodenum in combination with sodium cholate and aprotinin, there is a rapid increase in circulating levels of insulin followed by decreases in blood glucose concentration.[208] This raises the possibility for the clinical development of an oral preparation of insulin.

RADIATION DAMAGE

The small intestine is radiation sensitive. In humans there are early and late gastrointestinal symptoms produced by radiation. Acute injury is due to the loss of surface epithelium and damage to the intestinal crypts, which leads to ulceration and loss of proteins, blood, and electrolytes. Late symptoms are related to the dose of radiation and are the result of progressive occlusive vasculitis with fibrosis and collagen deposition. Exposure of rats to sublethal doses of radiation results in a reduction in tissue responsiveness to electrical field stimulation, to prostaglandin E_2, and to theophylline without associated changes in villus-crypt architecture.[209] The effect of ionizing radiation reducing the transport response to neural stimulation is temporarily correlated with a decrease in mast cells and in histamine. Abdominal radiation may influence small intestinal motor activity, and this may contribute to the development of diarrhea.[210]

SUMMARY

Major scientific advances have been made over the past year in the areas of small bowel physiology, pathology, microbiology, and clinical science. Over 1,000 papers have been reviewed, and a selected number are considered here. Wherever possible, the clinical relevance of these advances has been identified. There have been a number of important and/or interesting developments in the past year that may have clinical significance. For example, nucleotides added to the diet have been shown to alter intestinal morphology, and these may be important in infant nutrition. Macromolecules, including albumin, may be transported across the intestinal brush border membrane. This may be under the control of the enteric nervous system through cholinergic nerves acting on muscarinic receptors. Epidermal growth factor also modifies intestinal nutrient transport. Alcohol abolishes the circadian variation of the MMC, and this effect may be mediated by central rather than local mechanisms. Nitric oxide mediates inhibitory nerve input on smooth muscle in man and may play an important role in regulating MMC and cyclic motor activity during the fasting state as well as their disruption by a meal. Nitric oxide also plays a role in the regulation of gastrointestinal blood flow. Serotonin is a potent stimulant of intestinal fluid and electrolyte secretion, and a variety of antagonists to the 5-HT$_3$ receptor have been identified and appear to be effective in controlling cancer chemotherapy–induced emesis. The different 5-HT receptors may also be involved in stress-induced colonic motor activity, and a selective 5-HT re-uptake inhibitor, paroxetine, reduces MMC periodicity in healthy humans and has a prokinetic action in human small intestine. Protease inhibitors may improve mucosal hyperpermeability induced by ischemia/reperfusion injury. Celiac disease occurs in the elderly, particularly in patients with nonspecific gastrointestinal complaints and especially in the presence of unexplained anemia. Measuring the IgA to antireticulin antibody may be valuable in the assisting in the early recognition and treatment of occult celiac disease. Even the intake of small amounts of gliadin in children with celiac disease results in morphologic abnormalities in the intestine. A reduction in the number or loss of Kerkring's fold is the most sensitive and specific endoscopic change suggesting the presence of celiac disease. The D-xylose hydrogen breath test may be a useful and practical means for the post-treatment follow-up of celiac patients. The endoscopic findings of Whipple's disease include a combination of yellow-white plaques and an erythematous, erosive, or mildly friable mucosa. Central nervous system symptoms may rarely be the only initial manifestation in patients with Whipple's disease. Antibiotics such as trimethoprim-sulfamethoxazole have more reliable CNS penetration and should be used as first-line therapy. Increased intestinal permeability has been described in a variety of gastrointestinal diseases such as Crohn's disease, sprue, and NSAID-associated enteritis; administration of synthetic prostaglandin E analogue immediately preceding exposure to NSAIDs prevents the expected increase in epithelial permeability, as well as prevents the macroscopic lesions in the small intestine and in the stomach. The ^{14}C-D-xylose breath test has low sensitivity and specificity in detecting bacterial overgrowth syndrome, and there may also be a limitation in use of the measurement of H$_2$ excretion following lactulose injection to make this diagnosis. A long-acting analogue of somatostatin, octreotide, may be an effective antisecretory agent in patients with a variety of causes of secretory diarrhea such as intractable diarrhea of infancy. Giardiasis is the most common protozoal infection of the gastrointestinal tract, and treatment failures have been documented in both immunocompetent and immunodeficient patients. The gastrointestinal tract is a major target organ for disease associated with HIV infection, and diarrhea and weight loss are common even in community-based HIV-infected patients. Patients with lower CD4 counts are more prone to the development of gastrointestinal symptoms, and endoscopic abnormalities are common in HIV-infected adults, particularly those with low CD4 counts. Intestinal permeability is increased in HIV disease, and one must not forget that *Cryptosporidium* is a common cause of diarrhea in patients with AIDS. In type I diabetic patients with cardiac autonomic neuropathy, hyperactivity in the interdigestive state is common and correlates with symptoms.

The importance of these basic science developments in small bowel physiology are being recognized inasmuch as these are increasingly being applied to clinical situations.

REFERENCES

1. Tiruppathi C, Miyamoto Y, Ganapathy V, et al: Genetic evidence for role of DPP IV in intestinal hydrolysis and assimilation of prolyl peptides. *Am J Physiol* 265:G81–G89, 1993.

2. Suzuki Y, Erickson RH, Sedlmayer A, et al: Dietary regulation of rat intestinal angiotensin-converting enzyme and dipeptidyl peptidase IV. *Am J Physiol* 264:G1153–G1159, 1993.

3. Darmoul D, Lacasa M, Baricouilt L, et al: Dipeptidy/peptidase IV gene expression in enterocyte-like colon cancer cell lines HT-29 and Caco-2. *J Biol Chem* 267:4824–4833, 1992.

4. Baricault L, Garcia M, Cibert C, et al: Forskolin blocks the apical expression of dipeptidyl peptidase IV in Caco-2 cells and induces its retention in lamp-1–containing vesicles. *Exp Cell Res* 209:277–287, 1993.

5. Sanderson IR, He Y: Nucleotide uptake and metabolism by intestinal epithelial cells. *J Nutr* 124:1315–1375, 1994.

6. Carver JD: Dietary nucleotides: Cellular immune, intestinal and hepatic system effects. *J Nutr* 124:1445–1485, 1994.

7. Bustamante SA, Sanches N, Crosier J, et al: Dietary nucleotides: Effects on the gastrointestinal system in swine. *J Nutr* 124:1495–1565, 1994.

8. He Y, Chu S-HW, Walker WA: Nucleotide supplements alter proliferation and differentiation of cultured human (Caco-2) and rat (IEC-6) intestinal epithelial cells. *J Nutr* 123:1017–1027, 1993.

9. Grimble GK: Dietary nucleotides and gut mucosal defence. *Gut* 35:(suppl 1):46–51, 1994.

10. Terasaki T, Kadowaki A, Higashida H, et al: Expression of the Na^+-dependent uridine transport system of rabbit small intestine: Studies with mRNA-injected Xenopus laevis oocytes. *Biol Pharm Bull* 16:493–496, 1993.

11. Kim D-C, Burton PS, Borchardt RT: A correlation between the permeability characteristics of a series of peptides using an in vitro cell culture model (Caco-2) and those using an in situ perfused rat ileum model of the intestinal mucosa. *Pharm Res* 10:1710–1714, 1993.

12. Conradi RA, Wilkinson KF, Rush BD, et al: In vitro/in vivo models for peptide oral absorption: Comparison of Caco-2 cell permeability with rat intestinal absorption of renin inhibitory peptides. *Pharm Res* 10:1790–1792, 1993.

13. Burton PS, Conradi RA, Hilgers AR, et al: Evidence for a polarized efflux system for peptides in the apical membrane of Caco-2 cells. *Biochem Biophys Res Commun* 190:760–766, 1993.

14. Gustafsson B, Persson CGA: Allergen-induced mucosal exudation of plasma into rat ileum and its inhibition by budesonide. *Scand J Gastroenterol* 27:587–593, 1992.

15. Tanaka J-I, Fujimoto K, Sakata, et al: Effect of vagotomy on ornithine decarboxylase activity in rat duodenal mucosa. *Am J Physiol* 265:G1016–G1020, 1993.

16. Kobayashi M, Iseli K, Sugawara M, et al: The diversity of Na^+-independent uptake systems for polyamines in Mt intestinal brush-border membrane vesicles. *Biochim Biophys Acta* 1151:161–167, 1993.

17. Scemama J-L, Brabie V, Seidel ER: Characterization of univectorial polyamine transport in duodenal crypt cell line. *Am J Physiol* 265:G851–G856, 1993.

18. Munck LK, Munck, BG: Distinction between chloride-dependent transport systems for taurine and B-alanine in rabbit ileum. *Am J Physiol* 262:G609–G615, 1992.

19. Brandsch M, Miyamoto Y, Ganapathy V, et al: Regulation of taurine transport in human colon carcinoma cell lines (HT-29 and Caco-2) by protein kinase C. *Am J Physiol* 264:G939–G946, 1993.

20. Thwaites DT, Simmons NL, First BH: Thyrotropin-releasing hormone (TRH) uptake in intestinal brush-border membrane vesicles: Comparison with proton-coupled dipeptide and Na^+-coupled glucose transport. *Pharm Res* 10:667–673, 1993.

21. Thwaites DT, McEwan GTA, Cook MJ: H^+-coupled (Na^+-independent) proline transport in human intestinal (Caco-2) epithelial cell monolayers. *FEBS Lett* 333:78–82, 1993.

22. Thwaites DT, Hirst BH, Simmons HL: Direct assessment of dipeptide/H^+ symport in intact human intestinal (Caco-2) epithelium: A novel method utilizing continuous intracellular pH measurement. *Biochem Biophys Res Commun* 194:432–438, 1993.

23. Thwaites DT, Brown CDA, Hirst BH: H^+-coupled dipeptide (glycylsarcosine) transport across apical and basal borders of human intestinal Caco-2 cell monolayers display distinctive characteristics. *Biochim Biophys Acta* 1151:237–245, 1993.

24. Saito H, Inui K-I: Dipeptide transporters in apical and basolateral membranes of the human intestinal cell line Caco-2. *Am J Physiol* 265:G289–G294, 1993.

25. Nakanishi M, Tetsuka T, Kagawa Y: Solubilization and reconstruction of high- and low-affinity Na^+-dependent neutral L-α-amino acid transporters from rabbit small intestine. *Biochim Biophys Acta* 1151:193–200, 1993.

26. Pickel VM, Nirenberg MJ, Chan J: Ultrastructural localization of a neutral and basic amino acid transporter in rat kidney and intestine. *Proc Natl Acad Sci USA* 90:7779–7783, 1993.

27. Harvey CM, Muzyka WR, Yao SY-M: Expression of rat intestinal L-lysine transport systems in isolated oocytes of Xenopus laevis. *Am J Physiol* 265:G99–G106, 1993.

28. Magagnin S, Bertran J, Werner A: Poly (A)+ RNA from rabbit intestinal mucosa induces bt+ and y+ amino acid transport activities in Xenopus laevis oocytes. *J Biol Chem* 267:15384–15390, 1992.

29. Evans MA, Shronts EP: Intestinal fuels: Glutamine, short-chain fatty acids, and dietary fiber. *J Am Diet Assoc* 92:1239–1246, 1992.

30. Said HM, Morgan T, Hoefs J: Effect of chronic portal hypertension on glutamine transport across rat intestinal brush border and basolateral membranes. *J Lab Clin Med* 122:64–68, 1993.

31. Caillard I, Tomé D: Modulation of β-lactoglobulin transport in rabbit ileum. *Am J Physiol* 266:G1053–G1059, 1994.

32. Kimm MH, Curtis GH, Hardin JA, et al: Transport of bovine serum albumin across rat jejunum: Role of the enteric nervous system. *Am J Physiol* 266:G186–G193, 1994.

33. Crowe SE, Perdue MH: Anti–immunoglobulin E–stimulated ion transport in human large and small intestine. *Gastroenterology* 105:764–772, 1993.

34. Prigent SA, Lemonie NR, Hughes CM, et al: Expression of the c-erb B-3 protein in normal human adult and fetal tissues. *Oncogene* 7:1273–1278, 1993.

35. Salloum RM, Stevens BR, Schultz GS, et al: Regulation of small intestinal glutamine transport by epidermal growth factor. *Surgery* 113:552–559, 1993.

36. Bird AR, Croom WJ, Fan YK, et al: Jejunal glucose absorption is enhanced by epidermal growth factor in mice. *J Nutr* 124:231–240, 1994.

37. Sarna SK: Gastrointestinal longitudinal muscle contractions. *Am J Physiol* 265:G156–G164, 1993.

38. Gregersen H, Orvar K, Christensen J: Biomechanical properties of duodenal wall and duodenal tone during phase I and phase II of the MMC. *Am J Physiol* 263:G795–G801, 1992.

39. Staumont G, Dalvaux M, Fioramonti J, et al: Differences between jejunal myoelectric activity after a meal and during phase 2 of migrating motor complexes in healthy humans. *Dig Dis Sci* 37:1554–1561, 1992.

40. Zenilman ME, Parodi JE, Becker JM: Preservation and propagation of cyclic myoelectric activity after feeding in rat small intestine. *Am J Physiol* 263:G248–G253, 1992.

41. Husebye E, Hellstrom M, Midtvedt T: Intestinal microflora stimulates myoelectric activity of rat small intestine by promoting cyclic initiation and aboral propagation of migrating myoelectric complex. *Dig Dis Sci* 39:946–956, 1994.

42. Charles F, Evans DF, Castillo FD, et al: Daytime ingestion of alcohol alters nighttime jejunal motility in man. *Dig Dis Sci* 39:51–58, 1994.

43. De Boer SY, Masclee AAM, Lam WF, et al: Hyperglycemia modulates gallbladder motility and small intestinal transit time in man. *Dig Dis Sci* 38:2228–2235, 1993.

44. Lowenstein CJ, Dinerman JL, Snyder SH: Nitric oxide: A physiologic messenger. *Ann Intern Med* 120:227–237, 1994.

45. Stark ME, Bauer AJ, Sarr MG, et al: Nitric oxide mediates inhibitory nerve input in human and canine jejunum. *Gastroenterology* 104:398–409, 1993.

46. Timmermans J-P, Barbiers M, Scheuermann DW, et al: Nitric oxide synthase immunoreactivity in the enteric nervous system of the developing human digestive tract. *Cell Tissue Res* 275:235–245, 1994.

47. Kubes P: Nitric oxide modulates epithelial permeability in the feline small intestine. *Am J Physiol* 262:G1138–G1142, 1992.

48. Kanwar S, Wallace JL, Befus D, et al: Nitric oxide synthesis inhibition increases epithelial permeability via mast cells. *Am J Physiol* 266:G222–G299, 1994.

49. MacNaughton WK: Nitric oxide–donating compounds stimulate electrolyte transport in the guinea pig intestine in vitro. *Life Sci* 53:585–593, 1993.

50. Boughton-Smith NK, Evans SM, Laszlo F, et al: The induction of nitric oxide synthase and intestinal vascular permeability by endotoxin in the rat. *Br J Pharmacol* 110:1189–1195, 1993.

51. Daniel EE, Hough C, Woskowska Z: Role of nitric oxide–related inhibition in intestinal function: Relation to vasoactive intestinal polypeptide. *Am J Physiol* 266:G31–G39, 1994.

52. Grider JR, Jin JG: Vasoactive intestinal peptide release and L-citrulline production from isolated ganglia of the myenteric plexius: Evidence for regulation of vasaoactive intestinal peptide release by nitric oxide. *Neuroscience* 54:521–526, 1993.

53. Grider JR: Interplay of VIP and nitric oxide in regulation of the descending relaxation phase of peristalsis. *Am J Physiol* 264:G334–G340, 1993.

54. Baidan LV, Zholos AV, Shuba MF, et al: Patch-clamp recording in myenteric neurons of guinea pig small intestine. *Am J Physiol* 262:G1074–G1078, 1992.

55. Torihashi S, Kobayashi S, Gerthoffer WT, et al: Interstitial cells in deep muscular plexus of canine small intestine may be specialized smooth muscle cells. *Am J Physiol* 265:G638–G645, 1993.

56. Rossowski WJ, Zacharia S, Jiang N-Y, et al: Galanin: Structure-dependent effect on pancreatic amylase secretion and jejunal strip contraction. *Eur J Pharmacol* 240:259–267, 1993.

57. Chen CK, McDonald TJ, Daniel EE: Characterization of galanin receptor in canine small intestinal circular muscle synaptosomes. *Am J Physiol* 266:G106–G112, 1994.

58. Weber FH, Richards RD, McCallum RW: Erythromycin: A motilin agonist and gastrointestinal prokinetic agent. *Am J Gastroenterol* 88:485–490, 1993.

59. Wang X-B, Osugi T, Uchida S: Muscarinic receptors stimulate Ca^{2+} influx via phospholipase A_2 pathway in ileal smooth muscles. *Biochem Biophys Res Commun* 193:483–489, 1993.

60. Wade PR, Tamir H, Kirchgessner AL, et al: Analysis of the role of 5-HT in the enteric nervous system using anti-idiotopic antibodies to 5-HTYY receptors. *Am J Physiol* 266:G403–G416, 1994.

61. Dhasmana KM, Zhu YN, Cruz SL, et al: Gastrointestinal effects of 5-hydroxytryptamine and related drugs. *Life Sci* 53:1651–1661, 1993.

62. Siriwardena AK, Smith EH, Borum EH, et al: Identification of a 5-hydroxytryptamine (5-HT2) receptor on guinea pig small intestinal crypt cells. *Am J Physiol* 265:G339–G346, 1993.

63. Neya T, Mizutani M, Yamasato T: Role of 5-HT3 receptors in peristaltic reflex elicited by stroking the mucosa in the canine jejunum. *J Physiol* 471:159–173, 1993.

64. Kishibayashi N, Miwa Y, Hayashi H, et al: 5-HT3 receptor antagonists. 3. Quinoline derivatives which may be effective in the therapy of irritable bowel syndrome. *J Med Chem* 36:3286–3292, 1993.

65. Fiorica-Howells E, Wade PR, Gershon MD: Serotonin-induced increase in cAMP in ganglia isolated from the myenteric plexus of the guinea pig small intestine: Mediation by a novel 5-HT receptor. *Synapse* 13:333–349, 1993.

66. Broad RM, McDonald TJ, Cook MA: Adenosine and 5-HT inhibit substance P release from nerve endings in myenteric ganglia by distinct mechanisms. *Am J Physiol* 264:G454–G461, 1993.

67. Gue M, Alary C, Del Rio-Lacheze C, et al: Comparative involvement of 5-HT, 5-HT2 and 5-HT3 receptors in stress-induced colonic motor alterations in rats. *Eur J Pharmacol* 233:193–199, 1993.

68. Gorard DA, Libby GW, Farthing MJG: 5-Hydroxytryptamine and human small intestinal motility: Effect of inhibiting 5-hydroxytryptamine reuptake. *Gut* 35:496–500, 1994.

69. Kuemmerle JF, Makhlouf GM: Characterization of opioid receptors in intestinal muscle cells by selective radioligands and receptor protection. *Am J Physiol* 263:G269–G276, 1992.

70. Brown NJ, Rumsey DE, Read NW: The effect of the cholecystokinin antagonist/devazepide (L364718) on the ileal brake mechanism in the rat. *J Pharm Pharmacol* 245:1033–1036, 1993.

71. Pironi L, Stanghellini V, Miglioli M, et al: Fat-induced ileal break in humans: A dose-dependent phenomenon correlated to the plasma levels of peptide YY. *Gastroenterology* 105:733–739, 1993.

72. Armstrong DN, Krenz HK, Modlin IM, et al: Bile salt inhibition of motility in the isolated perfused rabbit terminal ileum. *Gut* 34:483–488, 1993.

73. Awouters F, Megens A, Verlinden M, et al: Loperamide survey of studies on mechanism of its antidiarrheal activity. *Dig Dis Sci* 38:977–995, 1993.

74. Keeling WF, Harris A, Martin BJ: Loperamide abolishes exercise-induced orocecal liquid transit acceleration. *Dig Dis Sci* 38:1783–1787, 1993.

75. Hardcastle, Hardcastle PT, Goldhill J: Comparision of the effects of loperamide and loperamide oxide on absorptive processes in rat small intestine. *J Pharm Pharmacol* 45:919–921, 1993.

76. De Luca A, Murray G, Coupar IM: Do antidiarrhoeal opiates accumulate in the rat 2 intestinal lumen? *J Pharm Pharmacol* 46:1082–1084, 1993.

77. McKee DP, Quigley MM: Intestinal motility in irritable bowel syndrome: Is IBS a motility disorder? Part 2. Motility of the small bowel, esophagus, stomach, and gallbladder. *Dig Dis Sci* 38:1773–1782, 1993.

78. McKee DP, Quigley EMM: Intestinal motility in irritable bowel syndrome: Is IBS a motility disorder? Part 1. Definition of IBS and colonic motility. *Dig Dis Sci* 38:1761–1772, 1993.

79. Gorard DA, Libby GW, Farthing MJG: Ambulatory small intestinal motility in 'diarrhoea' predominant irritable bowel syndrome. *Gut* 35:203–210, 1994.

80. Tada S, Iida M, Yao T, et al: Intestinal pseudo-obstruction in patients with amyloidosis: Clinicopathologic differences between chemical types of amyloid protein. *Gut* 34:1412–1417, 1993.

81. Camilleri M, Balm RK, Zinsmeister AR: Determinants of response to a prokinetic agent in neuropathic chronic intestinal motility disorder. *Gastroenterology* 106:916–923, 1994.

82. Troncon LEA, Oliveira RB, Romanello LMF, et al: Abnormal progression of a liquid meal through the stomach and small intestine in patients with Chagas' disease. *Dig Dis Sci* 38:1511–1517, 1993.

83. Stewart JJ, Battarbee HD, Farrar GE, et al: Intestinal myoelectrical activity and transit time in chronic portal hypertension. *Am J Physiol* 263:G474–G479, 1992.

84. Chesta J, DeFilippi C, DeFilippi C: Abnormalities in proximal small bowel motility in patients with cirrhosis. *Hepatology* 17:828–832, 1993.

85. Quigley EMM, Thompson JS: The motor response to intestinal resection: Motor activity in the canine small intestine following distal resection. *Gastroenterology* 105:791–798, 1993.

86. Benson MJ, Roberts JP, Wingate DL, et al: Small bowel motility following major intra-abdominal surgery: The effects of opiates and rectal cisapride. *Gastroenterology* 106:924–936, 1994.

87. Nilsson BO, Hellstrand P: Effects of polyamines on intracellular calcium and mechanical activity in smooth muscle of guinea-pig taenia coli. *Acta Physiol Scand* 148:37–43, 1993.

88. Nalini S, Ibrahim SA, Balasubramanian KA: Effect of oxidant exposure on monkey intestinal brush border membrane. *Biochim Biophys Acta* 1147: 169–176, 1993.

89. Gosche JR, Harris PD, Garrison RN: Age-related differences in intestinal microvascular responses to low-flow slates in adult and suckling rats. *Am J Physiol* 264:G447–G453, 1993.

90. Nowicki PT, Nankervis CA, Miller CE: Effects of ischemia and reperfusion on intrinsic vascular regulation in the post-natal intestinal circulation. *Pediatr Res* 33:400–404, 1993.

91. Salzman A, Wollert PS, Wang H, et al: Intraluminal oxygenation ameliorates ischemia/reperfusion-induced gut mucosal hyperpermeability in pigs. *Circ Shock* 40:37–46, 1993.

92. Murray MJ, Barbase JJ, Cobbs CF: Serum D(−)-lactate levels as a predictor of acute intestinal ischemia in a rat model. *J Surg Res* 54:507–509, 1993.

93. Hankey GL, Holmes GKT: Coeliac disease in the elderly. *Gut* 35:65–67, 1994.

94. Sategna-Guideffi C, Pulitano R, Grosso S, et al: Serum IgA antiendomysium antibody titers as a marker of intestinal involvement and diet compliance in adult celiac sprue. *J Clin Gastroenterol* 17:123–127, 1993.

95. Unsworth DJ, Brown DL: Serological screening suggests that adult coeliac disease is underdiagnosed in the UK and increases the incidence by up to 12%. *Gut* 35:61–64, 1994.

96. Uibo O, Uibo R, Kleimola V, et al: Serum IgA anti-gliadin antibodies in an adult population sample. *Dig Dis Sci* 38:2034–2037, 1993.

97. Arranz E, Bode J, Kingstone K, et al: Intestinal antibody pattern of coeliac disease: Association with γ/δ T cell receptor expression by intraepithelial lymphocytes, and other indices of potential coeliac disease. *Gut* 35:476–482, 1994.

98. Arranz E, Ferguson A: Intestinal antibody pattern of celiac disease: Occurrence in patients with normal jejunal biopsy histology. *Gastroenterology* 104:1263–1272, 1993.

99. Holm K, Savilahti E, Koskimies S, et al: Immunohistochemical changes in the jejunum in first degree relatives of patients with celiac and the coeliac disease marker DQ genes. HLA class II antigen expression, interleukin-2 receptor positive cells and dividing crypt cells. *Gut* 35:55–60, 1994.

100. Catassi C, Rossini M, Ratsch I-M, et al: Dose dependent effects of protracted ingestion of small amounts of gliadin in coeliac disease children: A clinical and jejunal morphometric study. *Gut* 34:1515–1519, 1993.

101. Dyduch A, Karczewska K, Grzybek H, et al: Transmission electron microscopy of microvilli of intestinal epithelial cells in celiac disease in remission and transient gluten enteropathy in children after a gluten-free diet. *J Pediatr Gastroenterol Nutr* 16:269–272, 1993.

102. Ensari A, Marsh MN, Loft DE, et al: Morphometric analysis of intestinal mucosa. V quantitative histological and immunocytochemical studies of rectal mucosae in gluten sensitivity. *Gut* 34:1225–1229, 1993.

103. Fluge O, Sletten K, Fluge G, et al: In vitro toxicity of purified gluten peptides tested by organ culture. *J Pediatr Gastroenterol Nutr* 18:186–192, 1994.

104. Marsh MN, Ensari A, Morgan S: Evidence that gluten sensitivity is an immunologic disease. *Curr Opin Gastroenterol* 9:994–1000, 1993.

105. Sollid LV, Thorsby E: HLA susceptibility genes in celiac disease: Genetic mapping and role in pathogenesis. *Gastroenterology* 105:910–922, 1993.

106. Lundin KEA, Scott H, Hansen T, et al: Gliadin-specific, HLA-DQ(α1*0501,β1*0201) restricted T cells isolated from the small intestinal mucosa of celiac disease patients. *J Exp Med* 178:187–196, 1993.

107. Roschmann E, Wienker TF, Gerok W, et al: T-cell receptor variable genes and genetic susceptibility to celiac disease: An association and linkage study. *Gastroenterology* 105:1790–1796, 1993.

108. Doyle GJ, Rose JDG, Kesteven PJL: Pleural lymphoma in a patient presenting with malabsorption: An illustration of the clinicopathological behaviour in a case of enteropathy associated T cell lymphoma. *Gut* 34:1463–1466, 1993.

109. Maurino E, Capizzano H, Niveloni S, et al: Value of endoscopic markers in celiac disease. *Dig Dis Sci* 38:2028–2033, 1993.

110. Alvarez D, Vazquez H, Bai JC, et al: Superior mesenteric artery blood flow in celiac disease. *Dig Dis Sci* 38:1175–1182, 1993.

111. Casellas F, Chichana L, Malogelada JR: Potential usefulness of hydrogen breath test with D-xylose in clinical management of intestinal malabsorption. *Dig Dis Sci* 38:321–327, 1993.

112. Lerner A, Gruener N, Iancu TC: Serum carnitine concentrations in coeliac disease. *Gut* 34:933–935, 1993.

113. Amer MH, El-Akkad S: Gastrointestinal lymphoma in adults: Clinical features and management of 300 cases. *Gastroenterology* 106:846–858, 1994.

114. Ruskone-Fourmestraux A, Aegerter P, Delmer A, et al: Primary digestive tract lymphoma: A prospective multicentric study of 91 patients. *Gastroenterology* 105:1662–1671, 1993.

115. Arista-Nasr J, Gonzalez-Romo MA, Mantilla-Morales A, et al: Immunoproliferative small intestinal disease in Mexico. *J Clin Gastroenterol* 18:67–71, 1994.

116. Gaist D, Ladefoged K: Whipple's disease. *Scand J Gastroenterol* 29:97–101, 1994.

117. Relman DA, Schmidt TM, MacDermott RP, et al: Identification of the uncultured bacillus of Whipple's disease. *N Engl J Med* 327:293–301, 1992.

118. Ectors NL, Geboes KJ, De Vos RM, et al: Whipple's disease: A histological, immunocytochemical, and electron microscopic study of the small intestinal epithelium. *J Pathol* 172:73–79, 1994.

119. Marth T, Roux M, van Herbay A, et al: Persistent reduction of complement receptor 3 alpha-chain expressing mononuclear blood cells and transient inhibitory serum factors in Whipple's disease. *Clin Immunol Immunopathol* 72:217–226, 1994.

120. Gillen CD, Coddington R, Monteith PG, et al: Extraintestinal lymphoma in association with Whipple' disease. *Gut* 34:1627–1629, 1993.

121. Feurle GE, Marth T: An evaluation of antimicrobial treatment for Whipple's disease. Tetracycline versus trimethoprim-sulfamethoxazole. *Dig Dis Sci* 39:1642–1648, 1994.

122. Cooper GS, Blades EW, Remler BF, et al: Central nervous system Whipple's disease: Relapse during therapy with trimethoprim-sulfamethoxazole and remission with cefixime. *Gastroenterology* 106:782–786, 1994.

123. Bjarnason I: Intestinal permeability. *Gut* 35(suppl 1):18–22, 1994.

124. Deitch EA: Bacterial translocation: The influence of dietary variables. *Gut* 35(suppl 1):23–27, 1994.

125. Spitz J, Hecht G, Taveras M, et al: The effect of dexamethasone administration on rat intestinal permeability: The role of bacterial adherence. *Gastroenterology* 106:35–41, 1994.

126. Runkel NSF, Moody FG, Smith GS, et al: Alterations in rat intestinal transit by morphine promote bacterial translocation. *Dig Dis Sci* 38:1530–1536, 1993.

127. Van Leeuwen PAM, Boermeester MA, Houdijk APJ, et al: Clinical significance of translocation. *Gut* 35(suppl 1):28–34, 1994.

128. Cynober L: Can arginine and ornithine support gut functions? *Gut* 35(suppl 1):42–45, 1994.

129. Krugliak P, Hollander D, Schlaepfer CC, et al: Mechanisms and sites of mannitol permeability of small and large intestine in the rat. *Dig Dis Sci* 39:796–801, 1994.

130. Zuckerman MJ, Watts MT, Bhatt BD, et al: Intestinal permeability to [^{51}Cr]EDTA infectious diarrhea. *Dig Dis Sci* 38:1651–1657, 1993.

131. Stenson WF, Eason RA, Reihl TE, et al: Regulation of paracellular permeability in Caco-2 cell monolayers by protein kinase C. *Am J Physiol* 265:G955–G962, 1993.

132. Hecht G, Robinson B, Koutsouris A: Reversible disassembly of an intestinal epithelial monolayer by prolonged exposure to phorbol ester. *Am J Physiol* 266:G214–G221, 1994.

133. See NA, Bass P: Nutrient-induced changes in the permeability of the rat jejunal mucosa. *J Pharm Sci* 82:721–724, 1993.

134. Mion F, Cuber J-C, Minaire Y, et al: Short term effects of indomethacin on rat small intestinal permeability. Role of eicosanoids and platelet activating factor. *Gut* 35:490–495, 1994.

135. Langer JC, Sohal SS, Mumford DA: Mucosal permeability in the immature rat intestine: Effects of ischemia-reperfusion, cold stress, hypoxia, and drugs. *J Pediatr Surg* 28:1380–1385, 1993.

136. Nygard G, Anthony A, Piasecki C, et al: Acute indomethacin-induced jejunal injury in the rat: Early morphological and biochemical changes. *Gastroenterology* 106:567–575, 1994.

137. Chmaisse HM, Antoon JS, Kvietys PR, et al: Role of leukocytes in indomethacin-induced small bowel injury in the rat. *Am J Physiol* 266:G239–G246, 1994.

138. Roumen RMH, van der Vliet JA, Wevers RA, et al: Intestinal permeability is increased after major vascular surgery. *J Vasc Surg* 17:734–737, 1993.

139. Ohri SK, Bjarnason I, Pathi V, et al: Cardiopulmonary bypass impairs small intestinal transport and increases gut permeability. *Ann Thorac Surg* 55:1080–1086, 1993.

140. Isolauri E, Majamaa H, Arvola T, et al: Lactobacillus casei strain GG reverses increased intestinal permeability induced by cow milk in suckling rats. *Gastroenterology* 105:1643–1650, 1993.

141. Isolauri E, Kaila M, Arvola T, et al: Diet during rotavirus enteritis affects jejunal permeability to macromolecules in suckling rats. *Pediatr Res* 33:548–533, 1993.

142. Velasquez OR, Tso P, Crissinger KD: Fatty acid–induced injury in developing piglet intestine: Effect of degree of saturation and carbon chain length. *Pediatr Res* 33:543–547, 1993.

143. Velasquez OR, Henninger K, Fowler M, et al: Oleic acid–induced mucosal injury in developing piglet intestine. *Am J Physiol* 264:G576–G582, 1993.

144. Velasquez OR, Place AR, Tso P, et al: Developing intestine is injured during absorption of oleic acid but not its ethyl ester. *J Clin Invest* 93:479–485, 1994.

145. Dias VC, Shaffer EA, Wallace JL, et al: Bile salts determine leukotriene B_4 synthesis in a human intestinal cell line (CaCo-2). *Dig Dis Sci* 39:802–808, 1994.

146. Valdovinos MA, Camilleri M, Thomforde, et al: Reduced accuracy of ^{14}C-D xylose breath test for detecting bacterial overgrowth in gastrointestinal motility disorders. *Scand J Gastroenterol* 28:963–968, 1993.

147. Corazza G, Strocchi A, Sorge M, et al: Prevalence and consistency of low breath H_2 excretion following lactulose ingestion. *Dig Dis Sci* 38:2010–2016, 1993.

148. Strocchi A, Corazza G, Ellis CJ, et al: Detection of malabsorption of low doses of carbohydrate: Accuracy of various breath H_2 criteria. *Gastroenterology* 105:1404–1410, 1993.

149. Shorvon P, Lamb G: Radiology of the small intestine. *Curr Opin Gastroenterol* 10:163–170, 1994.

150. Soper NJ, Brunt LM, Kerbl K: Laparoscopic general surgery. *N Engl J Med* 303:409–419, 1994.

151. Dixon PM, Roulston ME, Nolan DJ: The small bowel enema: A ten year review. *Clin Radiol* 47:46–48, 1993.

152. Gourtsoyiannis NC, Bays D, Papaioannou N, et al: Benign tumors of the small intestine: Preoperative evaluation with a barium infusion technique. *Eur J Radiol* 16:115–125, 1993.

153. Maglinte DDT, Gage SN, Harmon BH, et al: Obstruction of the small intestine: Accuracy and role of the CT in diagnosis. *Radiology* 188:61–64, 1993.

154. Buts J-P, De Keyser N, Romain N, et al: Response of rat immature enterocytes to insulin: Regulation by receptor binding and endoluminal polyamine uptake. *Gastroenterology* 106:49–59, 1994.

155. Gomez de Segura IA, de Miguel E, Mata A, et al: Plasma enteroglucagon levels in different models of intestinal resection in the rat. *Dig Dis Sci* 39:65–68, 1994.

156. Sharara AI, Bouras EP, Misukonis MA, et al: Evidence for indirect dietary regulation of cholecystokinin release in rats. *Am J Physiol* 265:G107–G112, 1993.

157. Yamanishi R, Kotera J, Fushiki T, et al: A specific binding of the cholecystokinin-releasing peptide (monitor peptide) to isolated rat small-intestinal cells. *Biochem J* 291:57–63, 1993.

158. Gyr KE, Meier R: Pharmacodynamic effects of Sandostatin in the gastrointestinal tract. *Digestion* 54(Suppl 1):14–19, 1993.

159. Reubi JC, Mazzucchelli L, Laissue JA: Intestinal vessels express a high density of somatostatin receptors in human inflammatory bowel disease. *Gastroenterology* 106:951–959, 1994.

160. Miller GV, Preston SR, Woodhouse LF, et al: Somatostatin binding in human gastrointestinal tissues: Effect of cations and somatostatin analogues. *Gut* 34:1351–1356, 1993.

161. Bisset WM, Jenkins H, Booth I, et al: The effect of somatostatin on small intestinal transport in intractable diarrhoea of infancy. *J Pediatr Gastroenterol Nutr* 17:169–175, 1993.

162. Zimmer T, Ziegler K, Bader M, et al: Localisation of neuroendocrine tumours of the upper gastrointestinal tract. *Gut* 35:471–475, 1994.

163. Thwaites DT, McEwan GTA, Brown CDA, et al: Na^+independent, H^+-coupled transepithelial β-alanine absorption by human intestinal Caco-2 cell monolayers. *J Biol Chem* 268:18438–18441, 1993.

164. Gan L-S, Niederer T, Eads C, et al: Evidence for predominantly paracellular transport of thyrotropin-releasing hormone across Caco-2 cell monolayers. *Biochem Biophys Res Commun* 197:771–777, 1993.

165. Thwaites DT, Brown CDA, Hirst BH, et al: H^+-coupled dipeptide (glycylsarcosine) transport across apical and basal borders of human intestinal Caco-2 cell monolayers display distinctive characteristics. *Biochim Biophys Acta* 1151:237–245, 1993.

166. Alison MR, Sarrof CE: The role of growth factors in gastrointestinal cell proliferation. *Cell Biol Int* 18:1–10, 1994.

167. Thompson JF, Lamprey RM, Stokkers PCF: Orogastric EGF enhances c-neu and EGF receptor phosphorylation in suckling rat jejunum in vivo. *Am J Physiol* 265:G63–G72, 1993.

168. Bilchik, AJ, Hines OJ, Adrian TE, et al: Peptide YY is a physiological regulator of water and electrolyte absorption in the canine small bowel in vivo. *Gastroenterology* 105:1441–1448, 1993.

169. Butcher PD, Cevallos AM, Carnaby S, et al: Phenotypic and genotypic variation in Giardia lamblia isolates during chronic infection. *Gut* 35:51–54, 1994.

170. Kelly D, King TP, McFadyen M, et al: Effect of preclosure colostrum intake on the development of the intestinal epithelium of artificially reared piglets. *Biol Neonate* 64:235–244, 1993.

171. Pothoulakis C, Karmeli F, Kelly CP, et al: Ketotifen inhibits Clostridium difficile toxin A–induced enteritis in rat ileum. *Gastroenterology* 105:701–707, 1993.

172. Croese J, Loukas A, Opdebeeck J, et al: Occult enteric infection by Ancylostoma caninum: A previously unrecognized zoonosis. *Gastroenterology* 106:3–12, 1994.

173. Simon D, Brandt LJ: Diarrhea in patients with the acquired immunodeficiency syndrome. *Gastroenterology* 105:1238–1242, 1993.

174. May GR, Gill MJ, Church DL: Gastrointestinal symptoms in ambulatory HIV-infected patients. *Dig Dis Sci* 38:1388–1394, 1993.

175. Thea DM, St Louis ME, Atido U, et al: A prospective study of diarrhea and HIV-1 infection among 429 Zairian infants. *N Engl J Med* 329:1696–1702, 1993.

176. Lim SG, Lipman MCI, Squire S, et al: Audit of endoscopic surveillance biopsy specimens in HIV positive patients with gastrointestinal symptoms. *Gut* 34:1429–1432, 1993.

177. Fontana M, Boldorini R, Zuin G, et al: Ultrastructural changes in the duodenal mucosa of HIV-infected children. *J Pediatr Gastroenterol Nutr* 17:255–259, 1993.

178. Lim SG, Menzies IS, Lee CA, et al: Intestinal permeability and function in patients infected with human immunodeficiency virus. *Scand J Gastroenterol* 28:573–580, 1993.

179. Asmuth DV, Hammer SM, Wanke CA: Physiological effects of HIV infection on human intestinal epithelial cells: An in vitro model for HIV enteropathy. *AIDS* 8:205–211, 1994.

180. Wiest PM, Johnson JH, Flanigan TP: Microtubule inhibitors block Cryptosporidium parvum infection of a human enterocyte cell line. *Infect Immun* 61:4888–4890, 1993.

181. Argenzio RA, Lecce J, Powell DW: Prostanoids inhibit intestinal NaCl absorption in experimental porcine cryptosporidiosis. *Gastroenterology* 104:440–447, 1993.

182. Genta RM, Chappell CL, White AC Jr, et al: Duodenal morphology and intensity of infection in AIDS-related intestinal cryptosporidiosis. *Gastroenterology* 105:1769–1775, 1993.

183. Rabeneck L, Gyorkey F, Genta RM, et al: The role of microsporidia in the pathogenesis of HIV-related chronic diarrhea. *Ann Intern Med* 119:895–899, 1993.

184. Field AS, Hing MC, Millikin ST: Microsporidia in the small intestine of HIV-infected patients. *Med J Aust* 158:390–394, 1993.

185. Toloza EM, Diamond J: Ontogenetic development of nutrient transporters in rat intestine. *Am J Physiol* 263:G593–G604, 1992.

186. Matsumoto K, Takao Y, Akazawa S, et al: Developmental change of facilitative glucose transporter expression in rat embryonal and fetal intestine. *Biochem Biophys Res Commun* 193:1275–1282, 1993.

187. Freeman TC, Wood IS, Sirinathsinghji DJS, et al: The expression of the Na^+/glucose cotransporter (SGLT1) gene in lamb small intestine during postnatal development. *Biochim Biophys Acta* 1146:203–212, 1993.

188. McDonald MC, Henning SJ: Synergistic effects of thyroxine and dexamethasone on enzyme ontogeny in rat small intestine. *Pediatr Res* 32:306–311, 1992.

189. Nanthakumar NN, Henning SJ: Ontogeny of sucrase-isomaltase gene expression in rat intestine: Responsiveness to glucocorticoids. *Am J Physiol* 264:G306–G311, 1993.

190. Meetze WH, Shenoy V, Martin G, et al: Ontogeny of small intestinal glutaminase and glutamine synthetase in the rat: Response to dexamethasone. *Biol Neonate* 64:368–375, 1993.

191. Horvath K, Blochin B, Hill I, et al: The pre- and postnatal development of Na^+/K^+-ATPase in gastrointestinal organs of the rat: Effect of betamethasone treatment. *J Pediatr Gastroenterol Nutr* 16:412–418, 1993.

192. Foltzer-Jourdainne C, Garaud J-C, Nsi-Emvo E, et al: Epidermal growth factor and the maturation of intestinal sucrase in suckling rats. *Am J Physiol* 265:G459–G466, 1993.

193. Buchmiller TL, Shaw KS, Chopourian HL, et al: Effect of transamniotic administration of epidermal growth factor on fetal rabbit small intestinal nutrient transport and disaccharidase development. *J Pediatr Surg* 28:1239–1244, 1993.

194. Marti A, Fernandez-Otero MP: Prostaglandin E_2 accelerates enzymatic and morphological maturation of the small intestine in suckling rats. *Biol Neonate* 65:119–125, 1994.

195. Wild G, Daly AS, Saurid N, et al: Effect of exogenously administered polyamine on the structural maturation and enzyme ontogeny of the postnatal rat intestine. *Biol Neonate* 63:246–257, 1993.

196. Kaouass M, Deloyer P, Dandrifosse G: Intestinal development in suckling rats: Direct or indirect spermine action? *Digestion* 55:160–167, 1994.

197. Shneider BL, Michaud A, West AB, et al: The effects of bile acid feeding on the development of ileal bile acid transport. *Pediatr Res* 33:221–224, 1993.

198. Holt PR, Balint JA: Effects of aging on intestinal lipid absorption. *Am J Physiol* 264:G1–G6, 1993.

199. Atillasoy E, Holt PR: Gastrointestinal proliferation and aging. *J Gerontol* 48:B43–B49, 1993.

200. Fleming SE, Kight CE: The TCA cycle as an oxidative and synthetic pathway is suppressed with aging in jejunal epithelial cells. *Can J Physiol Pharmacol* 72:266–274, 1994.

201. Ferraris RP, Vinnakota RR: Regulation of intestinal nutrient transport is impaired in aged mice. *J Nutr* 123:502–511, 1993.

202. Reville M, Gosse F, Kachelhoffer J, et al: Ileal compensation for age dependent loss of jejunal function in rats. *J Nutr* 121:498–503, 1991.

203. Ferraris RP, Hsiao J, Hernandez R: Site density of mouse intestinal glucose transporters declines with age. *Am J Physiol* 264:G285–G293, 1993.

204. Jebbink HJA, Bravenboer B, Akkermans LMA, et al: Relationships between dyspeptic symptoms and gastrointestinal motility in patients with type 1 (insulin-dependent) diabetes mellitus. *Diabetologia* 36:948–954, 1993.

205. Debnam ES, Chowrimootoo G: Insulin induced hypoglycaemia and sugar transport across the brush border and basolateral membranes of rat jejunal enterocytes. *Eur J Clin Invest* 23:480–485, 1993.

206. Burant CF, Flink S, De Paoli AM, et al: Small intestine hexose transport in experimental diabetes increased transporter mRNA and protein expression in enterocytes. *J Clin Invest* 93:578–585, 1994.

207. Feingold KR, Wilson DE, Wood LC, et al: Diabetes increases hepatic hydroxymethyl glutaryl coenzyme A reductase protein and mRNA levels in the small intestine. *Metabolism* 43:450–454, 1994.

208. Bendayan M, Ziv E, Gingras D, et al: Biochemical and morphocytochemical evidence for the intestinal absorption of insulin in control and diabetic rats. Comparison between the effectiveness of duodenal and colon mucosa. *Diabetologia* 37:119–126, 1994.

209. MacNaughton WK, Leach KE, Prud'Homme-Lalonde L, et al: Ionizing radiation reduces neurally evoked electrolyte transport in rat ileum through a mast cell–dependent mechanism. *Gastroenterology* 106:324–335, 1994.

210. Otterson MF, Sarna SK, Leming SC, et al: Effects of fractionated doses of ionizing radiation on colonic motor activity. *Am J Physiol* 263:G518–G526, 1992.

CHAPTER 4

The Colon

Martin Anthony Eastwood, M.B., Ch.B., M.Sc., F.R.C.P.E.
Consultant Gastroenterologist, Reader in Medicine, University of Edinburgh, Gastrointestinal Unit, Western General Hospital, Edinburgh, Scotland, United Kingdom

This chapter will review a selection of papers on the colon that have been published during 1994 and will include a personal view of the trends during the year. Areas covered include basic and clinical colonic physiology, aspects of diverticular disease and irritable bowel, colon polyps, and inflammatory bowel disease.

COLONIC FUNCTION

Absorption From the Colon

The colon has an important but not obligatory function as a salvage organ, not obligatory as shown by the good health of patients who have undergone colectomy. Nevertheless, the colon has an important role in the conservation of water and ions. Ion transport in the mammalian colon is dependent on colonic mucosal chloride secretion. The movement of water across the mucosal membrane depends on electrical and osmotic gradients. Such gradients are established by the opening of ion channels regulated by secretagogues through epithelial intracellular second message pathways or surface membrane–bound receptors. Secretagogues are released from cells within the lamina propria of the intestinal mucosa.[1] The large intestine secretes bicarbonate through a Cl^--HCO_3^- exchange mechanism in the colonic apical membrane. An additional transport system facilitates $HCO_3^-/(OH^-)$ entry or H^+ exit across the basolateral cell surface.[2] Net Na^+ colonic absorption is independent of Cl^- but partially (60%) dependent on the transport of HCO_3^--CO_2. Net Cl^- flux is partially dependent (70%) on Na^+ and totally dependent on HCO_3^- -CO_2 absorption.[3]

Hormone Control of Colon Ion Fluxes

The hormonal control of ionic and water absorption continues to be elucidated. Aldosterone stimulates colonic potassium secretion quicker than Na^+ absorption. Sodium absorption is inhibited by amiloride independently of K^+ secretion. The protein induced by aldosterone is not one of the membrane proteins responsible for K^+ secretion.[4] Several transport proteins are trafficked to the cell membrane in response to secretagogues. The secretion of Cl^- is dependent on an intact micro-tubular anatomy. There are more than one Cl^- secretory systems and includes an adenosine 3′,5′-cyclic monophosphate dependent and a Ca^{2+}-dependent Cl^- secretion system.[5] Interleukin-1β (IL-1β) regulates intestinal ion and water transport through prostaglandin release. This is nerve but not H_1 receptor mediated and involves mast cell degranulation and prostaglandin release.[6]

Corticotropin-releasing hormone (CRH) is produced by a range of tissues, including human colonic mucosal enterochromaffin cells. Corticotropin-releasing hormone regulates the hypothalamic pituitary adrenal axis, coordinates the gastrointestinal response to stress, and affects the immune system and other gut functions.[7]

Fatty Acids in the Colon

Short-chain fatty acids (SCFAs) are now regarded as important contributors to the well-being of colonic mucosal cells. Short-chain fatty acids are derived from the fermentation of dietary complex carbohydrates in the colon. The rate of absorption of SCFA varies along the intestine and the colon and may be linked to Na^+ absorption or an anion exchange mechanism.[8] Propionate absorption is controlled by colonic luminal pH or by coincidental electroneutral sodium absorption (Na^+-H^+ exchange) but not by the Cl^- or HCO_3^- gradient or electrogenic Na^+ absorption. Propionate absorption in the distal colon was not significantly affected by stimulation of electrogenic Na^+ absorption or presence of epinephrine or Cl^-.[9] The gastrointestinal tract is an important site of acetate utilization in the fasted state.[10]

The colon salvages Na^+ and water not absorbed in the jejunum and ileum. This absorption capacity depends on the metabolic well-being of colonic epithelial cells, a process that requires the presence of luminal SCFAs. Sodium absorption is dependent on HCO_3^- production from n-butyrate.[8]

Unabsorbed dietary unsaturated fatty acids increase net colonic water secretion and reduces NaCl absorption in a concentration-dependent manner.[11] The effect in order of magnitude is linolenic acid (18:3) > linoleic acid (18:2) > ricinoleic acid (18:1 OH) > oleic acid (18:1) > palmitoleic acid (16:1). In normal subjects,[12] the addition of SCFAs to enteral feeds increases net colonic water and electrolyte absorption. This may hold promise in preventing the diarrhea associated with enteric feeding support systems.

Primary Bile Acid Malabsorption

Bile acids are absorbed efficiently by the terminal ileum, with a spillover into the colon of less than 5%. Aqueous solutions of bile acids instilled into the colon of more than 3mM produce diarrhea. Reduced ileal absorption of bile acids follows ileal resection, bacterial colonization, and vagotomy. Idiopathic bile acid absorption is a congenital or an acquired defect in bile acid transport. No identifiable anatomic ileal lesion suggests a functional cause.[13]

Chemical Probes

A need for chemical probes allows the identification and characterization of intestinal and colonic absorption. One such probe is mannitol. The absorption of mannitol varies along the intestine.[14] A linear relationship between permeability rate and the luminal concentration of mannitol indicates that the absorption is by passive diffusion and solvent drag. Increasing luminal fluid osmolality (0.3–0.6 osm/L) resulted in decreased net water flux with a corresponding decrease in mannitol permeability in both jejunum (65%) and colon (89%). Chenodeoxycholate (5 mM) decreases water absorption and mannitol permeability. Colonic oxalate absorption is reduced by thiazides.[15] Such inhibition involves the oxalate transport system across the colonocyte basolateral membrane.

Studies that give promise for the colonic delivery of drugs have become of interest. Studies of colonic absorption of substances of therapeutic value are now being reported.[16] The delivery of drugs to the colon could use an azoaromatic hydrogel that protects peptide macromolecules (e.g., insulin) from digestive enzymes.[16] The mechanisms of colonic mucosal absorption are poorly understood and complicated. The interpretation of results from experiments under conditions wherein a sterile colon is perfused to the situation of a colon full of bacteria as in the normal colon is not easy or reasonable. Lysine and methionine are not absorbed in nutritionally significant amounts from the proximal colon of the milk-fed piglet.[17] Biologically active insulin and recombinant human insulin growth factor is absorbed by the intestinal mucosa in both the duodenum and colon.[18, 19] This insulin can cause a significant prolonged decrease in plasma glucose levels in rats and has promise for glucose homeostasis.

Mucus

The colonic mucosa is covered by a mucous gel layer (secretory mucins) that protects the underlying epithelium. These mucins are glycoproteins rich in oligosaccharides and responsible for the physical properties of the mucus. The mucins consist of repeated amino sequences in the polypeptide backbone. Serine and threonine are O-linked to attached sialic acid and sulfate groups. These regions are flanked by short nonrepetitive amino acid sequences that are less glycosylated and susceptible to proteolytic degradation. The major human colonic mucin is Muc2 synthesized as a N-glycosylated precursor protein (600 kD), subsequently processed into a mucin (molecular weight 550 kD) and secreted into the colonic lumen.[20]

IRRITABLE BOWEL SYNDROME

The cause of irritable bowel syndrome is unknown and now includes visceral perception and alterations in colonic motility and tone. The latter are presumably the mechanism of the symptoms rather than giving insights into cause. Theories abound. In such an uncertain situation, it is incumbent on clinicians to be kind and not to impose theories and treatments on these individuals who are fraught with distress. Support and reassurance are important.[21] The continued question is: Why are these individuals miserable? Abuse, whether physical, emotional, or sexual in childhood, can disfigure individuals for the remainder of their lives.[22] A postal survey in which 74% of 919 people responsed reported childhood abuse—physical, sexual, and verbal—in 26% of responders. Symptoms of irritable bowel syndrome were reported by 14% of responders, dyspepsia by 23%, and heartburn by 12%. Of responders with irritable bowel syndrome, a history of sexual or verbal abuse was recorded by 50%. Of responders with dyspeptic symptoms or heartburn, sexual abuse was reported by 42% and verbal abuse by 39%. Patients with functional symptoms are more likely to clinically manifest their symptoms than calm, unpressured, and happy irritable bowel syndrome patients.

Few clinicians have the time or expertise to treat patients in a holistic way. A simplistic medical approach involves explanation of causes of upset and of extended roles in the patient's life, a high-fiber cereal breakfast, and fruit twice daily. Another concept of relevence is the sleep pattern of irritable bowel syndrome sufferers. Sleep is the major determinant of diurnal variation of colonic motility.[23] The characteristic high–amplitude propagating contractions of the colon are less frequent at night during sleep and most prevalent during rapid eye movement and on early morning waking. Low-dose amitriptyline (5–40 mg/day) taken at bedtime to reduce sedative effects is very helpful. Amitriptyline has a range of actions on receptors that extend from the potent effects on norepinephrine reuptake at nerve endings, inhibition of serotonin, muscarinic cholinergic receptor blockade in the central nervous system (CNS), to relatively potent antagonism of H_1 receptors and weak blockade of dopamine. It is not clear whether one or combination or all of these effects are responsible for the effectiveness.

COLONIC DIVERTICULOSIS

Little has been added to our understanding of diverticulosis during 1994. Treatment of bleeding is still a problem; bleeding can be torrential in patients with known or suspected diverticulosis. Some guidance is given in a study of patients (N = 78) with chronic bleeding colonic diverticula whose bleeding stopped spontaneously or who rebled and who were analyzed after 4.5 years.[24] Bleeding stopped spontaneously in 80 episodes in patients who required no more than three transfusions. Of patients requiring four or more transfusions in 1 day, 60% required emergency operations. The subsequent rebleeding rate was almost 40% after discharge in patients who were managed nonoperatively; 80% of these again stopped bleeding spontaneously. Colectomy is not indicated when a source of bleeding cannot be identified. Patients with acute colonic diverticulitis admitted over a 5-year period were followed over a 2-year period for recurrence.[25] One third of patients, most of whom were older than 50, required surgery during their first hospitalizations. These authors suggest computed tomography (CT) and water-soluble barium enema are vital examinations but indicate that they do not specifically predict the need for surgery. In practice it is not easy to locate the actual bleeding diverticulum. Clinical judgment allied to endosocopic and radiographic studies are used to determine the site of bleeding point.

COLONIC DYSFUNCTION

Incontinence

Incontinence is a degrading symptom in the disabled and elderly. Incontinence is an exclusion symptom for some levels of care. Debate also continues as to the best way to assess the causes of incontinence before a treatment is recommended. The debate rages between the informed clinical judgment and pathophysiologic measurements. An absolute answer is far from clear.

Identification
Incontinence in an elderly person has profound implications for continued independence. When elderly persons are admitted, their bowel and urinary incontinence status is closely related to their performance on a dementia rating scale. Most estimates of the prevalence and incidence of incontinence rely on self-reporting. The value of self-report has been examined in a study with repeat telephone calls to elderly individuals living in the community.[26] Although the overall estimate of incontinence remained the same, the variability of individual responses was in the range for estimates of incidence and remission rates of incontinence.

Value of Anorectal Tests
Fecal incontinence is a disabling condition[27] caused by the following:

1. Sphincter damage through childbirth, anorectal surgery, trauma, fistulas, and abscesses.

2. Pudendal neuropathy caused by stretching by long-standing constipation or prolonged labor.
3. Diminished rectal compliance in proctitis, low anterior resection, or small pouches.
4. Fecal impaction causing paradoxical diarrhea.
5. Neurologic disease involving the pelvic floor and the CNS.
6. Diarrhea.

Clinical Histories

Patients with idiopathic chronic fecal incontinence have been studied to compare the relative value of history, examination, and anorectal physiology.[28] The conclusion was that a good history and digital examination can predict the manometric findings of specialist anorectal physiology studies.

Another view is that a medical history and physical examination will generally provide a reasonable diagnosis (Table 1).[27] A study based on an audit of the use of colorectal physiologic tests in patients with functional disorders of defecation came to different conclusions.[29] Diagnoses were made after history and physical examination alone in 8% with constipation, 11% with incontinence, and 23% with intractable rectal pain. After physiologic tests (colonic transit study and manometry cinedefecography, electromyography of the anal sphincter, and terminal motor latency of the pudendal nerves, the number of diagnoses improved to 75% for constipation, 66% for incontinence, and 42% for intractable rectal pain. The value of colorectal physiologic tests overall was seen to be greatest in patients with constipation or incontinence and of little value in chronic intractable rectal pain.

Testing

A variety of anorectal physiologic measurements are available (Table 2), but normal values differ, and there are no established or reproducible normal ranges. The development of the anal canal in children is age dependent.[43] Such an appreciation of normal anal canal development is a prerequisite for detecting pathologic condi-

TABLE 1.

Anorectal Function Tests

Anal manometry for low sphincter pressures, rectal compliance, small rectal volume, anal mucosal sensitivity measurements, and pudendal nerve motor latency.

Anal endosonography as a basis for sphincter repair.

Defecography as a basis for rectopexy in incontinent patients.

TABLE 2.

Colonic Function Tests

Manometric evaluation[30]
Ambulatory anorectal manometry[31]
Defecography measurements[32]
Simplified solid sphere test[33]
Endosonographic assessment of spincter[34]
Anal endosonography[35, 36]
Transanal ultrasound, manometry and pudendal
 nerve terminal motor latency[37]
Anal pressure vectography[38]
Cinefecography and position[39]
Neuropeptides in the internal anal sphincter[40]
Cough pressure and squeeze pressure[41]
Computed anal rectal manometry system[42]

---

tions of the anorectal region in children. In general, abnormal measurements do not correlate with disease entities or explain symptoms. The results are often of limited value for diagnosis and management. Clinical outcome after intervention does not correlate with alterations in the measurements obtained. The consensus view is that anorectal physiology may help in the care of constipation, anismus, Hirschsprung's disease, fecal incontinence, and tenesmus. Management based on biofeedback modification of physiologic responses may be helpful in anismus and solitary rectal ulcer syndrome.[44]

Bowel Dysfunction in Specific Diseases

A number of chronic debilitating diseases that destroy the individual's well-being lead to incontinence of feces or to constipation. Some understanding of the etiologies is developing.

Obstetric-Related Damage

Anal incontinence of gas or feces affects up to 11% of adults and occurs frequently in 2%.[45] The most common cause of anal incontinence is unrecognized damage to the anal sphincter during childbirth. Thirteen percent of women after their first vaginal delivery develop incontinence or urgency, and 30% have structural changes shown by anal endosonography, forceps being the most common cause of damage with a third-degree tear. Neurogenic fecal and urine incontinence can result from a stretch-induced injury to the pelvic nerves during difficult childbirth or chronic straining at stool. Such damage has been claimed to be less frequent in societies who defecate in the squatting position. The suggestion is that squatting minimizes pelvic floor descent. However, a study of squatting and defecation showed no reduction in pelvic floor descent during defecation.[46]

Spina Bifida

Patients with spina bifida have great problems with defecation and passing urine. Patients with spina bifida (N = 144) were asked about bladder and bowel control.[47] Of 108 replies, 28 had a urinary diversion; 71 were reliably dry, emptying their bladders by a variety of techniques. Most required assistance in defecation (e.g., manual evacuation, laxatives, suppositories, or enemas). Only 25 of 104 patients responding to these questions were reliably clean and dry.

Fecal incontinence is a major social problem in 90% of spina bifida patients.[48] Bowel continence involving one or fewer incontinent episodes per month increased from 13% to 60% after toileting intervention strategy. This program emphasized patient and family education and a regular consistently timed reflex triggered bowel evacuation. It was especially effective if started before the age of 7 years.

Multiple Sclerosis

Large bowel transit studies showed abnormally slow transit in the distal bowel in 80% of multiple sclerosis patients.[49] In such patients there is marked impairment of external anal sphincter function with moderate changes in pelvic floor musculature.

Diabetes Mellitus

Somatic neuropathy[50] is an important cause of fecal incontinence in diabetic patients. This is combined with sensation threshold impairment as a result of autonomic nerve involvement.

Benefits of Treatment

Continent services for the handicapped and elderly in the community require an active approach using protocols, management systems, and evaluation measures that cross community care team boundaries.[51] Continence in individuals with severe learning disabilities is important. A behavioral program, albeit prolonged for people with severe learning disabilities,[52] resulted in near normal bowel function. Another treatment strategy for obstructive defecation is relaxation training by domiciliary self-regulation biofeedback.[53] Patients with neurogenic fecal incontinence may benefit from an intensive 12-week electric stimulation course.[54]

Patients with anal incontinence attributable to trauma are usually treated by sphincter reconstruction. Failure because of incomplete reconstruction can be detected by anal endosonography.[34] The results do not always reflect the clinical state. In a retrospective series (5–8 years),[55] patients who had undergone post–anal repair for neurogenic fecal incontinence were assessed clinically and by anorectal physiology. Twenty eight had long-term improvement, but six had no change. Two of the patients were housebound because of incontinence, and one required a stoma.

Anal endosonography showed a clinically undetected sphincter defect in 19 of 30 patients examined but did not relate to clinical outcome.

Short-term results of post–anal repair for idiopathic fecal incontinence are encouraging.[56] Longer-term studies are important. Six months after surgery 83% of patients had benefited from post–anal repair. Only 53% maintained this improvement at 2 years. Patients with better squeezing pressures preoperatively did well, but other tests had little long-term predictive value. Overall the outcome for 178 of 326 patients who had had surgery for Hirschsprung's disease from 1957 to 1990[30] was good. Manometric assessment of anorectal function in 16 with persisting obstructive symptoms was not useful. The values were not significantly different from patients with normal bowel evacuation as an outcome.

ANAL FISSURE

Anal fissure is an unpleasant problem. The cause is not understood, which restricts rational treatment. In patients with an anal fissure, anodermal blood flow at the posterior midline is reduced compared with the other segments of the anal canal.[57] Increased anal pressure reduces such anodermal blood flow, suggesting that anal fissures are ischemic ulcers. On the other hand, internal anal sphincter relaxation occurs on fewer occasions in patients with chronic anal fissures that have failed to heal when compared with patients with hemorrhoids and with normal controls.[58] Internal sphincter hypertonia may be important in the pathogenesis of chronic anal fissure. Botulinum toxin has been used successfully in the treatment of achalasia[59] and now in chronic anal fissure.[60] Type A botulinum toxin injected into the muscles of the internal anal sphincter resulted in long-term improvement in 6 of 10 patients.

PRURITUS ANI

Patients with idiopathic pruritus ani have an abnormal rectoanal inhibitory reflex and a lower threshold for internal sphincter relaxation. Pruritus ani may result from occult fecal leakage because of abnormal and transient internal sphincter relaxation.[61]

CYSTIC FIBROSIS AND COMPLICATIONS OF TREATMENT

The prognosis for children with cystic fibrosis has gradually improved. This improvement is in part due to pancreatic replacement therapy. However, five children aged 2 to 13 years with cystic fibrosis required surgery for intestinal obstruction with ascending colon strictures.[62] All had been placed on high-strength pancreatic enzyme therapy 12 to 15 months earlier. High-strength enzyme replacement may alter gastrointestinal mucus, resulting in the formation of a mucoid mass that causes pressure-induced ischemic necrosis in the ascending colon.

COLONIC CANCER

Colonic Polyps

Appropriately, current thoughts for the prevention of colonic cancer emphasize risk factors, diet, and early detection of polyps.

Etiology
Risk factors for colonic neoplasms have been evaluated in 32,085 men and 87,033 women questioned in 1986 and every 2 years thereafter.[63] The age-adjusted risk of colorectal cancer is shown in Table 3 and increases with age. This study may have underestimated risk because patients with previous colonoscopy, sigmoidoscopy, polyps, or cancer were excluded. In another study crude dietary fiber, vitamin E

TABLE 3.
Relative Risk of Adenoma or Cancer

	Risk	
	Adenoma	Cancer
Family[63]		
No family history		1.00
One first-degree family member		
<45 yr		5.37
>45 yr		1.72
Two or more first-degree family members		2.75
Diet (lowest to highest quintile)		
Meat[65]		1.71
Beef, pork, lamb		3.57
Body mass, aspirin, or activity		1.00
Fiber, fruit		1.00
Aspirin		
2 weekly compared with control[66]		0.38
Screening		
First sigmoidoscopy[81]	80%	0
Subsequent colonoscopy	24%	0
Second endoscopy 3.4 yr after sigmoidoscopy	0%–6%	
Polypectomy		
After mean 5.9-yr reduction compared with control[84]	76%–80%	

and A intake, but not total energy intake or body mass reduced the risk of cancer or adenoma.[64] There is much discussion as to whether animal fat or red meat increases the risk of colon cancer and whether high intake of vegetables or fiber is protective.[65] This has been the basis of a study in 47,949 U.S. male health professionals (see Table 3). The putative risk of colonic cancer from eating red meat was not altered by other dietary factors, physical activity, body mass, alcohol intake, cigarette smoking, or aspirin use. Other sources of animal fat, fiber, or vegetable intake were only slightly and inversely related to a risk of colon cancer. Another review of case control and cohort studies (N = 15) examined egg consumption as a risk factor for cancer of the colon and rectum.[66] The results suggest an enhanced risk with increased egg intake.

Biology of Colonic Cancer

The adenoma-carcinoma sequence of colorectal cancer formation evolves through a series of steps.[67] What is not yet clear is if the changes described by molecular biology are a description and not an indication of the underlying cause, somewhat parallel to the information afforded by histology. Some colorectal cancers do not progress through a polyp phase. K-*ras* activation is infrequent in the flat-type colorectal tumors, which are possibly a subpopulation of colorectal tumors, which undergo a different set of genetic changes.

Familial Polyposis Coli

The first example of familial polyposis coli has been reported in Africa, namely, Peutz-Jeghers syndrome in Ethiopia.[68] Familial adenomatous polyposis is an autosomal dominant condition, with more than 90% penetrance characterized by multiple polyps in the colon.[69] The risk of colorectal cancer in untreated familial polyposis coli is 100%; therefore, screening is important in at-risk individuals. Most cases of familial polyposis coli result from mutations of the adenomatous polyposis coli gene chromosome 5q21.

Indirect genotyping of familial polyposis coli with a closely linked and highly polymorphic microsatellite marker is a rapid efficient and highly reliable method for presymptomatic diagnosis of familial polyposis coli.[70] The gene responsible for familial adenomatous polyposis coli has been identified and characterized.[71] Linkage studies using two polymorphic systems close to or at the adenomatous polyposis coli locus have been used. Linkage studies by RsaI site polymorphism, cytosine-adenine repeat length polymorphism, and polymerase chain reaction–based sequencing allow accurate and efficient tools for presymptomatic diagnosis of familial polyposis coli in families.

Early Diagnosis

The early diagnosis of polyps is a yet-to-be-resolved problem. Simple and acceptable investigations are required for those at risk by family history or age. Yet the unexpected (i.e., random) appearance of cancer must also be anticipated. Not everyone is prepared to have invasive colonic investigations. Screening involves analysis of fecal constituents such as blood, as well as direct visualization by radiographic and endoscopic methods. A simple acceptable investigation for risk or polyps has yet to be introduced.

Fecal Constituents

A Canadian Task Force has reviewed trials from 1966 to 1993 using fecal occult blood testing, sigmoidoscopy, and colonoscopy for colorectal cancer.[72] The result was a small but significant decrease in the death rate from colorectal cancer. They conclude that there is insufficient evidence for the inclusion or exclusion of fecal occult blood analyses, sigmoidoscopy, or colonoscopy in colonic cancer prevention. The American Cancer Society and National Cancer Institute disagree with these conclusions and recommend screening.

Colorectal polyps are an important cause of rectal bleeding in children.[74] A report of polyps (usually located on the left side of the colon and treated in young children older than 10 years) diagnosed 29 solitary polyps from 730 colonoscopies; 24 juvenile polyps, 2 inflammatory polyps, 2 Peutz-Jeghers syndrome polyps, and 1 adenomatous polyp.

An exciting diagnostic prospect is the use of the K-*ras* gene mutation found in more than 50% of patients with colon tumors.[73] A sensitive polymerase chain reaction–based assay detected one mutant K-*ras* allele in 10,000 normal alleles. K-*ras* gene mutation has been identified in colonic washings from patients at risk of colorectal cancer but not in patients with inflammatory bowel disorders or normal colonoscopic examinations.

Invasive Investigations

In an audit of diagnostic failures of colon cancer by either barium enema or colonoscopy,[76] barium enema errors were caused by poor preparation or errors in interpretation. Colonoscopic failures resulted from incomplete examinations or incorrect interpretation of identified lesions. Colonic diverticulosis makes the diagnosis of colonic cancer and adenoma difficult. Neither double-contrast barium enema nor sigmoidoscopy alone is sufficient to detect all lesions in the sigmoid colon in patients with sigmoid diverticulosis.[77]

Preparation for colon examinations could be easier and more pleasant than at present. Three oral solutions (a standard 4-L polyethylene glycol solution, a new sulfate-free 4-L polyethylene glycol solution, or a 90-mL oral sodium phosphate preparation) have been compared to determine patient compliance or cleansing ability.[78] The small-volume oral sodium phosphate preparation was preferred by patients and was effective in colonic cleansing.

Colonoscopy

Adequate sedation is important for colonoscopy. In a controlled trial, treated patients received flumazenil to allow wakefulness during withdrawal of the scope from the cecum.[79] Eighty percent of patients who were not awakened with flumazenil said they would have preferred to view the withdrawal phase. A further 40 consecutive patients underwent colonoscopy without sedation unless they encountered pain. Most patients preferred no sedation for future colonoscopy. The median time to complete the colonoscopy was 5 to 7 minutes! Another group of patients studied did not share this enthusiasm.[80] Patients rated colonoscopy (5.0) as more painful than barium enema (3.4) on a scale of 1 to 10.

Does the finding of adenoma on flexible sigmoidoscopy predict the finding of advanced adenomas on a subsequent colonoscopy?[81] This has been studied by recording the finding at flexible sigmoidoscopy, followed by a full colonoscopy. On initial sigmoidoscopy in asymptomatic and symptomatic patients, a single polyp less than 1 cm was found in 80%. A subsequent colonoscopy found 24% new adenomas but no cancer. An advanced lesion found during sigmoidoscopy was an accurate predictor of an advanced lesion found during colonoscopy (10% prevalence). Patients with tubular adenomas less than 1 cm found during sigmoidoscopy had less than a 1% occurrence of an advanced synchronous lesion. The accuracy of polyp size estimates in clinical studies was not known until recently.[75] Skilled endoscopists and medical students estimated the size of ball bearings in a latex colon model using a video colonoscope with and without forceps. The performance of experienced gastroenterologists, fellows in training, and untrained residents did not differ.

How long after an initial negative flexible sigmoidoscopy should the procedure be repeated?[82] After a mean of 3.4 years, a second examination demonstrated adenomas (<1 cm, without severe dysplasia or cancer) in 6% of patients (15 of 259 patients). Full colonoscopy showed proximal adenomas (<1 cm without cancer or dysplasia) in five patients. The authors suggest a 5-year interval after initial negative screening examination. Patients who have had an adenoma are likely to have another.[84] Patients whose adenomas have been removed have been found to have a 15% to 60% risk for a new metachronous or recurrent adenoma within 3 to 4 years. The U.S. National Polyp Study showed a recurrence rate of 32% at 3 years. The adenoma incident rate can be determined only by repeated examinations of the colon in a population without a history of colorectal neoplasia. The incidence of left-sided adenomas is 6% after 3 years.[82] A study of colonoscopy showed that for patients who had negative results on colonoscopy and no prior colorectal neoplasia, the cumulative incidence rate of adenomas at 36 months was 16%.[85]

Polyp Limitation Practices

A diet rich in fruit and vegetables may protect against colonic polyps. This possibility has been extended to vitamins with antioxidant properties in a clinical trial that lasted 3.5 years using either placebo, β-carotene (25 mg daily), vitamin C (1 g daily plus 400 mg of vitamin E daily) or all three. All participants had had a colorectal adenoma removed previously by colonoscopy, a procedure repeated at 1 and 4 years.[83] The antioxidant supplements gave no protection against adenoma. This underlies the logical risk of applying epidemiology data such as the protective effect of fruit and vegetables in the prevention of cancer to one property, namely, antioxidant activity. Why not enjoy fruits and vegetables as the original study suggests?

Evidence is accumulating that polyp removal reduces colon cancer risk. After colonoscopy removal of adenomas, patients were followed by colonoscopy for a mean of 5.9 years and compared with three reference groups.[84] Two reference groups were taken from the precolonoscopic era when polyps were not removed, and the third group represented patients at average risk in the population. Polyp removal reduced the incidence of colon cancer by 90%, 88%, and 76%, respectively, when compared with these reference groups.

In the Harvard Medical School Study, 51,529 male professionals were enrolled in 1986 to study risks in cardiovascular disease and cancer.[86] Patients who took aspirin at least twice per week over 6 years had a decreased risk (1.0–0.38) of developing a malignancy (see Table 2). This study excluded men with a prestudy diagnosis of adenomatous polyp. They are therefore a lower-risk group; nevertheless, the reduction is comparable with the National Polyp Study.

Sulindac (100 mg twice daily) and colectomy with ileorectal anastomosis on rectal mucosa proliferation and polyp occurrence appear to reduce the number but not size of rectal polyps in patients with familial adenomatous polyposis.[87]

The intake of aspirin is an exciting development in the prevention of polyps. This raises the interesting question of how aspirin and sulindac act. An immediate and reasonable possibility is antiprostaglandin activity. Other more subtle effects need to be considered. It is difficult to know whether having a regular colonoscopy, increasing the fiber or fruit and vegetable content of the diet, or taking aspirin twice per week is the most effective preventive strategy.

INFLAMMATORY BOWEL DISEASE

Etiology

The etiology of the various forms of inflammatory bowel disease probably includes a familial predisposition. Further evidence for such a predisposition comes in a study of perinuclear antineutrophil cytoplasmic antibodies (pANCAs) in patients with ulcerative colitis, Crohn's disease, or sclerosing cholangitis and first-degree relatives.[88] Seventy percent of patients with ulcerative colitis and 30% of their relatives were pANCA positive. Eighty-two percent of patients with sclerosing cholangitis and 25% of their relatives were pANCA positive. Only 27% of patients with Crohn's disease, 6% of their relatives, and none of the controls were pANCA positive. The pANCA titer did not correlate with disease activity because these titers remained increased after colectomy or liver transplantation.

Treatment

Patients with Crohn's disease frequently require surgery for complications, strictures, fistulas, and abscesses. Of patients with ileal involvement with Crohn's disease, 86% require surgery by 10 years after the first symptoms without lasting relief. Modest protection from further surgery is afforded by 3 g of mesalamine daily initiated within 1 month of surgery.[89]

A new corticosteroid, budesonide, has been unfavorably compared with prednisolone.[90] Prednisolone resulted in a greater decrease in mean Crohn's disease activity index but more corticosteroid side effects and a greater decrease in plasma cortisol levels. In a similar trial, patients received either placebo or oral doses of 15, 9, or 3 mg of budesonide for 8 weeks. Clinical remission (Crohn's disease activity index <150) occurred in 43% of patients receiving 15 mg of budesonide, 51% receiving 9 mg, 33% receiving 3 mg, and 20% using a placebo. An improvement in quality of life paralleled the remission rates. At an optimal oral dose of 9 mg daily, budesonide is effective and well tolerated but gives a remission rate of only 51%.[91] Metronidazole continues to play a tantalizing role in the treatment of Crohn's disease. Topical application of small doses of metronidazole (40–160 mg) into the reservoir is safe and effective in the treatment of pouchitis even when it is given on a continuous low-term basis.[92]

A new development is the use of intravenous cyclosporine in patients with severe ulcerative colitis refractory to intravenous corticosteroids. Eighty-two percent of patients treated with cyclosporine responded in 7 days compared with none of the placebo patients. In an uncontrolled trial, patients who had failed standard medical therapy and had active fistulas[93] were given 4 mg of intravenous cyclosporine/kg daily by continuous infusion; 88% improved, and there was complete fistula closure in 50% of patients. Oral cyclosporine was less successful; 36% of patients had relapses. In a further study, 60% of patients had relapses taking oral cyclosporine. The median time to deterioration was 338 days in the cyclosporine group and 492 days in the placebo group.[94]

5-Aminosalicylic acid (5-ASA) is always under review. A multicenter comparative trial examined the preferable form of 5-ASA enema.[96] For patients with either mild or moderate ulcerative colitis, 5-ASA foam is better tolerated and produces remission more quickly than 5-ASA in enema form. The disadvantage of salazopyrine is the released sulfapyridine. A novel alternative is sulfanilic acid linked to 5-ASA through an azolinkage.[97] Clinical trials are awaited.

Smokers have a reduced risk of developing ulcerative colitis compared with non-smokers. Patients with active ulcerative colitis were randomly assigned to a transdermal nicotine patch.[98] Remission was achieved in 48.5% compared with 24% using a placebo. Side effects occurred in 23 of 35 patients (66%) using a nicotine patch.

The etiology of Crohn's disease includes a tuberculosis-type organism. A double-blind randomized placebo-controlled trial of multidrug antimycobacterial therapy made up of ethambutol, dapsone, and clofazime was used in patients with refractory steroid-dependent Crohn's disease with little success.[99]

Outcome

There is an emotional and physical toll on patients with inflammatory bowel disease. Dyspareunia was more common among female patients with ulcerative colitis than controls. Fertility rates were similar between patients and controls. No difference in frequency of sexual intercourse was noted between patients and controls, although patients cited fear of incontinence and abdominal pain as reasons why their sexual activity might be impaired.[100]

The development of colonic cancer is a constant worry in the care of patients with inflammatory bowel disease. Patients with chronic ulcerative colitis of more than 10 years' duration underwent colonoscopy with biopsy every other year and in the intervening year rigid sigmoidoscopy with biopsy.[101] Colonic cancer was detected in 6% of all patients. The diagnostic yield was 1.6% for colonoscopy (66 colonoscopies for each cancer or significant dysplasia) and 0.7% for sigmoidoscopy. High-grade dysplasia predicted synchronous cancer in 67% of patients. The 5-year predictive value of low-grade dysplasia for subsequent high-grade dysplasia was 54%. Surveillance colonoscopy and sigmoidoscopy detected some cancers, but more than one third of cancers were not detected by screening. This screening scheme detected colonic cancer at an estimated cost of $100,000 per cancer.

The genetic changes associated with colonic malignancy may provide an answer for clinical practice. Mutations of adenomatous polyposis coli (APC) and K-*ras* genes are common in colitis-associated neoplasia[102] and can occur early in the neoplastic progression. Therefore, surveillance profiles of both morphologic features and molecular genetic changes are important.

Low bone mineral density (i.e., osteopenia) has been reported in 30% to 59% of patients with inflammatory bowel disease.[103, 104] Factors increasing low bone mineral density include corticosteroid therapy, reduced activity, inflammatory cytokines, small bowel disease or resection, sclerosing cholangitis, and vitamin D deficiency. Bone formation or bone resorption can be measured in various ways by serum concentrations of calcium, phosphate, parathyroid hormone, 25-hydroxyvitamin D_3, 1,25-dihydroxyvitamin D_3, and osteocalcin, a protein synthesized by the osteoblasts stimulated by 1,25-dihydroxyvitamin D_3. Bone turnover in inflammatory bowel disease is characterized by reduced bone formation in the presence of normal concentration of calcium-regulating hormones but high circulating concentrations of inflammatory factors that stimulate bone resorption. This may account for excessive bone loss in osteoporosis and other bone disease.

Proctocolectomy with ileal pouch anal anastomosis is regarded by some clinicians as a treatment of choice for patients with chronic ulcerative colitis.[105] The fear is of incontinence. This problem has been studied in individuals who had had a proctocolectomy 10 years earlier. Stool frequency 7 ± 3 times daily remained unchanged; of 50% of subjects with initially excellent daytime continence, 39% remained continent, 10% developed minor incontinence, and 1% developed poor control. Impairment of sphincter function in patients who undergo an ileoanal reservoir is usually most severe immediately after ileostomy closure.[106] Sphincter-strengthening exercises before ileostomy closure do not minimize the transient impairment and functional results.

Why Crohn's disease recurs primarily at the anastomotic site is not known.[107] The surgeon's concern is whether the resection is complete and whether apparently normal tissue is affected. A scanning electron microscope of Crohn's disease tissue at the resection margin showed mucosal architectural alterations, epithelial bridge formation, and goblet cell hyperplasia or hypertrophy. The epithelial bridges link either one territory to another or the opposite walls of a crypt. The epithelial bridge formation found close to the aphthoid ulcers may represent a morphologic phenomenon specific to Crohn's colitis. These early lesions may be initial morphologic changes and may lead to subsequent clinical Crohn's disease.

CONCLUSION

In many respects this has been a year of consolidation in colonic physiology and pathophysiologic studies. The need for an understanding of causes and, more important, treatment of incontinence in the increasing numbers of elderly and incapacitated continues. Tests are available, but a consensus of tests with defined norms is needed; no doubt one will soon be available. The etiology of the irritable syndrome is a major deficiency in our knowledge. The continued confusion between the scoring and measurement of signs and not the identification of cause retards progress. Exciting developments are occurring in the prevention and control of colonic polyps, with familial studies, diet, aspirin, and endoscopic investigations being front runners. The overall impression is that the colon is ceasing to be the unknown in gastroenterology and is the center of interesting findings.

REFERENCES

1. Baird AW: Regulation of chloride secretion in mammalian colon. *Ir J Med Sci* 163:277–281, 1994.
2. Feldman GM: HCO_3^- Secretion by rat distal colon: Effects of inhibitors and extracellular Na^+. *Gastroenterology* 107:329–338, 1994.

3. Hyun CS, Ahn J, Minhas BS, et al: Ion transport in rabbit proximal colon: Effects of sodium, amiloride, cAMP, and epinephrine. *Am J Physiol* 266:G1071–G1082, 1994.

4. Halm DR, Halm ST: Aldosterone stimulates K secretion prior to onset of Na absorption in guinea pig distal colon. *Am J Physiol* 266:C552–C558, 1994.

5. Fuller CM, Bridges RJ, Benos DJ: Forskolin—but not ionomycin—evoked Cl⁻ secretion in colonic epithelia depends on intact microtubules. *Am J Physiol* 266:C661–C668, 1994.

6. Theodorou V, Eutamene H, Fioramonti J, et al: Interleukin 1 induces a neurally mediated colonic secretion in rats: Involvement of mast cells and prostaglandins. *Gastroenterology* 106:1493–1500, 1994.

7. Kawahito Y, Sano H, Kawata M, et al: Local secretion of corticotropin-releasing hormone by enterochromaffin cells in human colon. *Gastroenterology* 106:859–865, 1994.

8. Roediger WE: Famine, fiber, fatty acids, and failed colonic absorption: Does fiber fermentation ameliorate diarrhea? *J Parenter Nutr* 18:4–8, 1994.

9. Sellin JH, DeSoignie R, Burlingame S: Segmental differences in short-chain fatty acid transport in rabbit colon: Effect of pH and Na. *J Membr Biol* 136:147–158, 1993.

10. Freeman K, Foy T, Feste AS, et al: Colonic acetate in the circulating acetate pool of the infant pig. *Paediatr Res* 34:318, 1993.

11. Ramakrishna BS, Mathan M, Mathan VI: Alteration of colonic absorption by long-chain unsaturated fatty acids: Influence of hydroxylation and degree of unsaturation. *Scand J Gastroenterol* 29:54–58, 1994.

12. Bowling TE, Raimundo AH, Grimble GK, et al: Reversal by short-chain fatty acids of colonic fluid secretion induced by enteral feeding. *Lancet* 342:1266–1268, 1993.

13. Sciarretta G, Furno A, Morrone B, et al: Absence of histopathological changes of ileum and colon in functional chronic diarrhea associated with bile acid malabsorption, assessed by SeHCAT test: A prospective study. *Am J Gastroenterol* 89:1058–1061, 1994.

14. Krugliak P, Hollander D, Schlaepfer CC, et al: Mechanism and sites of mannitol permeability of small and large intestine in the rat. *Dig Dis Sci* 39:796–801, 1994.

15. Hatch M, Vaziri ND: Do thiazides reduce intestinal oxalate absorption? A study in vitro using rabbit colon. *Clin Sci* 86:353–357, 1994.

16. Cheng CL, Gehrke SH, Ritschel WA: Development of an azopolymer based colonic release capsule for delivering proteins/macromolecules. *Exp Clin Pharmacol* 16:271–278, 1994.

17. Darragh AJ, Cranwell PD, Moughan PJ: Absorption of lysine and methionine from the proximal colon of the piglet. *Br J Nutr* 71:739–752, 1994.

18. Bendayan M, Ziv E, Gingras D, et al: Biochemical and morpho-cytochemical evidence for the intestinal absorption of insulin in control and diabetic rats: Comparison between the effectiveness of duodenal and colon mucosa. *Diabetologia* 37:119–126, 1994.

19. Quadros E, Landzert NM, LeRoy S, et al: Colonic absorption of insulin-like growth factor I in vitro. *Pharmacol Res* 11:226–230, 1994.

20. Tytgat KM, Buller HA, Opdam FJ, et al: Biosynthesis of human colonic mucin: Muc2 is the prominent secretory mucin. *Gastroenterology* 107:1352–1363, 1994.

21. Eldridge GD, Walker JR, Holborn SW: Cognitive-behavioral treatment for panic disorder with gastrointestinal symptoms: A case study. *J Behav Ther Exp Psychiatry* 24:367–371, 1993.

22. Talley NJ, Fett SL, Zinsmeister AR, et al: Gastrointestinal tract symptoms and self-reported abuse: A population-based study. *Gastroenterology* 107:1040–1049, 1994.

23. Furukawa Y, Cook IJ, Panagopoulos V, et al: Relationship between sleep patterns and human colonic motor patterns. *Gastroenterology* 107:1372–1381, 1994.

24. McGuire HH Jr: Bleeding colonic diverticula: A reappraisal of natural history and management. *Ann Surg* 220:653–656, 1994.

25. Ambrosetti P, Robert JH, Witzig JA, et al: Acute left colonic diverticulitis: A prospective analysis of 226 consecutive cases. *Surgery* 115:546–550, 1994.

26. Seidel GK, Millis SR, Lichtenberg PA, et al: Predicting bowel and bladder continence from cognitive status in geriatric rehabilitation patients. *Arch Phys Med Rehabil* 75:590–593, 1994.

27. Felt-Bersma RJ, Cuesta MA: Faecal incontinence 1994: Which test and which treatment? *Neth J Med* 44:182–188, 1994.

28. Hill J, Corson RJ, Brandon H, et al: History and examination in the assessment of patients with idiopathic fecal incontinence. *Dis Colon Rectum* 37:473–477, 1994.

29. Wexner SD, Jorge JM: Colorectal physiological tests: Use or abuse of technology? *Eur J Surg* 160:167–174, 1994.

30. Moore SW, Millar AJ, Cywes S: Long-term clinical manometric, and histological evaluation of obstructive symptoms in the postoperative Hirschsprung's patient. *J Paediatr Surg* 29:106–111, 1994.

31. Ferrara A, Pemberton JH, Grotz RL, et al: Prolonged ambulatory recording of anorectal motility in patients with slow-transit constipation. *Am J Surg* 167:73–79, 1994.

32. Hiltunen KM, Kolehmainen H, Matikainen M: Does defecography help in diagnosis and clinical decision making in defecation disorders? *Abdominal Imaging* 19:355–358, 1994.

33. Hiltunen KM, Matikainen M: Simplified solid sphere test to investigate anal sphincter strength in patients with anorectal diseases. *Dis Colon Rectum* 37:564–567, 1994.

34. Neilsen MB, Dammegaard L, Pedersen JF: Endosonographic assessment of the anal sphincter after surgical reconstruction. *Dis Colon Rectum* 37:434–438, 1994.

35. Eckardt VF, Jung B, Fischer B, et al: Anal endosonography in healthy subjects and patients with idiopathic fecal incontinence. *Dis Colon Rectum* 37:235–242, 1994.

36. Emblem R, Diseth T, Morkrid L, et al: Anal endosonography and physiology in adolescents with corrected low anorectal anomalies. *J Paediatr Surg* 29:447–451, 1994.

37. Falk PM, Blatchford GJ, Cali RL, et al: Transanal ultrasound and manometry in the evaluation of fecal incontinence. *Dis Colon Rectum* 37:468–472, 1994.

38. Yang YK, Wexner SD: Anal pressure vectography is of no apparent benefit for sphincter evaluation. *Int J Colorectal Dis* 9:92–95, 1994.

39. Jorge JM, Ger GC, Gonzalez L, et al: Patient position during cinedefecography. Influence on perineal descent and other measurements. *Dis Colon Rectum* 37:927–931, 1994.

40. Speakman CT, Hoyle CH, Kamm MA, et al: Neuropeptides in the internal anal sphincter in neurogenic faecal incontinence. *Int J Colorectal Dis* 8:201–205, 1993.

41. Meagher AP, Lubowski DZ, King DW: The cough response of the anal sphincter. *Int J Colorectal Dis* 8:217–219, 1993.

42. Farouk R, Duthie GS, MacGregor AB, et al: Rectoanal inhibition and incontinence in patients with rectal prolapse. *Br J Surg* 81:743–746, 1994.

43. Benninga MA, Wijers OB, van der Hoeven CW, et al: Manometry, profilometry, and endosonography: Normal physiology and anatomy of the anal canal in healthy children. *J Paediatr Gastroenterol Nutr* 18:68–77, 1994.

44. Carty NJ, Moran B, Johnson CD: Anorectal physiology measurements are of no value in clinical practice. True or false? *Ann R Coll Surg Engl* 76:276–280, 1994.

45. Kamm MA: Obstetric damage and faecal incontinence. *Lancet* 344:730–733, 1994.

46. Lam TC, Islam N, Lubowski DZ, et al: Does squatting reduce pelvic floor descent during defaecation. *Aust NZ J Surg* 63:172–174, 1993.

47. Malone PS, Wheeler RA, Williams JE: Continence in patients with spina bifida: Long term results. *Arch Dis Child* 70:107–110, 1994.

48. King JC, Currie DM, Wright E: Bowel training in spina bifida: Importance of education, patient compliance, age and anal reflexes. *Arch Phys Med Rehabil* 75:243–247, 1994.

49. Waldron DJ, Horgan PG, Patel FR, et al: Multiple sclerosis: Assessment of colonic and anorectal function in the presence of faecal incontinence. *Int J Colorectal Dis* 8:220–224, 1993.

50. Pinna Pintor M, Zara GP, Falletto E, et al: Pudendal neuropathy in diabetic patients with faecal incontinence. *Int J Colorectal Dis* 9:105–109, 1994.

51. Swaffield J: The management and development of continence services within the framework of the NHS and Community Care Act (1990). *J Clin Nurs* 3:119–124, 1994.

52. Smith LJ, Franchetti B, McCoull K, et al: A behavioural approach to retraining bowel function after long-standing constipation and faecal impaction in people with learning disabilities. *Dev Med Child Neurol* 36:41–49, 1994.

53. Papachrysostomou M, Smith AN: Effects of biofeedback on obstructive defecation—reconditioning of the defecation reflex? *Gut* 35:252–256, 1994.

54. Scheuer M, Kuijpers HC, Bleijenberg G: Effect of electrostimulation on sphincter function in neurogenic fecal continence. *Dis Colon Rectum* 37:590–593, 1994.

55. Setti Carraro P, Kamm MA, Nicholls RJ: Long-term results of postanal repair for neurogenic faecal incontinence. *Br J Surg* 81:140–144, 1994.

56. Jameson JS, Speakman CT, Darzi A, et al: Audit of postanal repair in the treatment of fecal incontinence. *Dis Colon Rectum* 37:369–372, 1994.

57. Schouten WR, Briel JW, Auwerda JJ: Relationship between anal pressure and anodermal blood flow. The vascular pathogenesis of anal fissures. *Dis Colon Rectum* 37:664–669, 1994.

58. Farouk R, Duthie GS, MacGregor AB, et al: Sustained internal sphincter hypertonia in patients with chronic anal fissure. *Dis Colon Rectum* 37:424–429, 1994.

59. Pasricha PJ, Ravich WJ, Hendrix TR, et al: Treatment of achalasia with intrasphincteric injection of botulinum toxin: A pilot trial. *Ann Intern Med* 121:590–591, 1994.

60. Gui D, Cassetta E, Anastasio G, et al: Botulinum toxin for chronic anal fissure. *Lancet* 344:1127–1128, 1994.

61. Farouk R, Duthie GS, Pryde A, et al: Abnormal transient internal sphincter relaxation in idiopathic pruritus ani: Physiological evidence from ambulatory monitoring. *Br J Surg* 81:603–606, 1994.

62. Smyth RL, van Velzen D, Smyth AR, et al: Strictures of ascending colon in cystic fibrosis and high strength pancreatic enzymes. *Lancet* 343:85–86, 1994.

63. Fuchs CS, Giovannucci EL, Colditz GA, et al: A prospective study of family history and the risk of colorectal cancer. *N Engl J Med* 331:1669–1674, 1994.

64. Olsen J, Kronborg O, Lynggaard J, et al: Dietary risk factors for cancer and adenomas of the large intestine. A case-control study within a screening trial in Denmark. *Eur J Cancer* 30A:53–60, 1994.

65. Giovannucci E, Rimm EB, Stampfer MJ, et al: Intake of fat, meat and fiber in relation to risk of colon cancer in men. *Cancer Res* 54:2390–2397, 1994.

66. Steinmetz KA, Potter JD: Egg consumption and cancer of the colon and rectum. *Eur J Cancer Prev* 3:237–245, 1994.

67. Yamashita N, Minamoto T, Ochiai A, et al: Frequent and characteristic K-ras activation and absence of p53 protein accumulation in aberrant crypt foci of the colon. *Gastroenterology* 108:434–440, 1995.

68. Mengesha B, Johnson O, Negussie Y: Familial polyposis in two Ethiopians. *Ethiop Med J* 32:49–55, 1994.

69. Petersen GM: Knowledge of the adenomatous polyposis coli gene and its clinical application. *Ann Med* 26:205–208, 1994.

70. Park JG, Han HJ, Kang MS, et al: Presymptomatic diagnosis of familial adenomatous polyposis coli. *Dis Colon Rectum* 37:700–707, 1994.

71. Eckert WA, Jung C, Wolff G: Presymptomatic diagnosis in families with adenomatous polyposis

using highly polymorphic dinucleotide CA repeat markers flanking the APC gene. *J Med Genet* 31:442–447, 1994.

72. Solomon MJ, McLeod RS: Periodic health examination, 1994 update: 2. Screening strategies for colorectal cancer. Canadian Task Force on the periodic health examination. *Can Med Assoc J* 150:1961–1970, 1994.

73. Tobi M, Luo FC, Ronai Z: Detection of K-ras mutation in colonic effluent samples from patients without evidence of colorectal carcinoma. *J Natl Cancer Inst* 86:1007–1010, 1994.

74. Latt TT, Nicholl R, Domizio P, et al: Rectal bleeding and polyps. *Arch Dis Child* 69:144–147, 1993.

75. Margulies C, Krevsky B, Catalano MF: How accurate are endoscopic estimates of size? *Gastrointest Endosc* 40:174–177, 1994.

76. Brady AP, Stevenson GW, Stevenson I: Colorectal cancer overlooked at barium enema examination and colonoscopy: a continuing perceptual problem. *Radiology* 192:373–378, 1994.

77. Stefansson T, Bergman A, Ekbom A, et al: Accuracy of double contrast barium enema and sigmoidoscopy in the detection of polyps in patients with diverticulosis. *Acta Radiol* 35:442–446, 1994.

78. Cohen SM, Wexner SD, Binderow SR, et al: Prospective, randomized, endoscopic-blinded trial comparing precolonoscopy bowel cleansing methods. *Dis Colon Rectum* 37:689–696, 1994.

79. Seow-Choen F, Leong AF, Tsang C: Selective sedation for colonoscopy. *Gastrointest Endosc* 40:661–664, 1994.

80. Steine S: Which hurts the most? A comparison of pain rating during double-contrast barium enema examination and colonoscopy. *Radiology* 191:99–101, 1994.

81. Zarchy TM, Ershoff D: Do characteristics of adenomas on flexible sigmoidoscopy predict advanced lesions on baseline colonoscopy? *Gastroenterology* 106:1501–1504, 1994.

82. Rex DK, Lehman GA, Ulbright TM, et al: The yield of a second screening flexible sigmoidoscopy in average-risk persons after one negative examination. *Gastroenterology* 106:593–595, 1994.

83. Greenberg ER, Baron JA, Tosteson TD: A clinical trial of antioxidant vitamins to prevent colorectal adenoma. Polyp Prevention Study Group. *N Engl J Med* 331:141–147, 1994.

84. Winawer SJ, Zauber AG, Ho MN, et al: Prevention of colorectal cancer by colonoscopic polypectomy. The National Polyp Study Workgroup. *N Engl J Med* 329:1977–1981, 1993.

85. Neugut AI, Jacobson JS, Ahsan H, et al: Incidence and recurrence rates of colorectal adenomas: A prospective study. *Gastroenterology* 108:402–408, 1995.

86. Giovannucci E, Rimm EB, Stampfer MJ, et al: Aspirin use and risk for colorectal cancer and adenoma in male health professionals. *Ann Intern Med* 121:241–246, 1994.

87. Spagnesi MT, Tonelli F, Dolara P, et al: Rectal proliferation and polyp occurrence in patients with familial adenomatous polyposis after sulindac treatment. *Gastroenterology* 106:362–366, 1994.

88. Seibold F, Slametschka D, Gregor M, et al: Neutrophil auto-antibodies: A genetic marker in primary sclerosing cholangitis and ulcerative colitis. *Gastroenterology* 107:532–536, 1994.

89. Brignola C, Cottone M, Pera A, et al: Mesalamine in the prevention of endoscopic recurrence after intestinal resection for Crohn's disease. Italian Co-operative Study Group. *Gastroenterology* 108:345–349, 1995.

90. Rutgeerts P, Lofberg R, Malchow H, et al: A comparison of budesonide with prednisolone for active Crohn's disease. *N Engl J Med* 331:842–845, 1994.

91. Greenberg GR, Feagan BG, Martin F, et al: Oral budesonide for active Crohn's disease. Canadian Inflammatory Bowel Disease Study Group. *N Engl J Med* 331:836–841, 1994.

92. Nygaard K, Bergan T, Bjorneklett A, et al: Topical metronidazole treatment in pouchitis. *Scand J Gastroenterol* 29:462–467, 1994.

93. Lichtiger S, Present DH, Kornbluth A, et al: Cyclosporine in severe ulcerative colitis refractory to steroid therapy. *N Engl J Med* 330:1841–1845, 1994.

94. Present DH, Lichtiger S: Efficacy of cyclosporine in treatment of fistula of Crohn's disease. *Dig Dis Sci* 39:374–380, 1994.

95. Feagan BG, McDonald JW, Rochon J, et al: Low-dose cyclosporine for the treatment of Crohn's disease. The Canadian Crohn's Relapse Prevention Trial Investigators. *N Engl J Med* 330:1846–1851, 1994.

96. Campieri M, Paoluzi P, D'Albasio G, et al: Better quality of therapy with 5-ASA colonic foam in active ulcerative colitis: A multicenter comparative trial with 5-ASA enema. *Dig Dis Sci* 38:1843–1850, 1993.

97. Yamaguchi T, Sasaki K, Kurosaki Y, et al: Biopharmaceutical evaluation of salicylazosulfanilic acid as a novel colon-targeted prodrug of 5-aminosalicyclic acid. *J Drug Target* 2:123–131, 1994.

98. Pullan RD, Rhodes J, Ganesh S, et al: Transdermal nicotine for active ulcerative colitis. *N Engl J Med* 330:811–815, 1994.

99. Prantera C, Kohn A, Mangiarotti R, et al: Antimycobacterial therapy in Crohn's disease: Results of a controlled, double-blind trial with a multiple antibiotic regimen. *Am J Gastroenterol* 89:513–518, 1994.

100. Moody GA, Mayberry JF: Perceived sexual dysfunction amongst patients with inflammatory bowel disease. *Digestion* 54:256–260, 1993.

101. Connell WR, Lennard-Jones JE, Williams CB, et al: Factors affecting the outcome of endoscopic surveillance for cancer in ulcerative colitis. *Gastroenterology* 107:934–944, 1994.

102. Redston MS, Papadopoulos NN, Caldas C, et al: Common occurrence of APC and K-ras gene mutations in the spectrum of colitis-associated neoplasias. *Gastroenterology* 108:383–392, 1995.

103. Ghosh S, Cowen S, Hannan WJ, et al: Low bone mineral density in Crohn's disease, but not in ulcerative colitis, at diagnosis. *Gastroenterology* 107:1031–1039, 1994.

104. Abitbol V, Roux C, Chaussade S, et al: Metabolic bone assessment in patients with inflammatory bowel disease. *Gastroenterology* 108:417–422, 1995.

105. McIntyre PB, Pemberton JH, Wolff BG, et al: Comparing functional results one year and ten years after ileal pouch-anal anastomosis for chronic ulcerative colitis. *Dis Colon Rectum* 37:303–307, 1994.

106. Jorge JM, Wexner SD, Morgado PJ Jr, et al: Optimization of sphincter function after the ileoanal reservoir procedure. A prospective, randomized trial. *Dis Colon Rectum* 37:419–423, 1994.

107. Nagel E, Bartels M, Pichlmayr R: Scanning electron-microscopic lesions in Crohn's disease: Relevance for the interpretation of postoperative recurrence. *Gastroenterology* 108:376–382, 1995.

CHAPTER 5

Gastrointestinal Hormones and Neuropeptides

Stephan Böhm, M.D.

Postdoctoral Research Fellow, Departments of Surgery and Physiology, University of California, San Francisco, School of Medicine, San Francisco, California

Nigel W. Bunnett, Ph.D.

Associate Professor, Departments of Surgery and Physiology, University of California, San Francisco, School of Medicine, San Francisco, California

Eileen F. Grady, Ph.D.

Assistant Professor, Departments of Surgery and Physiology, University of California, San Francisco, School of Medicine, San Francisco, California

Neuropeptides form one of the largest and most functionally diverse groups of regulatory molecules. Their numbers grow yearly. They are widely distributed and are produced by endocrine glands and neurons of the central and peripheral nervous systems, where they are frequently secreted with other neurotransmitters. Neuropeptides interact with cell-surface receptors, which have seven hydrophobic, membrane-spanning domains and are functionally coupled to the heterotrimeric G-proteins. Just as the number of peptides grows steadily, so does the number of identified receptors. Indeed, there are probably more known receptors than peptides, and it is well established that a single neuropeptide can interact with a family of related receptors with varying affinity. All the peptides have multiple and often unrelated biologic actions on numerous different cell types, and some peptides are associated with disease processes. Specific peptide and nonpeptide antagonists are available for many peptide receptors, some of which are useful for treating disease and elucidating physiologic function.

However, the remarkable recent progress in this area poses more questions than it answers, and neuropeptides remain one of the least-understood groups of regulators. We know that neurons produce and secrete multiple neurotransmitters, but what is the functional relevance of this behavior? Peptides bind to extracellular domains of their receptors, but how does binding to an extracellular domain affect interaction of intracellular domains with G-proteins? Almost all peptides are produced in several forms of varying size and interact with multiple receptors, but what is the physiologic significance of this multiplicity of ligand and receptor? Cells express numerous different receptors and are continuously bombarded with information, so how do cells sort through numerous forms of information to give a tightly controlled response? Although many effects of peptides are known, which of their actions occur at physiologic levels?

This review focuses on progress made during 1994 and 1995 in the field of gastrointestinal hormones and neuropeptides and attempts to address some of the aforementioned questions. Where possible we will discuss peptides in the digestive system. However, we will also cover major advances that have been made in other systems for signaling molecules other than peptides. Rather than discuss each peptide in detail, the review highlights important advances made in three general areas: (1) investigations of the function of neuronal and hormonal peptides; (2) investigations of receptor structure, function, and signal transduction; and (3) investigations of the involvement of peptides in disease.

INVESTIGATIONS OF THE FUNCTION OF NEURONAL AND HORMONAL PEPTIDES

Usually many complementary approaches are required to define the biologic significance of a particular peptide and to determine precisely how they are achieved. On a molecular level, examination of transcriptional regulatory sites may suggest responsive elements and thus identify proteins or hormones that can modify expression of the peptide. Localization of message and peptide during development and disease states may suggest a specific site and sequence of action. However, the extracellular milieu must not be overlooked, because neuropeptides could be released on stimulus and rapidly degraded. Responsiveness in specific tissues may be tightly regulated, so that certain tissues are exquisitely sensitive to a given neuropeptide. In other tissues, a neuropeptide may encounter low numbers of receptors, receptors of a nonpreferred subtype, or high levels of proteases such that higher concentrations of neuropeptides are required to exert effects. Often neuropeptides have opposing effects, and it is the sum of these actions that produces the observed response. Here, use of receptor agonists, receptor antagonists, antisense oligonucleotides, and antibodies specific for the neuropeptide are useful to isolate individual events in the phenomena observed. In summary, multiple approaches must be used to analyze the function of any given neuropeptide.

Localization of Neuropeptides Provides a Clue to Their Physiologic Functions

Localization of neuropeptides can suggest at what time during development and in what processes they are likely to function. For example, calcitonin gene-related peptide was detected in cholinesterase-positive motor end plates of epithelial cells of cat esophagus.[1] This suggests it functions as a neurotransmitter or neuromodulator in this tissue.

Gene knockout and transgenic methods to eliminate expression of a neuropeptide are valuable for determining the physiologic actions of specific peptides. Elimination of a neuropeptide can also be used to identify cell lineages. The pancreatic polypeptide gene promoter was coupled to diphtheria toxin A chain in transgenic mice to ablate cells expressing pancreatic polypeptide.[2] This resulted in embryos lacking pancreatic insulin- and somatostatin-containing cells. This suggests that development of the insulin- and somatostatin-secreting cells requires pancreatic polypeptide or that they derive from a pancreatic polypeptide-expressing stem cell. Transgenic mice can also be used to study the localization and promoter region of a neuropeptide. Part of the 5′ flanking region (1.6 kb) of the secretin gene was linked to the human growth hormone or simian virus 40 large T antigen reporter gene. The distribution of growth hormone expression was similar to that of secretin in normal mice, suggesting that most *cis*-regulatory elements leading to tissue-specific expression occur within 1.6 kb from the transcriptional start site. With the use of double immunofluorescence staining, enteroendocrine cells in the small intestine were determined to contain secretin, cholecystokinin, substance P, and serotonin but not peptide YY, neurotensin, somatostatin, or gastrin. In contrast, in the colon, secretin-containing cells also contained glucagon, peptide YY, and neurotensin but not substance P or somatostatin.[3]

Localization of neurotransmitters can provide important clues to their functions. For example, galanin-immunoreactive neurons and a small subset of vasoactive intestinal polypeptide and neuropeptide Y–immunoreactive neurons in the myenteric plexus of rat stomach and duodenum contained reduced nicotinamide adenine dinucleotide phosphate (NADPH)–diaphorase (nitric oxide synthetase) activity. These peptides may function with nitric oxide as neurotransmitters within the myenteric plexus. Bombesin and 5-hydroxytryptamine were not colocalized with NADPH-diaphorase activity. In the connective tissue between the duodenum and the pancreas, nerve fibers with NADPH-diaphorase activity ramified the adventitia of blood vessels.[4]

Species variation in localization of neuropeptides must also be considered. For instance, in contrast to neuropeptide Y mRNA and peptide, galanin mRNA and peptide were found to be intensely expressed in the celiac ganglion of dogs, but less than one fourth of this amount was found in monkey celiac ganglion, and none was found in rats.[5]

Regulation of Expression and Processing of Neuropeptides

Peptide Sequences

Closely related peptides may exist in a species specific or tissue specific form. For example, the mouse secretin complementary DNA (cDNA) encodes a protein of 133 amino acids, with the 27 amino acid secretin peptide located at positions 32 and 58.[6] Comparison with genomic DNA revealed that the mouse secretin gene consists of four exons, with most of the peptide being encoded by the second exon. The mouse secretin differs from the rat and porcine secretin at position 5 (of mature secretin), with a Met substitution for Thr.

A peptide YY variant isolated from the skin of frog *Phyllomedusa bicolor* has 94% identity to intestinal peptide YY of the frog *Rana ridibunda* and a 72% sequence homology with intestinal neuropeptide Y.[7] A synthetic version of the peptide inhibited secretion of α-melanocyte-stimulating hormone in vitro. Whether this peptide is an alternative form of peptide YY in this species or is a tissue specific isoform is unclear.

Genetic analysis of phenotypic mutant *Drosophila* is proving to be a valuable tool for identification of proteins regulating physiologic functions. For example, screening of candidate genes involved in learning and memory in *Drosophila* resulted in the identification of a novel amnesiac neuropeptide.[8] This peptide bears sequence homology to mammalian adenylate cyclase–activating peptide and growth hormone–releasing hormone. Detection of phenotypic changes in organisms carrying mutations in polypeptide genes could clarify the function of neuropeptides.

Analysis of Gene Promoters

Analysis of the promoter region of a neuropeptide gene can lead to an understanding of how growth factors through their signaling mechanisms alter gene expression in a positive or negative fashion. This requires (1) scrutiny of the sequence to identify putative binding sites for regulatory factors, (2) experimental identification of important regions by analysis of deletion constructs, and (3) determination of whether regulatory factors bind to these sites and thus control transcription. The immediate proximal promoter for the bovine galanin gene was sequenced and the transcriptional start site was mapped to two sites 27 to 31 base pairs (bp) downstream from an atypical TATA box.[9, 10] The galanin promoter and deletion constructs were linked to a luciferase receptor gene and transfected into the neuroblastoma cell SH-SY5Y.[9] Positive regulatory elements were detected within 131 bp from the transcriptional start site, and repressor elements were detected more than 900 bp upstream from the transcriptional start site. A TPA responsive element was located at positions -66 to -62 upstream from the transcriptional start site.[10] Analysis of the 5' flanking region of the human galanin gene using the CAT reporter gene and transient transfections in NG 108-15 and Chinese hamster ovary (CHO) cells revealed a negative modulator between positions -1891 and -207.[11] Elements were identified by sequence analysis that could be activated by protein kinase C and protein kinase A. Similar regulatory elements exist in the preprotachykinin gene. For example, a 25-bp element located at position -200 from the major start of transcription of the rat preprotachykinin A promoter activated CAT transcription in HeLa cells when one copy was placed in conjunction with the minimal c-*fos* promoter.[12]

Specific sequences in the gene promoter and enhancer act as binding sites for proteins that regulate transcription. In addition, gene expression can be regulated at the posttranscriptional level. For example, nerve growth factor stimulates neuropeptide Y expression by stabilizing messenger RNA (mRNA) and by increasing transcription rates. *cis*-Acting promoter elements in the human neuropeptide Y gene responsible for nerve growth factor–induced transcription were located to residues -87 and -36.[13] Gel retardation analysis revealed tissue specific interaction of three putative transcription factors with this fragment (AP-2 and two unknown proteins). Nerve growth factor also stimulates substance P and calcitonin gene-related peptide expression in dorsal root ganglia neuronal cultures and inhibits vasoactive intestinal peptide expression.[14]

Splice Variants

Certain neuropeptides occur in different isoforms that are generated by alternate splicing of the RNA, which results in alternate mRNA species. In this way tissue-specific mRNA variants can be generated. Preprotachykinin mRNA is known to occur in three forms; α, β, and γ. These isoforms are generated by omission of exon 4 in γ and exon 6 in α. A fourth isoform of preprotachykinin mRNA was sequenced and found to be most closely related to β-preprotachykinin mRNA, because it was generated by exclusion of both exon 4 (as in γ) and exon 6 (as in α). It was present in ileal smooth muscle and mucosa of rat ileum, in brain, and in colon.[15] A highly repeated TGCATG motif in the intron downstream of exon 4 was determined to be important for cell type–specific recognition of this exon.[16] Because similar sequences occur downstream of alternatively spliced exons of the gene for calcitonin gene-related peptide, they may function generally in tissue-specific alternative splicing.[17, 18] Tissue-specific variants may lead to expression of one number of a neuropeptide family as a specific site.

Posttranslational and Postsecretory Processing of Neuropeptides

Peptides are synthesized as large precursors, which then undergo posttranslational processing within the cell to form biologically active molecules destined for secretion. Intracellular processing involves proteolytic cleavage, as well as modifications of specific residues, for example, by sulfation. It is important to identify sites within the cell where this processing occurs. For example, cholecystokinin is sulfated at a tyrosine residue before secretion. This is required for full biologic activity. In Cos7 cells, this sulfation step occurs before the peptide reaches the Golgi apparatus.[19]

Processing of neuropeptides also occurs after peptide secretion. This may serve to alter the activity or inactivate a peptide. For example, removal of the amino terminal dipeptide Tyr-Pro of rabbit peptide YY-I changes an unselective Y_1/Y_2 receptor agonist into a peptide that selectively interacts with the Y_2 receptor.[20] Dipeptidyl peptidase-IV clips these residues from human peptide YY-I, whereas endopeptidase-24.11 cleaves peptide YY at the Asn^{29}-Leu^{30} bond, which inactivates the peptide.[21] Different tissues have different relative amounts of these enzymes, which would alter receptor affinity and levels of functional peptide.

Release of endogenous peptides can also be modified, thus affecting their availability. For example, several neuropeptides, including substance P, contribute to inflammation. Bradykinin stimulates the release of substance P and calcitonin gene-related peptide from sensory neurons in culture. Prostaglandin E_2 enhances this release, and preexposure to indomethacin attenuates it.[22] Thus, bradykinin and prostaglandin E_2 may contribute to inflammation by release of neuropeptides. Electrical stimulation of the rat peroneal nerve below a tetrodotoxin block (7 days prior) caused a rapid release of the accumulated calcitonin gene-related peptide.[23] Therefore, nerve impulse activity can deplete even extensive intracellular stores of neuropeptides.

Structural Analysis of Neuropeptides and Development of Receptor-Specific Agonists and Antagonists

Analysis of the three-dimensional structure of peptides is important for several reasons: (1) it provides insight into peptide domains that interact with receptors, (2) it gives information about receptor subtype specificity, and (3) it facilitates the design of specific agonists and antagonists of receptors that may be used to probe peptide function and as therapeutic agents.

In some cases the peptide may have a random structure. Circular dichroism measurements of human galanin showed that in aqueous solution it had the conformation of a completely random coil peptide.[24] Galanin may assume a short-range structural motif to enable receptor recognition and may fold to a more stable conformation on binding to the receptor. Besides helical stability, another factor that must be considered is the temperature and pH dependence of folding of helical peptides.[25]

Once the three-dimensional structure has been determined by nuclear magnetic resonance and molecular dynamics simulations, it is possible to design analogues of the peptide to determine which conformations are required to retain binding. For example, a model of neuropeptide Y predicts a compact tertiary structure, consisting of N-terminal polyproline type II helix in residues 1 to 9, a β-turn in residues 9 to 12, an amphiphilic α-helix in residues 14 to 31, and a C-terminal, structurally undefined tail. This brings the N-terminus and C-terminus in proximity, and the polyproline helix and β-turn are thought to stabilize the α-helix. The effects of different residues on this structure were determined by synthesizing a series of Nα-acetyl N-terminal deletion fragments, and analyzing their solution structure by circular dichroism spectroscopy.[26] Removal of residues around Pro^5 prevented aggregation and decreased the helical content, resulting in a twofold to threefold drop in receptor binding. Deletions beyond Glu^{15} destabilized the α-helix, suggesting that Asp^{16} participates in its stabilization.[27] It has been suggested that rather than the α-helix, folding of the N- and C-termini may be more important to binding. Examination of more than 50 analogues of neuropeptide Y revealed that changes in the C-terminus affected the Y_2 receptor affinity.[28] Although the C-terminal pentapeptide amide (32–36) was important for binding to the receptor, Arg^{33} and Arg^{35} were required for specific Y_1 receptor recognition, and Arg^{35} and Tyr^{36} were required for specific Y_2 receptor recognition.[27, 28] In a different approach, substitutions were made using nonproteinogenic, conformationally restricted amino acids that could induce turns similar to those present in the native peptide.[29] This yielded several neuropeptide Y analogues that reacted with both the Y_1 and Y_2 receptors. Novel C-terminal analogues of NPY were developed that acted as agonists and antagonists of Y_2 and Y_1 receptors.[30]

The overlay of the three-dimensional structure of several analogues of a neuropeptide can predict the minimal residues required to generate a binding site. Thus, conformational analysis of the neurokinin 2 receptor agonists [β-Ala^8]neurokinin A(4–10) and GR-64349 with the polycyclic peptide derivative MEN-10627, a neurokinin 2 receptor antagonist, revealed a superimposition in the low-energy conformations of the agonists to MEN-10627 in three residues, Phe, Leu, and Met. This suggests that the recognition sites of these three molecules on the neurokinin 2 receptor overlap, with MEN-10627 having only one diaminopropoionic acid residue between the Phe and the Leu rather than two amino acids as in the agonists.[31] Similarly, analysis of low-energy structures of several cholecystokinin peptide analogues that bind the cholecystokinin B receptor revealed a common conformation for receptor-bound agonists.[32]

Analysis of the three-dimensional structure of a peptide may suggest the spatial requirements for peptide antagonist activity, because in some cases peptide antagonists may bind in similar pockets as agonists. Nonpeptide antagonists are known to bind deeper in the transmembrane segments of G-protein coupled receptors. Previous peptide antagonists have been designed using D amino acid substitutions or residues with specific conformational properties, such as Pro, which signals a tight turn. Thus, replacement of the Lys residue in the cholecystokinin A tetrapeptide agonist Boc-Trp-Lys(Tac)-Asp-Met-Phe-NH_2 (A71623) with L-4 or D or L-3 aminophenylalanine generated analogue that were specific antagonists of the cholecystokinin A receptor.[33] The replacement of Leu for Pro at position 4 of neuropeptide Y generated a potent Y_1 antagonist.[30] Antagonists may be quite small molecules, and slight modifications can enhance their activity. For example, the opioid dipeptide Tyr-L-tetrahydro-3-isoquinoline carboxylic acid(=Tic)-NH_2 is a δ-specific opioid receptor antagonist, and Tyr-D-Tic is a nonselective agonist.[34] Lengthening the peptide to Tyr-Tic-Ala-NH_2 increased δ-specific opioid receptor antagonist activity. Modification of cholecystokinin A receptor selective tetrapeptides by methylation markedly increased their in vivo ability to suppress eating in rats.[35, 36]

In summary, understanding of the three-dimensional configurations of a neuropeptide can lead to an understanding of the interactions between a given neuropeptide and its receptor.

Use of Receptor-Specific Agonists and Antagonists to Probe Neuropeptide and Receptor Function

Species Specificity of Receptor-Specific Agonists and Antagonists

Specific peptide and nonpeptide agonists and antagonists are available for the tachykinin family of receptors (neurokinin [NK]1, NK2, and NK3 receptors). It is well known that some antagonists are species specific. For example, the NK1 receptor antagonist FK888 showed a 320-fold higher affinity for the human NK1 receptor than for the rat NK1 receptor when transiently expressed in monkey kidney Cos7 cells.[37] A potent nonpeptide antagonist of the NK3 receptor, SR-142801, inhibited [MePhe[7]]neurokinin B binding to human NK3 receptor expressed in CHO cells and to guinea pig and gerbil cerebral cortex but was less active on the rat receptor.[38] It effectively antagonized [MePhe[7]]neurokinin B–induced contractions of guinea pig ileum.

Although agonists and antagonists are invaluable for determining the physiologic functions of particular peptides, care must be taken to ensure that they are appropriate for a given species. This may be difficult, because species-specific nonpeptide antagonists, which are not degraded as quickly as peptides, may not be available. For example, substance P and neurokinin A stimulate contraction of isolated segments of canine ileum. The substance P response was found to be unaffected by CP-96345 (a nonpeptide human NK1 receptor–preferring antagonist), RP-67580 (a nonpeptide rat NK1 receptor–preferring antagonist) either alone or together with SR-48968 (a nonpeptide NK2 receptor–preferring antagonist) and R-487 (an NK3 receptor–preferring antagonist).[39] Thus, an unknown tachykinin receptor may mediate substance P–induced contractions in this tissue. Neurokinin A–induced contractions were decreased 50% by SR-48968, suggesting that these contractions are mediated by the NK2 receptor. However, SR-48968 also interacts with human NK3 receptors ($IC_{50} = 350nM$) and with rat NK3 receptors ($IC_{50} > 10\mu M$).[40] If the canine NK3 receptor behaves similarly to the human NK3 receptor, there may be cross reactivity. Moreover, it is difficult to clearly identify additional receptor subtypes when the species specificity of the antagonist is less than ideal. At present, specific nonpeptide antagonists exist only for human NK1 and NK3 receptors and for rat NK1 and NK2 receptors. Additional nonpeptide antagonists will probably be forthcoming.

Analysis of Complex Physiologic Interactions in vitro and in vivo

Basic insights can be drawn from studies on neuropeptide function in vitro. Thus, high concentrations of substance P derivatives inhibited the growth of peptide-sensitive small cell lung carcinoma lines.[41] Use of a combination of receptor agonists and antagonists could identify how this response is mediated. Transfected cells have been used extensively for biochemical studies on receptors and to examine signaling mechanisms. However, results with transfected cells may be artifacts due to high levels of expression of the receptor or due to unique properties of the transfected cell. To analyze highly differentiated functions such as regulated secretion, primary cultures are especially useful. For example, exposure of dispersed guinea pig chief cells to cholecystokinin-8 or the cholecystokinin receptor agonist A-71378 decreased the affinity of somatostatin receptors, a process mediated by the cholecystokinin A receptor, because it was blocked by the antagonist L-364718.[42]

A limitation of in vitro studies is that integrated functions such as blood flow, central effects of neuropeptides, alterations in other organs, and neuronal effects cannot be studied. Thus, it is difficult to dissect the exact points of action and the neuropeptides required to yield the observed physiologic response. Another limitation of in vitro studies is that isolation and dispersion of primary cultures may be considered an injured state and evoke inflammatory responses.

Localization of neuropeptides is a good starting point for analysis. For example, peripheral inflammation induces upregulation of opioids, substance P, calcitonin gene-related peptide, and galanin. Injection of Freund's adjuvant into the hind paw of a rat induces an upregulation of neuropeptide Y mRNA and immunoreactivity in ipsilateral dorsal horn neurons and an increase in neuropeptide Y (Y_1) receptor mRNA.[43] This suggests that neuropeptide Y may be involved in nociception.

Several approaches are best combined to analyze neuropeptide physiology in vivo. Intraduodenal administration of oligopeptide and a mixed amino acid solution resulted in a dose-related increase in pancreatic juice volume, bicarbonate, amylase, and trypsin secretion in rats.[44] An antisecretin serum blocked volume flow and HCO_3^-, output, whereas the cholecystokinin receptor antagonist loxiglumide decreased amylase and trypsin output. Thus, pancreatic secretion under these conditions results from endogenous secretin and cholecystokinin.

INVESTIGATIONS OF RECEPTOR STRUCTURE, FUNCTION, AND SIGNAL TRANSDUCTION

In the past 5 years the major focus of neuropeptide research has been in the receptors rather than in the peptides themselves. All the regulatory peptides in the gastrointestinal tract exert their multiple biologic actions by interacting with cell-surface receptors that are anchored to cells with seven domains of hydrophobic residues and that are functionally coupled to G-proteins. The primary structure of many of these receptors has been deduced by molecular cloning, allowing detailed examination of structure and function. Despite their obvious differences in primary structure, ligand affinity, and sites of expression, it is their similarity that is remarkable. For example, all peptide receptors bind ligand in the extracellular and transmembrane domains, all interact with G-proteins by their intracellular loops and tail, and ligand binding often causes activation of the same effector molecules. Furthermore, there is remarkable structural and functional similarity between the peptide receptors and other G-protein-coupled receptors such as rhodopsin and receptors for biogenic amines. Therefore, we will discuss the important principles of receptor function for both peptide and nonpeptide receptors.

Binding Domains for Agonists and Antagonists

Agonists and antagonists interact with the receptors by binding to domains in the extracellular loops and transmembrane domains. Strategies that have been used to identify binding domains include generating receptor chimeras, point mutation of specific residues, molecular modeling, and cross-linking-labeled ligands and sequencing receptor fragments to which they are bound (for review see Strader et al.[45]). Some of these approaches have been used with great success for the receptors for the tachykinin family of peptides, which includes substance P, neurokinin A, and neurokinin B. The accumulation of information about this family was triggered partly by the development of therapeutically promising receptor antagonists. There are at least three tachykinin receptors, NK1, NK2, and NK3 receptors. Each peptide interacts with all three receptors, albeit with varying affinity. The high-affinity receptor for substance P is the NK1 receptor.

Two genetic strategies that have been commonly used to identify binding domains of receptors are generation of chimeric receptors and point mutant receptors. Chimeric receptors are formed by splicing together sequences of two different receptors that have distinctly different binding characteristics. However, the results of domain-exchange experiments require careful interpretation because the effects of these manipulations on ligand binding may be caused by (1) widespread conformational changes in the receptor, (2) local conformational changes in the binding pocket, or (3) disruption of direct interactions between the receptor and the ligand.[46] Substitution of the second or third extracellular loop between the NK1 receptor (which has high affinity for substance P) and the NK3 receptor (which has low affinity for substance P) affected binding affinities for both agonists and antagonists.[46] The aforementioned uncertainties about the interpretation of domain-swapping experiments were resolved by replacing residues in these segments of the NK1 receptor with corresponding residues from the NK2 or NK3 receptors. Single residue mutations in the third but not the second extracellular loop were able to recreate changes in binding affinities obtained with chimeric receptors.

Therefore, results obtained with domain swapping should be confirmed by exchange of individual residues between related receptors.

Point mutations of residues in the second and seventh transmembrane domain of the NK1 receptor also identified specific residues in these regions that are important for interacting with substance P (e.g., Asn^{85} may interact with the C-terminus of substance P).[47] Some of the critical residues that bind substance P are close to residues that interact with competitive antagonists, indicating that volume exclusion may partly explain the competitive antagonism of high-affinity substance P binding by nonpeptide antagonists.

Mutational experiments with the NK1 receptor indicate that natural peptide agonists bind to residues scattered throughout the extracellular regions, whereas nonpeptide antagonists interact with residues in the transmembrane domain. Different residues are important for interaction with different antagonists. For example, His^{197} in the fifth transmembrane domain of the human NK1 receptor is critical for binding to CP-96345 but not RP-67580 (nonpeptide NK1 receptor–preferring antagonists).[48] However, His^{265} in the sixth transmembrane domain is required for binding of RP-67580 but not CP-96345. There are also species differences. Thus, in contrast to the human receptor, in the rat receptor both His residues interact with both antagonists. These experiments predict that a binding pocket for nonpeptide antagonists of the NK1 receptor is composed of His residues located on opposing faces of the outer portions of the fifth and sixth transmembrane domain. Although involving different residues, the binding pocket for epinephrine in the β-adrenergic receptor is similarly located. Thus, there may be conservation of binding pockets for small molecules in G-protein-coupled receptors.

The importance of other residues in the putative binding pocket for nonpeptide antagonists of the NK1 receptor was further explored by the systematic mutation of nearby residues to His to create a metal ion–binding domain (Fig 1).[49] Substitution of Glu^{193} to His increased the affinity for Zn^{2+} by 44-fold. A double mutation of Glu^{193} and Tyr^{272} to His increased the affinity for Zn^{2+} by 794-fold by creating a pocket of four His residues to bind Zn^{2+}. Remarkably, the creation of a high affinity–binding pocket for Zn^{2+} in this region inhibited binding of labeled substance P and inhibited substance P–induced generation of inositol triphosphate. Therefore, binding of Zn^{2+} ions to the mutated receptor may cause an allosteric alteration that mimics that of nonpeptide antagonists and stabilizes it in a conformation that cannot bind substance P. Thus, the introduction of metal ion binding sites into receptors is a novel way to examine structure-function relationships.

Two new classes of structurally dissimilar antagonist (dicylpiperazine compounds and acyclic 2-benzhydryl-2-aminoethyl ethers) for the human NK1 receptor have been described.[50] Both classes showed reduced affinity for mutants involving residues Gln^{165}, His^{197}, and His^{265}, indicating that they interact with the same residues as the quinuclidine amide CP-96345 and the perhydroisoindole RP-67580. Therefore, chemically distinct antagonists must adopt a similar structure to fit into the antagonist–binding pocket of the NK1 receptor, which has important implications for rational drug design.

An alternate biochemical strategy has been used to map residues of the NK1

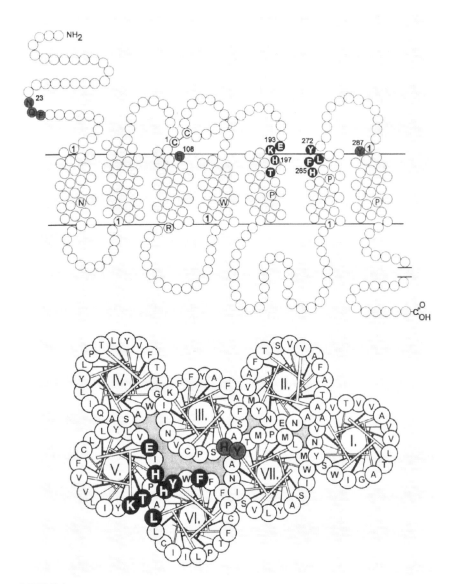

FIGURE 1.

Diagram of the human NK1 receptor showing putative binding sites for the nonpeptide antagonist CP-96345 and Zn^{2+} ions. The upper panel shows a serpentine model and the lower a helical wheel (viewed from outside) model of the NK1 receptor indicating His[197] *(helix or transmembrane domain V)*, His[265] *(helix VI)*, and Glu[193] *(helix V)* and Tyr[272] *(helix VI)*, which were mutated to His to create the high-affinity binding site for Zn^{2+} (Reprinted with permission from *Nature* from Elling CE, Nielsen SM, Schwartz TW: Conversion of antagonist-binding site to metal-ion site in the tachykinin NK-1 receptor. *Nature* 374:74–77, 1995. Copyright 1995 Macmillan Magazines Limited.)

receptor that interact with specific residues of substance P.[51] Photoactivatable forms of substance P were generated by replacing residues in positions 3 and 8 of the peptide with p-benzoyl-L-phenylalanine. These peptides were fully bioactive and were radioactively labeled. Peptides were covalently linked to the NK1 receptor by photolysis, and the receptor was enzymatically digested. Fragments were purified and sequenced to identify binding motifs. The third and eighth positions of substance P interacted with the extracellular tail (residues 1–21) and the second extracellular loop (residues 173–183), respectively, of the NK1 receptor. This approach allows identification of binding sites of both the peptide and its receptor and avoids problems with altered protein folding that may be artifacts of receptor mutation or generation of receptor chimeras.

A novel spectrofluorometric approach was used to investigate the interaction of fluorescent peptide ligands with the NK2 receptor.[52] Several heptapeptide antagonists were labeled with the nitrobenzoxadiazole (NBD) probe, the fluorescence of which is strongly sensitive to the medium, with higher fluorescence in a hydrophobic environment. The heptapeptide antagonists differed in the length of the spacer between the NBD group and the peptide. On antagonists binding to the receptor, an increase in NBD fluorescence was observed when the spacer length was less than 10 Å. Collisional quenching of fluorescence using iodide and Co^{2+} ions helped to further define the binding pocket for antagonists: The N-terminal portion of antagonists bound into a hydrophobic pocket shielded from the solvent and located at a depth of 5 to 10 Å in the protein or membrane. In contrast, the N-terminal region of agonist peptides were accessible to the solvent when bound to NK2 receptors.

A unique opportunity for studying sites in the NK1 receptor responsible for substance P binding was raised by the presence of a noninterrupted pentapeptide homology between the NK1 receptor and the anti–substance P antibody NC1, which recognizes the C-terminus of substance P.[53] The common sequence Gly-Tyr-Tyr-Ser-Thr is located in the outer portion of helix 4 of the NK1 receptor and in the third hypervariable region of the heavy chain of the antibody. Both locations are consistent with a potential role in recognition of the C-terminal substance P pentapeptide, which is highly conserved among all three tachykinins (consensus Phe-Gly-X-Leu-Met). To test the relevance of the consensus sequence as a common molecular determinant in substance P binding, residues Gly^{166} and Tyr^{167} in the NK1 receptor were replaced by the corresponding amino acids of the NK2 receptor (Cys and Phe). The double mutation increased receptor affinity for substance P twofold and increased it 11-fold for neurokinin A and 21-fold for neurokinin B. The C-terminal hexapeptides of substance P and neurokinin A demonstrated a mutation-induced increase in binding affinity of 35- and 57-fold, respectively. A hybrid tachykinin consisting of the C-terminal hexapeptide of neurokinin A and the N-terminal pentapeptide of substance P was bound with 30-fold higher affinity by the mutant receptor compared with the wild-type NK1 receptor. These results suggest that the consensus sequence between receptor and antibody is involved in binding to the common core element of tachykinins. In addition, they further refine the "address-message" model for interaction of tachykinins with their receptors. It predicts that the common C-terminal half (message) of tachykinins interacts with subsites of the receptor that are common to all tachykinin receptors and plays a role in activation of the receptor, whereas the diverse N-terminus (address) interacts with sites that differ among different NK receptor subtypes and provide the molecular basis for selectivity. Address and message parts of tachykinins do not bind independently of each other to their respective receptor binding sites, but binding of the N-terminal half constrains the degree of freedom of the C-terminal half.

As long as attempts to crystallize G-protein-coupled receptors do not succeed, diverse molecular and biochemical approaches will have to contribute to refine our understanding of agonist and antagonist interactions with peptide receptors and to move us closer to rational drug design and new powerful therapeutic options.

Receptor Modifications: Splice Variants and Proteolytic Cleavage

For many neuropeptides multiple receptors are products of different genes. Another form of receptor heterogeneity is the modification of a single gene product to produce receptor subtypes. This may be achieved in many ways, including alternative splicing of the gene and proteolytic cleavage of the receptor protein.

Splice variants have been described for several neuropeptide receptors in which a single gene is alternately spliced to form several forms of mRNA and thus several receptor proteins. Two forms of the human gastrin/cholecystokinin B receptor, which differed by the presence or absence of a pentapeptide sequence in the third intracellular loop, were reported to arise by differential splicing.[54] A truncated form of the cholecystokinin. A receptor was identified in rat pancreas by photoaffinity labeling, which may represent a splice variant or a cleaved receptor.[55] Five splice variants of rat pituitary adenylyl cyclase–activating peptide (PACAP) receptor were identified with insertions in the third intracellular loop.[56] The functional significance of such splice variants is unknown. However, domains in the third intracellular loop are important for G-protein coupling, and the PACAP splice variants showed altered patterns of adenylyl cyclase and phospholipase C activation, suggesting that splice variants signal differently.

Proteolytic cleavage also modifies G-protein-coupled receptors. Many single transmembrane domain receptors are shed from the plasma membrane by proteolytic cleavage close to the cell surface. This forms a soluble receptor that may act as a receptor antagonist by mopping up ligand in the extracellular fluid. Far less is known about cleavage of seven transmembrane receptors. Cleavage of these receptors may cause inactivation and contribute to downregulation of cellular responses to peptides. The renal vasopressin V_2 receptor, with an apparent molecular weight of 58,000, was found to be cleaved by a metalloproteinase in the plasma membrane to a fragment of 30,000.[57] Cleavage occurred between the Gln[92] and Val[93] residues of the second transmembrane domain, close to the extracellular agonist binding site. Remarkably, cleavage occurred rapidly only when the receptor was occupied by ligand, and, as expected, cleavage resulted in a loss of ligand binding. Cleavage may inactivate the receptor and contribute to downregulation of cellular responses, whereas splice variants may show altered intracellular signaling. It will be important to determine if other receptors are cleaved by cell-surface proteinases in an agonist-dependent manner, to identify the enzymes involved, and to determine if proteolysis is a general mechanism of downregulation.

Multiple Affinity States

A single neuropeptide can interact with multiple receptors with varying affinities. For example, the order of affinity of the tachykinin receptors for substance P is NK1 > NK2 > NK3. Another layer of complexity is the observation that a single receptor molecule can exist in multiple affinity states. This is best exemplified by the cholecystokinin A and B receptors, which exist in high-affinity, low-affinity, and very low–affinity states with respect to binding their natural ligands, cholecystokinin-8, and gastrin.[58] This is physiologically important because the ability of a receptor to interact with its ligand will be determined by the affinity state of the receptor. Therefore, it is important to understand the factors responsible for conversion of one affinity state to another because they will govern how a cell responds to a receptor agonist.

The three affinity states of the cholecystokinin A and B receptors have been identified by ligand binding experiments using labeled agonists and antagonists capable of interacting with the different states of the receptors.[58, 59] The ability of the cholecystokinin A receptor to exist in these states is an intrinsic property of the receptor because the three states were observed in cells transfected with cDNA encoding the receptor and in pancreatic acini, which naturally express the cholecystokinin A receptor.[59] The very low–affinity state of the cholecystokinin A receptor predominated in both transfected cells and pancreatic acini. Thus, in pancreatic acini only 1% of receptors were found in high-affinity state (K_d for cholecystokinin-8 = 985pM), 19% in a low-affinity state (K_d for cholecystokinin-8 = 30nM), and 80% in a very low affinity state (K_d for cholecystokinin-8 = 13μM). Furthermore, each state of the cholecystokinin A receptor in pancreatic acini had a characteristic spectrum of affinities for various agonists and antagonists. For example, the high-affinity state interacted with cholecystokinin-8 with high affinity, whereas gastrin had a 100-fold lower affinity than cholecystokinin-8 for this state.

What is the possible physiologic relevance of multiple affinity states of a single receptor? Under physiologic circumstances cholecystokinin-8 would be at high enough concentrations to interact with only the high- and the low-affinity states of the cholecystokinin A receptor. In addition, the different states of the cholecystokinin A receptor are functionally coupled to different transduction pathways in pancreatic acini.[60] Occupation of low-affinity receptors caused stimulation of enzyme secretion, oscillations in $[Ca^{2+}]_i$, and increased diacylglycerol formation. Occupation of the very low–affinity receptors inhibited enzyme secretion and caused a large, transient increase in $[Ca^{2+}]_i$. As yet there is no known action of cholecystokinin that is mediated by the high-affinity state of the cholecystokinin A receptor, although the tools are available to address this issue because treatment with carbachol abolishes the high-affinity state of the cholecystokinin receptor. Thus, actions of cholecystokinin-8 that persist in carbachol-treated acini cannot be attributed to the high-affinity state.

Alterations in the proportion of cholecystokinin A receptors in a particular affinity state will govern how a cell responds to cholecystokinin and are thus physiologically important. Indeed, these proportions are physiologically regulated in pancreatic acini. For example, carbachol, bombesin, secretin, and vasoactive intestinal peptide (VIP), each with distinct receptors on pancreatic acini, affected binding of cholecystokinin-8 to acini.[61] Carbachol, secretin, and VIP inhibited high-affinity binding, whereas bombesin inhibited both high- and low-affinity binding. Binding was also affected by activation of protein kinase C, which inhibited the high-affinity state, and activation of G-proteins with NaF, which affected high- and low-affinity states. Interaction with the high-affinity state was also inhibited by some agents that interfere with microtubules. Exactly how these agents alter the affinity state and what specific chemical factors are responsible for the existence of these states are unknown.

New Models of Ligand-Receptor Interaction

A central issue of pharmacology is the interaction of receptors with agonists and antagonists. In the classical model, receptors are inactive when they are unoccupied by agonist. Agonist binding to an extracellular domain of a 7 transmembrane domain receptor somehow activates the receptor, permitting its interaction with G-proteins and triggering a biologic response. Almost nothing is known about how agonist binding allows G-protein coupling. However, peptide fragments of intracellular receptor domains can bind and stimulate G-proteins in vitro. This suggests that the receptor is physically incapable of binding to G-proteins until it interacts with an agonist, which causes an allosteric transition and initiates signal transduction. A partial agonist is a compound that binds the receptor but is less efficacious than a full agonist in eliciting a biologic response. A competitive antagonist binds to a receptor in a reversible manner but fails to activate the receptor. The agonist and antagonist are presumed to compete with a single class of receptors, and the antagonist has no biologic effects on the tissue. These simple concepts have been invaluable to our understanding of the actions between hormones and neurotransmitters with their receptors.

A basic principal of molecular pharmacology is that agonists but not antagonists bind and stabilize active conformations of receptors. This has led to the ternary

Moving?

I'd like to receive my *Current Gastroenterology* without interruption.
Please not the following change of address, effective:

Name: _____

New Address: _____

_____

City: _____ State: _____ Zip: _____

Old Address: _____

_____

City: _____ State: _____ Zip: _____

Reservation Card

Yes, I would like my own copy of *Current Gastroenterology*. Please begin my subscription with the current edition according to the terms described below.* I understand that I will have 30 days to examine each annual edition. If satisfied, I will pay just $80.95 plus sales tax, postage and handling (price subject to change without notice).

Name: _____

Address: _____

City: _____ State: _____ Zip: _____

Method of Payment
○ Visa   ○ Mastercard   ○ AmEx   ○ Bill me   ○ Check (in US dollars, payable to Mosby, Inc.)

Card number: _____ Exp date: _____

Signature: _____

ls-0909

*Your *Current* Service Guarantee:

When you subscribe to *Current*, we'll send you an advance notice of future volumes about two months before they publish. This automatic notice system is designed to take up as little of your time as possible. If you do not want *Current*, the advance notice makes it quick and easy for you to let us know your decision, and you will always have at least 20 days to decide. If we don't hear from you, we'll send you the new volume as soon as it's available. And, of course, *Current* is yours to examine free of charge for 30 days (postage, handling and applicable sales tax are added to each shipment.).

BUSINESS REPLY MAIL
FIRST CLASS MAIL   PERMIT No. 762   CHICAGO, IL

POSTAGE WILL BE PAID BY ADDRESSEE

Chris Hughes
Mosby-Year Book, Inc.
200 N. LaSalle Street
Suite 2600
Chicago, IL 60601-9981

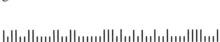

BUSINESS REPLY MAIL
FIRST CLASS MAIL   PERMIT No. 762   CHICAGO, IL

POSTAGE WILL BE PAID BY ADDRESSEE

Chris Hughes
Mosby-Year Book, Inc.
200 N. LaSalle Street
Suite 2600
Chicago, IL 60601-9981

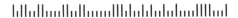

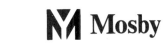

M Mosby
Dedicated to publishing excellence

model of receptor activation, in which the active form of the receptor is a complex of the hormone, the receptor, and a G-protein.[62–64] However, a new model of receptor activation, the allosteric ternary or two-state model has been developed to describe results obtained with constitutively active receptors and of experiments in which wild-type receptors are overexpressed.

Point mutations in the third intracellular loop of β_2-adrenergic receptors and peptide receptors have been described that result in constitutive activation-signaling even in the absence of agonist. The basal signaling activity of these receptors is greatly enhanced to levels normally observed only after full stimulation of the wild-type receptor with agonist. Presumably these mutations result in a conformational change in the receptor that mimics that seen after agonist binding to the wild-type receptor. In addition, overexpression of wild-type β_2-adrenergic receptors in cultured cells and in transgenic animals results in activation in the absence of agonist. For example, the hearts from transgenic mice in which the β_2-adrenergic receptor is overexpressed by 200-fold behave as if they are being maximally stimulated even in the absence of an agonist.[63, 64] Together, the observations made on constitutively active receptors and the overexpressing wild-type receptors indicate that unoccupied receptors can exist in an active form. Thus, G-protein-coupled receptors may exist in equilibrium between an inactive conformation (R) and a spontaneously active conformation (R*), which is able to couple to G-proteins in the absence of agonist (Fig 2). In this model, agonists do not activate receptors. Rather, they bind to already activated receptors, and their agonist activity is caused by an alteration in the equilibrium between inactive and active receptors. Some ligands previously classified as competitive antagonists are capable of switching off spontaneously active β_2-adrenergic receptors overexpressed in the heart. These compounds are now termed "inverse agonists," which bind inactive receptors, pulling the equilibrium from activated to inactivated receptors. Competitive antagonists bind to both receptor states with equal affinity and do not disturb the equilibrium. If correct, the terms agonist and antagonist may no longer be applicable; they are simply ligands that bind to active or inactive forms of a receptor. Results of experiments with agonists and antagonists of neuropeptide receptors may require reinterpretation in light of this two-stage model of receptor-ligand interactions.

Signal Transduction by G-Proteins

The heterotrimeric G-proteins, which are composed of α, β, and γ subunits, are the molecular switches for signal transduction (Fig 3). In the inactive state, the α subunit binds to GDP, and all three subunits are associated as α-GDP.$\beta\gamma$. Agonist binding to a seven transmembrane domain receptor is thought to cause a conformational change in the receptor that allows it to interact with the G-proteins. This interaction catalyzes the release of GDP from the guanine-nucleotide-binding site of G_α. Now GTP binds to this site, triggering dissociation of G_α from $G_{\beta\gamma}$ and

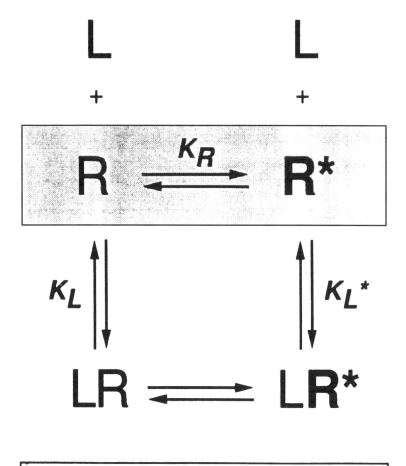

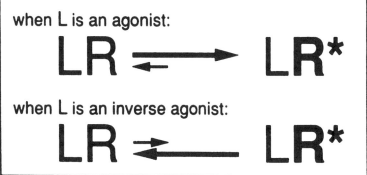

FIGURE 2.
Two-state model of receptor activation depicting the receptor in an inactive *(R)* and active *(R*)* conformation. L = ligand; K_R = equilibrium constant for distribution of receptor between R and R^*; K_L and K_L^* = equilibrium constants for ligand at the two receptor states. (From Bond RA, Leff P, Johnson TD, et al: *Nature* 374:272–276, 1995. Used by permission.)

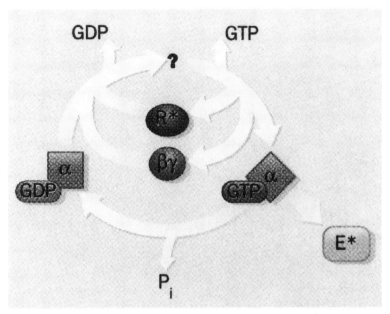

FIGURE 3.
Guanosine triphosphatase (GTPase) cycle of a trimeric G-protein. After the guanosine diphosphate (GDP)–bound form of G_α bind to $G_{\beta\gamma}$, an activated receptor R* triggers dissociation of GDP; GTP binds, and then receptor and $G_{\beta\gamma}$ dissociate from G_α, which can activate an effector E*. Hydrolysis of GTP converts α.GTP back to α.GDP, and the cycle repeats. (From Bourne HR: *Nature* 369:611–612, 1994. Used by permission.)

from the receptor. The dissociated G_α and $G_{\beta\gamma}$ subunits are now free to stimulate effector molecules such as enzymes and channels. This cycle is reversed when G_α hydrolyzes the bound GTP and returns to its inactive state as α-GDP.$\beta\gamma$. How does a ligand binding to its receptor trigger the molecular switch (the G-protein) for the signaling cascade?

It is not known how ligand binding alters the conformation of a receptor molecule and allows it to interact with and activate G-proteins, a central issue in signal transduction. However, through a combination of genetic mutation, biochemical analysis, and protein crystallography, we are beginning to understand how the G-protein switch is activated and inactivated during signal transduction. The crystal structure of the α-subunit ($G_{t\alpha}$ or $G_{\alpha t}$) of the trimeric G-protein for retinal transducin has been described both when it is inactive and bound to GDP and when it is activated and bound to GTP.[65–68] (The analogue GTP-γS was used as it resists hydrolysis.) The GTPase domain of $G_{t\alpha}$ is similar to that of other GTPases, composed of β-sheets and α-helices. A second domain, which is conserved in other G_α molecules but not found in other GTPases and is composed of α-helices, appears to be crucial in turning the protein on (GDP release and GTP binding) and off (GTP hydrolysis). The GTPase core and the helical domain surround the bound guanine nucleotide. The helical domain hinges to restrict movement to and from the

GTPase domain. Thus, receptor activation must flip open the helical domain, possibly by weakening hydrogen bonds and van der Waals forces that connect these two domains, allowing GTP to replace GDP and thereby initiate the signaling event. How does binding to GTP allow $G_{t\alpha}$ to dissociate from $G_{\beta\gamma}$ and stimulate effector molecules? When $G_{t\alpha}$ is bound to GTP, there are structural changes in three regions of the protein (designated switch I, II, and III), forming a hump across the face of the molecule. $G_{\beta\gamma}$ interacts with residues in or close to the switch II domain of $G_{t\alpha}$, suggesting that conformational changes in this region trigger dissociation of $G_{t\alpha}$ and $G_{\beta\gamma}$. Presumably alterations in the conformation of $G_{t\alpha}$ after binding GTP also allow it to stimulate effector molecules, although mutational experiments have identified residues outside the switch regions as important for activating effectors. Unfortunately, these structures of activated and inactivated $G_{t\alpha}$ do not provide information about how G_{α} and $G_{\beta\gamma}$ interact with the activated receptor molecule. Binding of GTP to G_{α} is important because it triggers dissociation of the receptor from the G-proteins, allowing the receptor to bind to and activate other G-proteins and thereby amplify the extracellular signal.

Although most of the progress in this area has focused on G-proteins that couple to rhodopsin, it is likely that much of this information will be directly applicable to the neuropeptide receptors.

Turning off the Signal: Desensitization of G-Protein-Coupled Receptors

A common feature of cellular responses to agonists of G-protein-coupled receptors is that they are short lived even in the continued presence of agonist and that repeated application of agonist results in an attenuation or desensitization of the signal. It is important to understand these mechanisms because they prevent the uncontrolled stimulation of cells, which may otherwise lead to disease. Mechanisms of desensitization have been most thoroughly studied for rhodopsin and the β_2-adrenergic receptor, although similar mechanisms almost certainly exist for the neuropeptide receptors.[69] The β_2-adrenergic receptor desensitizes by agonist-dependent phosphorylation. Agonist binding promotes phosphorylation of the receptor by G-protein receptor kinases 2 and 3 (formerly called β-adrenergic receptor kinases 1 and 2).[70, 71] This permits binding of the β-arrestins 1 and 2, which interdicts interaction with G-proteins and thus turns off the signal. Reversal of this pathway would then permit resensitization of the receptor. The β_2-adrenergic receptor is rapidly internalized after ligand binding. This may contribute to desensitization by depleting the cell surface of receptors available to bind hydrophilic ligands in the extracellular fluid. However, internalization is not the mechanism of rapid receptor desensitization, because desensitization persists if internalization is inhibited. However, resensitization does require internalization of the receptor and recycling to the plasma membrane, suggesting that the receptor is dephosphorylated in endosomes.

Ligand-induced internalization and recycling of the NK1 receptor has been directly observed in transfected cell lines and in vivo by using specific receptor antibodies, highly fluorescent peptides, and confocal microscopy.[72–76] In transfected rat kidney epithelial cells (KNRK), the NK1 receptor is confined to the plasma membrane with minimal intracellular stores. Within minutes of interacting with substance P at 37°C, the peptide and its receptor are internalized into the same superficial vesicles, and surface labeling is markedly reduced (Fig 4). The first-formed vesicles are labeled with a clathrin antibody, and inhibitors of clathrin-mediated endocytosis inhibit the internalization of substance P and the NK1 receptor, indicating that endocytosis is mediated by clathrin. The vesicles containing substance P and the NK1 receptor are early endosomes because they also contain the transferrin receptor, a well-known recycling receptor. Endosomes containing substance P and the NK1 receptor move to a perinuclear region, where the ligand and receptor are sorted into different compartments. Substance P enters prelysosomes and lysosomes, where it is degraded. In contrast, NK1 receptor reappears at the plasma membrane. This is because of recycling of the receptor rather than trafficking of newly synthesized receptors to the plasma membrane because the reappearance is unaffected by the protein synthesis inhibitor cycloheximide. Sorting of the NK1 receptor and substance P into recycling and degradative compartments requires endosomal acidification because receptor recycling and substance P degradation are inhibited by acidotropic agents, including bafilomycin A1, an inhibitor of vacuolar H^+–adenosine triphosphatase (ATPase). The gastrin-releasing peptide receptor is similarly internalized in transfected KNRK cells by a clathrin-dependent mechanism. However, it recycles fourfold more quickly than the NK1 receptor expressed in the same cell line.[77] The cholecystokinin A receptor is rapidly internalized in CHO cells and also recycles.[78] However, in these cells a portion of the receptor is internalized by a caveolin-dependent mechanism in addition to a clathrin-mediated mechanism. The functional implications of these two different routes of internalization is unknown.

There is considerable interest in identifying domains of G-protein-coupled receptors that interact with components of the clathrin or caveolin endocytosis machinery. This has been studied in detail for several single transmembrane domain receptors but far less is known about receptors with seven transmembrane regions. A sequence, Asn-Pro-X-X-Tyr, which is found in the seventh transmembrane domain of most G-protein-coupled receptors and resembles internalization motifs of single transmembrane receptors, is important for endocytosis of the β_2-adrenergic receptor.[79] Although mutation of the Tyr to Phe reduces internalization of the NK1 receptor, it has no effect on internalization of the gastrin-releasing peptide receptor.[80] Therefore, highly conserved motifs may function differently in different receptors. The carboxyl-tail also contains regions that are required for endocytosis of receptors. For example, deletion of portions of the tail of the parathyroid hormone receptor reduce internalization.[81] Remarkably this receptor also contains motifs in the tail that inhibit endocytosis because mutation of Glu-Val-Gln to Ala-Ala-Ala accelerated internalization by 40%. Thus, there are positive and negative signals for internalization of certain receptors.

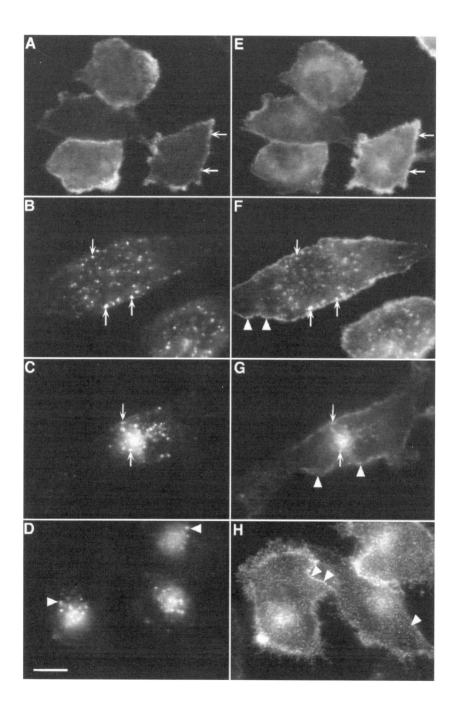

Observations of endocytosis in transfected cells could be artifacts of overexpression of receptors or unique to the chosen cell type. Therefore, it is important to study cells that naturally express peptide receptors. Intravenous injection of substance P into rats induces rapid internalization of the NK1 receptor by endothelial cells of postcapillary venules in the tracheal mucosa.[74] Here, as in transfected cells, internalization and recycling are correlated with desensitization and resensitization of cellular responses to substance P. Substance P also causes internalization of the receptor by neurons in the enteric nervous system and the central nervous system.[82]

Newly Characterized Receptors

The discovery of novel receptors offers new insights into control mechanisms. Of particular interest is the recent discovery of a receptor for the Gly-extended form of gastrin. Peptide α-amidation is necessary to produce many active peptides from their Gly-extended precursors. It is well established that only amidated gastrin stimulates gastric acid secretion. However, Gly-gastrin is also secreted with amidated gastrin, and both forms of the peptide were found to stimulate proliferation of the pancreatic tumor cell line AR4-2J.[83] The effects of amidated gastrin but not Gly-gastrin were inhibited by cholecystokinin/gastrin B receptors (Fig 5). This suggests that Gly-gastrin exerts its effects by interacting with a receptor that is distinct from the cholecystokinin/gastrin B receptor. We await the molecular cloning of this receptor. It is not known if there are receptors for Gly-extended forms of other regulatory peptides.

INVESTIGATIONS OF THE ROLE OF PEPTIDES IN DISEASE

Abnormalities in expression of peptides, their receptors, or other regulatory components may contribute to the etiology of several gastrointestinal diseases. In ad-

---

FIGURE 4.
Simultaneous detection of cy3-SP *(left panels)* and NK1-R immunoreactivity *(right panels)* in KNRK Flag NK1-R cells at various times after warming to 37°C. Cells were incubated with 100-nM cy3-SP for 60 minutes at 4°C, washed, and incubated in SP-free medium at 37°C for 0 minute (**A** and **E**), 10 minutes (**B** and **F**), 30 minutes (**C** and **G**) or 120 minutes (**D** and **H**). Cells were fixed and incubated with the NK1-R antibody and a FITC-labeled secondary antibody. Note the colocalization *(arrows)* of cy3-SP and NK1-R immunoreactivity at 0, 10, and 30 minutes after warming. By 120 minutes cy3-SP and NK1-R immunoreactivity are in different cellular compartments *(arrowheads)*. Scale bar = 10 μm. (Reproduced from *Molecular Biology of the Cell*, 1995, vol 6, pp 509-524 by copyright permission of the American Society for Cell Biology. Grady EF, Garland AG, Gamp PD, et al: *Mol Biol Cell* 6:509–524, 1995.)

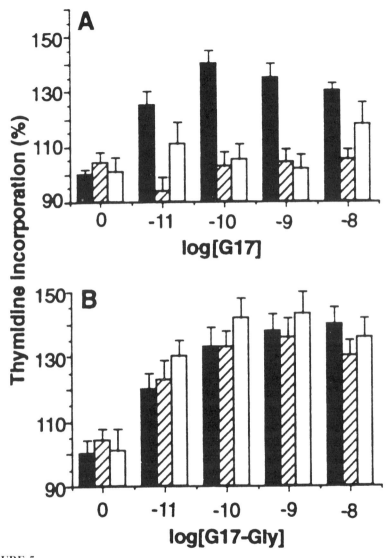

FIGURE 5.
Effects of gastrin/cholecystokinin B receptor antagonists L365260 and PD-134308 on incorporation of [³H]thymidine stimulated by (**A**) gastrin-17 and (**B**) Gly-extended gastrin-17 in AR4-2J cells. Cells were treated with either gastrin-17 or Gly-gastrin-17 alone *(black bars)* in the presence of L365260 (100nM, *hatched bars*) or PD-134308 (100nM, *white bars*). Results are expressed as a percent of control, unstimulated incorporation. Mean ± SE, n = 6 experiments in triplicate. (Reprinted with permission from Seva C, Dickinson CJ, Yamada T: Growth-promoting effects of glycine-extended progastrin. *Science* 265:410–412, 1994. Copyright 1994, American Association for the Advancement of Science.)

dition, agonists and antagonists of neuropeptide receptors may be used for imaging tumors that express these receptors and as therapeutic agents.

Gastrointestinal Peptides and Their Receptors in Tumor Imaging

There are several pharmacokinetic advantages to using small biologically active peptides rather than much larger antibodies or antibody fragments for tumor imaging: (1) the affinity of peptides for their receptors is significantly greater than that of monovalent antibody fragments, (2) peptides display a high target-to-background ratio, and (3) peptides are rapidly cleared.[84] A wide variety of malignant human tumor cell lines and human primary tumors overexpress high-affinity peptide receptors that can be identified using radioligands.[85]

Somatostatin as Prototype for a Peptide-Based Radiopharmaceutical

Somatostatin and its synthetic analogue octreotide, which is more resistant to degradation, are prototypes for a peptide-based radiopharmaceutical since the initial use of iodine [123]Tyr-3-octreotide for in vivo imaging of endocrine tumors in 1990. Recently the improved indium [111]labeled octreotide analogue, pentetreotide, has been used to localize metastatic gastroenteropancreatic neuroendocrine tumors, which are often difficult to visualize using other methods.[86, 87] The value of somatostatin-receptor scintigraphy (SRS) for visualization of those tumors was compared with conventional radiologic techniques. ^{111}In-pentetreotide scintigraphy detected tumor tissue not seen by computed tomography (CT), magnetic resonance imaging, and ultrasonography in 16 of 40 patients (40%). The study was extended to 74 patients, and the results of SRS for 60 were positive, indicating that about 20% of patients with endocrine tumors of the gastroenteropancreatic system will be negative by this imaging procedure. Tumors negative by SRS were mainly insulinomas and nonfunctional tumors. The resolution of SRS was excellent with lesions smaller than 5 mm detected in some cases. Overall, the sensitivity for tumors larger than 2 cm was approximately 90%, and it decreased to about 50% when tumors were smaller than 2 cm. Thus, because SRS allows imaging of the whole body with a single procedure, it is a very effective method of localizing and staging neuroendocrine tumors of the gastroenteropancreatic system. A smaller study came to similarly favorable results, with SRS displaying a considerably higher sensitivity compared with conventional radiologic methods (91% vs. 68%) in a series of histologically proved lesions.[88] Although prospective studies are needed to prove that SRS has actually a beneficial impact on patient outcome, it certainly has the promise to do so. The added sensitivity compared with conventional radiologic methods should result in a higher cure rate from surgery with curative intent and enable the physician to make better therapeutic decisions. In addition, SRS defines the somatostatin receptor status of the tumor, which has therapeutic implications on whether to expect the tumor to respond to octreotide therapy.

Somatostatin-receptor scintigraphy has also been evaluated and found to be a promising diagnostic tool in patients with neuroblastoma, lymphoma, and recurrent medullary carcinoma of the thyroid gland.[89–93] Somatostatin receptor imaging has also been tested for inflammatory conditions, including rheumatoid arthritis and acute infectious disease.[94, 95]

Future Developments in Somatostatin-Based Radiopharmaceuticals

One future direction is the development of somatostatin analogues selective for the five cloned receptor subtypes. The well-characterized analogues octreotide (SMS201-995, Sandostatin), somatuline (BIM 23014), and vapreotide (RC-160), although having slightly different profiles, are very similar in that they bind subtypes 2 and 5 with high affinity, subtype 3 with moderate affinity, and subtypes 1 and 4 with low affinity. Subtype-specific radioligands would allow use of SRS for tumors that cannot be detected with octreotide. Earlier reports of the development of subtype-selective somatostatin analogues[96] have been cautioned by a study in which 32 synthetic somatostatin analogues were tested.[97] Relative selectivity was achieved only for subtype 2 with compounds DC23-60 and EC5-21 at modest levels of 19- and 35-fold preference for this subtype compared with the four other subtypes. Another compound, NC8–12, demonstrated a high degree of selectivity for subtypes 2 and 3 compared with the other three subtypes. The study identified some structural features of somatostatin agonists that contribute to subtype selective binding properties.

Studies to determine the regions in the somatostatin receptor subtypes responsible for agonist selectivity and affinity will help in rational drug design. The two natural somatostatins, somatostatin-14 and somatostatin-28, have similar binding affinities to receptor subtypes 1 and 2, whereas many synthetic analogues, including MK-678, bind subtype 2 with much higher affinity (IC_{50} = 0.1nM) than subtype 1 (IC_{50} > 1mM). Chimeric receptors, formed from two receptors with different binding characteristics, are often generated to define binding domains for agonists and antagonists. A series of somatostatin receptor chimeras were created in which increasing portions of the mouse somatostatin receptor subtypes 1 and 2 were exchanged and transfected into HEK293 cells.[98] The results showed that receptor determinants responsible for MK-678 specificity reside in regions located in the second and third extracellular loops.

Radiolabeled octreotide has recently been evaluated as a radiotherapeutic agent.[99, 100] The rapid plasma clearance of radiolabeled peptides promises a much lower total body irradiation than treatment with radiolabeled antibodies and therefore a very localized and specific therapeutic irradiation of somatostatin-positive tumors. This therapeutic approach may be especially useful for somatostatin-positive tumors, which do not respond to octreotide treatment, and for widely disseminated unresectable disease, which is currently treated by systemic chemotherapy or conventional radiotherapy.

Vasoactive Intestinal Peptide Receptor Imaging

Vasoactive intestinal peptide is the second gastrointestinal hormone to be used for scintigraphic tumor imaging.[101] High-affinity receptors for VIP have been demonstrated in gastric, pancreatic, and colonic carcinomas, small cell lung carcinomas, carcinoid tumors, insulinomas, and lymphomas.[85, 101] Synthetic VIP was labeled with ^{123}I, high-power liquid chromatography (HPLC) purified and administered as a single injection to 79 patients. The fall in blood pressure due to the vasodilating effect of VIP was mild and transient. No other side effects were noted. Primary or recurrent tumor, organ or lymph node metastases were detected in 31 of 35 patients with colorectal adenocarcinomas (89%), in 17 of 19 patients with pancreatic adenocarcinomas (89%), in 8 of 8 patients with gastric adenocarcinomas (100%), in 13 of 16 patients with intestinal carcinoid tumors (81%), and in 4 of 4 patients with insulinomas (100%). The VIP scan was able to detect endocrine tumor lesions less than 2 cm in diameter. Vasoactive intestinal peptide receptor scanning was superior to CT scanning in patients with small carcinoid tumors: CT scanning detected tumors in only 2 of 10 patients, whereas VIP receptor scanning was positive in 9 of 10 patients. In 38 patients the results with the VIP receptor scan were directly compared with octreotide scans. The results were similar for carcinoid tumors and, surprisingly, for insulinomas, but the VIP receptor scan offered a considerable advantage in colonic and pancreatic adenocarcinomas. No positive VIP receptor scans were seen in 16 patients where the primary tumors had been resected, and no metastases were known.

In the near future other radiolabeled gastrointestinal peptides such as substance P and bombesin will become available, with the promise to further open new diagnostic and therapeutic dimensions.[93]

Gastrointestinal Peptides in the Treatment of Cancer

Somatostatin in the Treatment of Endocrine and Epithelial Tumors

Gastrointestinal hormones and neuropeptides control the proliferation of normal gastrointestinal mucosa and affect the growth of both gastrointestinal and extragastrointestinal tumors.[102, 103] Again, it is somatostatin, with its inhibitory effect on endocrine and exocrine secretions, as well as tumor cell growth, that leads the way for a therapeutic use of gastrointestinal peptides. Octreotide has been used for several nonmalignant conditions, including pituitary hypersecretion (especially acromegaly), polycystic ovary, variceal bleeding, gastrointestinal fistulas, and diarrhea.[104]

A study published in 1986 demonstrated that octreotide markedly improved the severe symptoms of patients with functional carcinoid and islet tumors, which were refractory to most treatments.[105] The drug was approved for controlling the symptoms caused by excessive hormone secretion in those malignancies in 1988. However, whether octreotide was also able to exert antiproliferative actions on such tumors remained controversial. A prospective multicenter study including 47 patients with endocrine gastroenteropancreatic tumors addressed this issue.[106] The patients demonstrated CT-documented tumor progression within a preobservation period of 3 to 6 months. After treatment with octreotide, 40% of the patients experienced stabilization of tumor growth. Stable disease continued in 25% of patients by month 12 and in 13% of patients by month 36. No tumor regressions occurred. Preliminary studies indicate that a combination of octreotide with interferon-α might improve these results.[106]

The importance of identifying subtypes of the somatostatin receptor for effective treatment of endocrine tumors by octreotide was highlighted by a recent study.[107] Receptor subtypes on two glucagonomas, four insulinomas, three pheochromocytomas, and one carcinoid were determined by reverse transcriptase polymerase chain reaction (PCR). Octreotide binds with highest affinity to type 2 somatostatin receptor. The glucagonoma, which expressed this subtype, responded to octreotide therapy. However, the carcinoid, which did not express this subtype, was unresponsive to octreotide therapy.

Although several studies have demonstrated that octreotide is able to inhibit growth of gastrointestinal carcinomas in vitro and in vivo, the results of many early clinical trials have been disappointing. One recent randomized trial compared octreotide with the best supportive care in 107 patients with advanced gastrointestinal cancer who were refractory to chemotherapy, using survival duration as the primary end point.[108] Patients treated with octreotide (15 stomach, 16 pancreas, and 24 colon and rectum carcinomas) had a significantly longer medium survival time (20 weeks) than the controls (11 weeks). Forty-five percent of patients given octreotide had stable disease compared with only 15% in the control group. The contradiction with earlier studies may be explained by the lower octreotide dose and the differing end points (response rate or survival) used in previous trials. However, a separate trial with octreotide in 24 patients with advanced hormonal-refractory prostatic cancer led to the conclusion that octreotide accelerated tumor growth.[109] Among 20 patients who could be evaluated, 12 developed new osseous and 4 new visceral metastases. Differences in outcome may be related to the dose of octreotide and the location and characteristics of the tumor.

Mechanisms of Growth Inhibition by Somatostatin

Both direct and indirect mechanisms have been postulated to explain the anticancer effects of somatostatin analogues. Direct growth inhibition may be exerted by stimulating signal transduction pathways that negatively control cell growth. Somatostatin analogues may also inhibit proliferation indirectly by downregulating stimuli of tumor growth, such as hormones and growth factors, or by affecting angiogenesis.

It has been reported that somatostatin mediates its actions on growth by interacting with a pertussis toxin–sensitive guanosine triphosphate (GTP)–binding protein (G_i) to inhibit adenylyl cyclase and activate phosphotyrosine phosphatases.[102] The role of phosphotyrosine phosphatases in somatostatin action has been further expanded in several studies. In rats, octreotide treatment rapidly induced pancreatic tyrosine phosphatase activity at the basolateral membrane but not in zymogen granules.[102, 110] In contrast, pancreatic tyrosine kinase activity was reduced by octreotide. This is the first in vivo demonstration of tyrosine phosphatase induction by somatostatin or an analogue.

Several groups have studied cells transfected with somatostatin receptor subtypes or tumor cell lines naturally expressing somatostatin receptors to elucidate the second messenger pathways involved in somatostatin receptor activation. Some controversy emerges concerning second messenger pathways, even when the same cell line was used for transfections. For example, one group found that the somatostatin 1 receptor expressed in CHO cells was linked to increased tyrosine phosphatase activity and to inhibition of adenylyl cyclase.[111] In contrast, the somatostatin 2 receptor subtype was coupled only to the inhibition of adenylyl cyclase. Both pathways were sensitive to pertussis toxin. Another group reported that stimulation of the somatostatin 2 receptor expressed in CHO cells by RC-160 inhibited growth by inducing tyrosine phosphatase activity.[112] The growth response was inhibited by orthovanadate, a phosphatase inhibitor. The same group also examined the somatostatin 1 and 2 receptors expressed in Cos7 cells.[113] Here they found that the induction of tyrosine phosphatase activity by activation of the somatostatin 2 receptor was not pertussis toxin sensitive.

Pathways different from tyrosine kinase activation and adenylyl cyclase inhibition were reported for somatostatin 1, 4, and 5 receptors. Somatostatin-14 stimulated formation of 1,4,5-triphosphate formation in CHO cells expressing the somatostatin 1 receptor. This pathway was blocked by pertussis toxin.[114] The somatostatin 4 receptor was found to couple to arachonidate release and activation of the mitogen-activated protein kinase cascade in addition to adenylyl cyclase inhibition.[115] Activation of the somatostatin 5 receptor expressed in CHO cells by RC-160 inhibited cholecystokinin-stimulated intracellular Ca^{2+} mobilization, suggesting that the inositol phospholipid/calcium pathway could be involved in the antiproliferative effect.[112]

A tyrosine phosphatase was copurified with a somatostatin receptor from rat pancreatic acinar membranes by affinity chromatography using immobilized antibodies raised against the N-terminal portion of somatostatin-28.[116] The purified somatostatin receptor preparations exhibited an elevated tyrosine phosphatase activity that dephosphorylated phosphorylated epidermal growth factor receptor. The activity was inhibited by orthovanadate. A polyclonal antibody directed against the SH2 domain containing tyrosine phosphatase SHPTP1 identified a protein of 66 kD. The anti-SHPTP1 antibody also immunoprecipitated somatostatin receptors from both somatostatin-pretreated and untreated pancreatic membranes. These data indicate that a 66-kD tyrosine phosphatase related to SHPTP1 is associated with somatostatin receptors at the membrane level.

Downstream events leading to somatostatin-induced growth inhibition were examined on a cellular and molecular level. Octreotide was shown to exert a direct antiproliferative effect by inducing apoptosis.[117] Octreotide was added to cell cycle synchronized mouse pituitary AtT-20 tumor cells in the G1 or in the G2 phase. Apoptosis was induced and became manifest in the subsequent cell cycle. Apoptosis was not observed in cells that were arrested in the G1 or the G2 phase. Octreotide did not induce detectable apoptosis in unsynchronized cells, which remained predominantly in G1 phase.

The proto-oncogene c-*fos* is a member of a family of transcription factors that are known to be expressed within minutes of cell stimulation and are therefore called "early response genes." They appear to play a critical role in the cellular response to external stimuli. The regulatory DNA elements that control the expression of c-*fos* are under the control of both Ca^{2+} and cyclic adenosine monophosphate (cAMP) signaling pathways. The c-*fos* gene product interacts with another early response gene product c-*jun* to form the heterodimeric transcription factor AP-1 that binds to specific AP-1 binding sites in gene promoters. The effect of somatostatin on c-*fos* expression and binding of AP-1 to its specific DNA element has been examined.[118] In isolated gastric parietal cells and the GH_3 pituitary cell line, c-*fos* mRNA was increased by cAMP and Ca^{2+}-dependent signaling pathways. Octreotide inhibited this response significantly in a pertussis toxin–sensitive manner. Similarly AP-1 binding as assessed by gel shift assays was stimulated by activation of adenyl cyclase and serum and inhibited by octreotide. These results suggest that somatostatin may mediate its inhibitory action by inhibition of expression of early response genes by a pertussis sensitive pathway.

Blood vessels surrounding various human cancer tissue were examined for expression of somatostatin receptors.[119] High expression of somatostatin receptors was found on the smooth muscle layer of peritumoral veins of colon adenocarcinomas and to a lesser degree in malignant lymphomas and renal cell carcinomas. The tumor tissue itself was receptor negative in many cases. Indeed, the receptor status of peritumoral vessel and neoplastic tissue seemed almost to be reciprocal. Intestinal carcinoid tumors demonstrated high receptor levels, whereas the corresponding peritumoral veins expressed low or undetectable receptor levels. Vessels of normal human intestine or lymphatic organs expressed few receptors, suggesting that the massive overexpression of receptors is a tumor-induced host response. However, high levels of somatostatin receptors were detected in vessels from nonmalignant diseases such as inflammatory bowel disease, lymphadenopathy, and granulomatous disease, including tuberculosis.[120] It is therefore likely that high-level expression of receptors for the vasoconstrictive peptide somatostatin is a general defense mechanism.

Development of Other Peptide Receptor Agonists/Antagonists for Tumor Therapy

Somatostatin is unique among gastrointestinal peptides because it inhibits growth. Many other peptides stimulate growth. Here, antagonists must be developed so that autocrine or paracrine growth loops can be interrupted. For example, a bombesin/gastrin–releasing peptide antagonist RC-3095 has now been demonstrated to inhibit the growth of MKN45 human gastric xenografts in nude mice.[121]

Role of Gastrointestinal Peptides in Inflammatory Bowel Disease

Anatomic and physiologic studies of neurons with cell bodies located in dorsal root ganglia suggest that sensory neurons containing substance P and calcitonin gene-related peptide are involved in conveying nociceptive information to the spinal cord and in regulating the inflammatory and immune responses in the peripheral tissues they innervate. Thus, substance P released by a sensory neuron may signal tissue damage in the spinal cord and may participate in regulating the inflammation, immune responses, and wound healing in the affected peripheral tissue (for review, see Mantyh et al.[122]). Over the last 5 years it was established that the neurogenic inflammation mediated by sensory neurons and their neurotransmitters substance P and calcitonin gene-related peptide play an important role in inflammatory bowel disease. However, it is unclear whether these neuropeptides fuel the chronic inflammation or have a protective function on the intestine. Thus, we do not know if substance P receptor antagonists would be useful or harmful in the treatment of inflammatory bowel disease. This question was addressed in an experimental acute colitis model in rabbits.[123] The neurotoxin capsaicin was used to ablate sensory neurons before induction of inflammation in the colon. Capsaicin treatment reduced substance P and calcitonin gene-related peptide levels in dorsal root ganglia. The colitis was more severe in the capsaicin-treated group than in the control group. In both control animals and capsaicin-treated animals substance P and calcitonin gene-related peptide immunoreactivity was markedly decreased in inflamed tissue compared with uninflamed colon. These data suggest that neurotransmitters are released from sensory nerves during inflammation and that they have a protective effect in an acute colitis model.

Role of Gastrointestinal Peptides in Functional Bowel Disorders

Patients who have chronic abdominal pain or discomfort constitute up to 50% of the clientele seeking the care of a gastroenterologist. The symptoms share the mechanism of altered sensory perception of visceral sensations and may arise in the form of heartburn, chest pain, dyspepsia, bloating, abdominal cramps, and the sensation of incomplete rectal evacuation. Recent breakthroughs in the neurophysiology of somatic and visceral sensation suggest that chronic hyperalgesia in the human gastrointestinal tract results from the development of hyperexcitable neurons in the dorsal horn (for review, see Mayer and Gebhart[124]). These can develop in response to either peripheral tissue irritation or descending influences originating in the brain stem. The release of excitatory amino acids and the neuropeptides substance P and calcitonin gene-related peptide from the terminals of primary afferent fibers appears to play an important role in the development of central or spinal hyperexcitability.[124]

Role of Gastrointestinal Peptides in Obesity

Twenty percent of Western European and North American adults are affected by obesity, which may shorten life expectancy. Two different gastrointestinal peptides, which are also found in the brain, have been implicated in the regulation of food intake.

Neuropeptide Y

Neuropeptide Y stimulates feeding, reduces energy expenditure, and thus induces weight gain. Neuropeptide Y is synthesized in the arcuate nucleus, which projects neuropeptide Y–containing axons to the paraventricular nucleus of the hypothalamus. The receptors that mediate the effects of neuropeptide Y on feeding and energy metabolism are not fully characterized. Thus, a variant of the Y_1 receptor was postulated to mediate the stimulation of food intake, and an unidentified neuropeptide Y receptor was thought to be responsible for inhibition of brown fat thermogenesis. Advances in understanding the important role that neuropeptide Y plays in the control of energy balance in rodents make it a promising candidate for therapeutic exploitation.[125, 126]

Neuropeptide Y injection in the paraventricular nucleus of rats both downregulated the mRNA for the enzyme responsible for thermogenesis from brown fat and upregulated mRNA for the key white fat storage enzyme.[127] This underscores the critical role of neuropeptide Y in coordinating energy metabolism.

Hypothalamic neuropeptide Y mRNA and neuropeptide Y protein content were elevated in genetically obese rats (fa/fa-strain = Zucker rats).[128, 129] A longitudinal study showed that hypothalamic mRNA levels were normal in 13-day-old preobese fa/fa rats and increased in the 28-day-old rats, which display overt obesity. Intracerebroventricular neuropeptide Y administration to normal rats for 7 days produced a marked hyperphagia, increased body weight gain, increased basal insulinemia, and a much greater insulin response to meal feeding than that of controls. Neuropeptide Y administration also resulted in a marked increase in the in vivo insulin-stimulated glucose uptake by adipose tissue but in a marked decrease in uptake by different muscle types. The increased insulin-responsive glucose uptake was accompanied by increases in both the mRNA and the protein level of the insulin-dependent glucose-transporter GLUT4. In contrast, insulin resistance in the muscle tissue was not related to GLUT4 expression. When neuropeptide Y was discontinued, all abnormalities were normalized.[129] The hormonal-metabolic situation caused by neuropeptide Y administration resembled very closely the dynamic phase of the genetic obesity in the fa/fa strain, suggesting that neuropeptide Y could be of primary importance in obesity syndromes with incipient insulin resistance (non-insulin-dependent diabetes mellitus).

In both normal rats and Zucker rats, intracerebroventricular neuropeptide Y injections stimulated food intake in a dose-dependent manner.[130] However, the minimal effective dose was three to four times greater in the obese animals. Meal size, meal duration, and time spent eating increased significantly in the normal rats; the latter two parameters increased also in obese animals, although only with the highest dose. The obese Zucker rats were therefore less sensitive to neuropeptide Y than the lean ones. The changed eating behavior indicates that neuropeptide Y is able to overcome a potential satiety signal.

Cholecystokinin

Another peptide hormone linked to satiety is cholecystokinin. In contrast to neuropeptide Y, cholecystokinin is thought to exert its effect on satiety in the gastrointestinal tract. Cholecystokinin is secreted by cells in the duodenal epithelium in response to luminal lipid, peptides, and trypsin inhibitor. Intravenous infusion of cholecystokinin octapeptide significantly reduces food intake, and administration of cholecystokinin antagonists increases food intake in rats. Although it has been suggested that cholecystokinin sensitizes the stomach to distension by increasing vagal afferent activity, the mechanism of cholecystokinin action on satiety is not really understood.

Studies on the effect of both cholecystokinin and cholecystokinin antagonists in humans have produced controversial results.[131] Two closely related studies describe the effect of physiologic doses of cholecystokinin-33 on healthy obese and lean volunteers.[132, 133] Cholecystokinin reduced food intake, as well as subjective assessments of hunger, in both normal and obese subjects. These results suggest that physiologic levels of cholecystokinin induce satiety in humans.

CONCLUSION

Although many aspects of the function of regulatory peptides remain to be determined, recent advances in cell and molecular biology have provided new information about these signaling molecules. The genes for many peptides have been sequenced, and in some cases regulatory elements have been identified. Similarly, the receptors have been cloned for most peptides. Advances in molecular modeling of peptides and in structure-function analysis of receptors have allowed binding sites for receptor agonists and antagonists to be identified, which have facilitated the development of increasingly potent and specific ligands. Receptor agonists and antagonists have been widely used to define the physiologic functions of neuropeptides, and some have been used clinically.

What advances in our understanding on regulatory peptides can we expect in the future? Transgenic and gene knockout methods will permit the development of animals that either overexpress or lack a specific peptide, so that its role in development and normal physiology can be assessed. Gene knockout animals will also be developed for neuropeptide receptors, providing another strategy, in addition to using receptor antagonists, to examine the function of peptides. The pharmaceutical industry will continue to develop receptor antagonists and agonists with improved selectivity and potency for use as therapeutic agents and as tools for physiologic investigations. Our knowledge about mechanisms that regulate neuropeptide receptors and their interaction with signaling mechanisms will also advance. Information from these diverse areas will help us to understand the role of these fascinating molecules in health and disease states.

Acknowledgement

We would like to thank Dr. Adella Garland for insightful discussions.

REFERENCES

1. Rodrigo J, Pedrosa JA, Alvarez FJ, et al: Presence of calcitonin gene-related peptide in intraepithelial nerve fibers and motor end-plates of the cat esophagus: A light and electron microscopic study. *J Auton Nerv Syst* 49:21–31, 1994.

2. Herrera P-L, Huarte J, Zufferey R, et al: Ablation of islet endocrine cells by targeted expression of hormone-promoter-driven toxigenes. *Proc Natl Acad Sci USA* 91:12999–13003, 1994.

3. Lopez MJ, Upchurch BH, Rindi G, et al: Studies in transgenic mice reveal potential relationships between secretin-producing cells and other endocrine cell types. *J Biol Chem* 270:885–891, 1995.

4. Kirchgessner AL, Liu M-T, Gershon MD: NADPH diaphorase (nitric oxide synthase)–containing nerves in the enteropancreatic innervation: Sources, co-stored neuropeptides, and pancreatic function. *J Comp Neurol* 342:115–130, 1994.

5. Verchere CB, Kowalyk S, Shen GH, et al: Major species variation in the expression of galanin messenger ribonucleic acid in mammalian celic ganglion. *Endocrinology* 135:1052–1059, 1994.

6. Lan MS, Kajiyama W, Donadel G, et al: cDNA sequence and genomic organization of mouse secretin. *Biochem Biophys Res Commun* 200:1066–1071, 1994.

7. Mor A, Chartrel N, Vaudry H, et al: Skin peptide tyrosine-tyrosine, a member of the pancreatic polypeptide family: Isolation, structure, synthesis, and endocrine activity. *Proc Natl Acad Sci USA* 91:10295–10299, 1994.

8. Feany MB, Quinn WG: A neuropeptide gene defined by the *Drosophila* memory mutant *amnesiac*. *Science* 268:869–873, 1995.

9. Rokaeus A, Waschek JA: Primary sequence and functional analysis of the bovine galanin gene promoter in human neuroblastoma cells. *DNA Cell Biol* 13:845–855, 1994.

10. Anouar Y, MacArthur L, Cohen J, et al: Identification of a TPA-responsive element mediating preferential transactivation of the galanin gene promoter in chromaffin cells. *J Biol Chem* 269:6823–6831, 1994.

11. Kofler B, Evans HF, Liu ML, et al: Characterization of the 5'-flanking region of the human pre-progalanin gene. *DNA Cell Biol* 14:321–329, 1995.

12. Morrison CF, McAllister J, Dobson SP, et al: An activator element within the preprotachykinin-A promoter. *Mol Cell Neurosci* 5:165–175, 1994.

13. Minth-Worby CA: Transcriptional regulation of the human neuropeptide Y gene by nerve growth factor. *J Biol Chem* 269:15460–15468, 1994.

14. Mulderry PK: Neuropeptide expression by newborn and adult rat sensory neurons in culture: Effects of nerve growth factor and other neurotrophic factor. *Neuroscience* 59:673–688, 1994.

15. Khan I, Collins SM: Fourth isoform of preprotachykinin messenger RNA encoding for substance P in the rat intestine. *Biochem Biophys Res Commun* 202:796–802, 1994.

16. Huh GS, Hynes RO: Regulation of alternative pre-mRNA splicing by a novel repeated hexanuclotide element. *Genes Dev* 8:1561–1574, 1994.

17. Liu H, Brown JL, Jasmin L, et al: Synaptic relationship between substance P and the substance P receptor: Light and electron microscopic characterization of the mismatch between neuropeptides and their receptors. *Proc Natl Acad Sci USA* 91:1009–1013, 1994.

18. van Oers CCM, Adema GJ, Zandberg H, et al: Two different sequence elements within exons 4 are necessary for calcitonin-specific splicing of the human calcitonin/calcitonin gene-related peptide I Pre-mRNA. *Mol Cell Biol* 14:951–960, 1994.

19. Leitinger B, Brown JL, Spiess M: Tagging secretory and membrane proteins with a tyrosine sulfation site. *J Biol Chem* 269:8115–8121, 1994.

20. Grandt D, Schimiczek M, Struk K, et al: Characterization of two forms of peptide YY, PYY(1–36) and PYY(3–36), in the rabbit. *Peptides* 15:815–820, 1994.

21. Medeiros MS, Turner AJ: Processing and metabolism of peptide-YY: Pivotal roles of dipeptidylpeptidase-IV, aminopeptidase-P, and endopeptidase-24.11. *Endocrinology* 134:2088–2093, 1994.

22. Vasko MR, Campbell WB, Waite KJ: Prostaglandin E$_2$ enhances bradykinin-stimulated release of neuropeptides from rat sensory neurons in culture. *J Neurosci* 14:4987–4997, 1994.

23. Sala C, Andreose JS, Fumagalli G, et al: Calcitonin gene-related peptide: Possible role in formation and maintenance of neuromuscular junctions. *J Neurosci* 15:520–528, 1995.

24. Morris MB, Ralston GB, Biden TJ, et al: Structural and biochemical studies of human galanin: NMR evidence for nascent helical structures in aqueous solution. *Biochemistry* 34:4538–4545, 1995.

25. Munoz V, Serrano L: Elucidating the folding problem of helical peptides using empirical parameters: III. Temperature and pH dependence. *J Mol Biol* 245:297–308, 1995.

26. Hu L, Balse P, Doughty MB: Neuropeptide Y N-terminal deletion fragments: Correlation between solution structure and receptor binding activity at Y$_1$ receptors in rat brain cortex. *J Med Chem* 37:3622–3629, 1994.

27. Fournier A, Gagnon D, Quirion R, et al: Conformational and biological studies of neuropeptide Y analogs containing structural alterations. *Mol Pharmacol* 45:93–101, 1994.

28. Beck-Sickinger AG, Wieland HA, Wittneben H, et al: Complete L-alanine scan of neuropeptide Y reveals ligands binding to Y1 and Y2 receptors with distinguished conformations. *Eur J Biochem* 225:947–958, 1994.

29. Beck-Sickinger AG, Hoffmann E, Paulini K, et al: High-affinity analogues of neuropeptide Y containing conformationally restricted non-proteinogenic amino acids. *Biochem Soc Trans* 22:145–149, 1994.

30. Leban JJ, Heyer D, Landavazo A, et al: Novel modified carboxy terminal fragments of neuropeptide Y with high affinity for Y_2-type receptors and potent functional antagonism at a Y_1-type receptor. *J Med Chem* 38:1150–1157, 1995.

31. Giolitti A, Maggi CA: Structural comparison of NK_2 receptor agonists and antagonists. *J Comput Aided Mol Des* 8:341–344, 1994.

32. Kolodziej SA, Nikiforovich GV, Skeean R, et al: Ac-[3- and 4-alkylthioproline[31]]-CCK_4 analogs: Synthesis and implications for the CCK-B receptor-bound conformation. *J Med Chem* 38:137–149, 1995.

33. Sugg EE, Kimery MJ, Sing JM, et al: CCK-A receptor selective antagonists derived from the CCK-A receptor selective tetrapeptide agonist Boc-Trp-Lys(Tac)-Asp-MePhe-NH_2 (A-71623). *J Med Chem* 38:207–211, 1995.

34. Temussi PA, Salvadori S, Amodeo P, et al: Selective opioid dipeptides. *Biochem Biophys Res Commun* 198:933–939, 1994.

35. Holladay MW, Kopecka H, Miller TR, et al: Tetrapeptide CCK-A agonists: Effect of backbone N-methylation on *in vitro* and *in vivo* CCK activity. *J Med Chem* 37:630–635, 1994.

36. Bennett MJ, Nikkel AL, Bianchi BR, et al: CCK-A-selective tetrapeptides containing Lys(N^ϵ)-amide residues: Favorable *in vivo* and *in vitro* effects of N-methylation as the aspartyl residue. *J Med Chem* 37:1569–1571, 1994.

37. Aramori I, Morikawa N, Zenkoh J, et al: Subtype- and species-selectivity of a tachykinin receptor antagonist, FK888, for cloned rat and human tachykinin receptors. *Eur J Pharmacol* 269:277–281, 1994.

38. Emonds-Alt X, Bichon D, Ducoux JP, et al: SR 142801, the first potent nonpeptide antagonist of the tachykinin NK_3 receptor. *Life Sci* 56:PL27–PL32, 1995.

39. Daniel EE, Parrish MB, Watson EG, et al: The tachykinin receptors inducing contractile responses of canine ileum circular muscles. *Am J Physiol* 268:G161–G170, 1995.

40. Chung F-Z, Wu L-H, Vartanian MA, et al: The non-peptide tachykinin NK_2 receptor antagonist SR 48968 interacts with human, but not rat, cloned tachykinin NK_3 receptors. *Biochem Biophys Res Commun* 198:967–972, 1994.

41. Bunn PA Jr, Chan D, Stewart J, et al: Effects of neuropeptide analogues on calcium flux and proliferation in lung cancer cell lines. *Cancer Res* 54:3602–3610, 1994.

42. Felley CP, O'Dorisio TM, Howe B, et al: Chief cells possess somatostatin receptors regulated by secretagogues acting through the calcium or cAMP pathway. *Am J Physiol* 266:G789–G798, 1994.

43. Ji R-R, Zhang X, Wiesenfeld-Hallin Z, et al: Expression of neuropeptide Y and neuropeptide Y (Y1) receptor mRNA in rat spinal cord and dorsal root ganglia following peripheral tissue inflammation. *J Neurosci* 14:6423–6434, 1994.

44. Shimizu K, Shiratori K, Watanabe S, et al: Effect of protein derivatives on pancreatic secretion and release of secretin and CCK in rats. *Am J Physiol* 267:G508–G514, 1994.

45. Strader CD, Fong TM, Tota MR, et al: Structure and function of G protein–coupled receptors. *Annu Rev Biochem* 63:101–132, 1994.

46. Huang R-RC, Yu H, Strader CD, et al: Localization of the ligand binding site of the neurokinin-1 receptor: Interpretation of chimeric mutations and single-residue substitutions. *Mol Pharmacol* 45:690–695, 1994.

47. Huang R-RC, Yu H, Strader CD, et al: Interaction of substance P with the second and seventh transmembrane domains of the neurokinin-1 receptor. *Biochemistry* 33:3007–3013, 1994.

48. Fong TM, Yu H, Cascieri MA, et al: The role of histidine 265 in antagonist binding to the neurokinin-1 receptor. *J Biol Chem* 269:2728–2732, 1994.

49. Elling CE, Nielsen SM, Schwartz TW: Conversion of antagonist-binding site to metal-ion site in the tachykinin NK-1 receptor. *Nature* 374:74–77, 1995.

50. Cascieri MA, Shiao L-L, Mills SG, et al: Characterization of the interaction of diacylpiperazine

antagonists with the human neurokinin-1 receptor: Identification of a common binding site for structurally dissimilar antagonists. *Mol Pharmacol* 47:660–665, 1995.

51. Li Y-M, Marnerakis M, Stimson ER, et al: Mapping peptide-binding domains of the substance P (NK-1) receptor from P388D$_1$ cells with photolabile agonists. *J Biol Chem* 270:1213–1220, 1995.

52. Turcatti G, Vogel H, Chollet A: Probing the binding domain of the NK2 receptor with fluorescent ligands: Evidence that heptapeptide agonists and antagonists bind differently. *Biochemistry* 34:3973–3980, 1995.

53. Werge TM: Identification of an epitope in the substance P receptor important for recognition of the common carboxyl-terminal tachykinin sequence. *J Biol Chem* 269:22054–22058, 1994.

54. Song I, Brown DR, Wiltshire RN, et al: The human gastrin/cholecystokinin type B receptor gene: Alternative splice donor site in exon 4 generates two variant mRNAs. *Proc Natl Acad Sci USA* 90:9085–9089, 1993.

55. Poirot SS, Escriieut C, Dufresne M, et al: Photoaffinity labeling of rat pancreatic cholecystokinin type A receptor antagonist binding sites demonstrates the presence of a truncated cholecystokinin type A receptor. *Mol Pharmacol* 45:599–607, 1994.

56. Spengler D, Waeber C, Pantaloni C, et al: Differential signal transduction by five splice variants of the PACAP receptor: *Nature* 365:170–175, 1993.

57. Kojro E, Fahrenholz F: Ligand-induced cleavage of the V$_2$ vasopressin receptor by a plasma membrane metalloproteinase. *J Biol Chem* 270:6476–6481, 1995.

58. Huang S-C, Fortune KP, Wank SA, et al: Multiple affinity states of different cholecystokinin receptors. *J Biol Chem* 269:26121–26126, 1994.

59. Talkad VD, Fortune KP, Pollo DA, et al: Direct demonstration of three different states of the pancreatic cholecystokinin receptor. *Proc Natl Acad Sci USA* 91:1868–1872, 1994.

60. Talkad VD, Patto RJ, Metz DC, et al: Characterization of the three different states of the cholecystokinin (CCK) receptor in pancreatic acini. *Biochim Biophys Acta* 1224:103–116, 1994.

61. Pandya PK, Huang S-C, Talkad VD, et al: Biochemical regulation of the three different states of the cholecystokinin (CCK) receptor in pancreatic acini. *Biochim Biophys Acta* 1224:117–126, 1994.

62. Lefkowitz RJ, Cotecchia S, Samama P, et al: Constitutive activity of receptors coupled to guanine nucleotide regulatory proteins. *TIPS* 14:303–307, 1993.

63. Bond RA, Leff P, Johnson TD, et al: Physiological effects of inverse agonists in transgenic mice with myocardial overexpression of the β$_2$-adrenoceptor. *Nature* 374:272–276, 1995.

64. Black JW, Shankley NP: Inverse agonists exposed. *Nature* 374:214–215, 1995.

65. Noel JP, Hamm HE, Sigler PB: The 2.2 A crystal structure of transducin-α complexed with GTP$_\gamma$S. *Nature* 366:654–663, 1993.

66. Bourne HR: A turn-on and a surprise. *Nature* 366:628–629, 1993.

67. Lambright DG, Noel JP, Hamm HE, et al: Structural determinants for activation of the α-subunit of a heterotrimeric G protein. *Nature* 3369:621–628, 1994.

68. Bourne HR: The importance of being GTP. *Nature* 369:611–612, 1994.

69. Hausdorff WP, Caron MG, Lefkowitz RJ: Turning off the signal: Desensitization of β-adrenergic receptor function: *FASEB J* 4:2881–2889, 1990.

70. Lefkowitz RJ: G-protein-coupled receptors: Regulatory role of receptor kinases and arrestin proteins. *Cold Spring Harb Symp Quant Biol* 57:127–133, 1992.

71. Lefkowitz RJ: G protein–coupled receptor kinases. *Cell* 74:409–412, 1993.

72. Garland AM, Grady EF, Payan DG, et al: Agonist-induced internalization of the substance P (NK1) receptor expressed in epithelial cells. *Biochem J* 303:177–186, 1994.

73. Garland AM, Grady EF, Bowden JJ, et al: Mechanisms regulating the responsiveness of cells to substance P (SP): Cell-surface SP degradation and NK1 receptor (NK1R) endocytosis. *Biomed Res* 15(suppl 2): 5–13, 1994.

74. Bowden JJ, Garland AM, Baluk P, et al: Direct observation of substance P–induced internalization of NK1 receptor at sites of inflammation. *Proc Natl Acad Sci U S A* 91:8964–8968, 1994.

75. Bunnett NW, Dazin PF, Payan DG, et al: Characterization of receptors using cyanine 3-labeled neuropeptides. *Peptides* 16:733–740, 1995.

76. Grady EF, Garland AG, Gamp PD, et al: Delineation of the endocytic pathway of substance P and the seven transmembrane domain NK1 receptor. *Mol Biol Cell* 6:509–524, 1995.

77. Grady EF, Slice LW, Brant WO, et al: Direct observation of endocytosis of gastrin releasing peptide and its receptor in epithelial cells. *J Biol Chem* 270:4603–4611, 1994.

78. Roettger BF, Rentsch RU, Pinon D, et al: Dual pathways of internalization of the cholecystokinin receptor. *J Cell Biol* 128:1029–1041, 1995.

79. Barak LS, Tiberi M, Freedman NJ, et al: A highly conserved tyrosine residue in G protein–coupled receptors is required for agonist-mediated β_2-adrenergic receptor sequestration. *J Biol Chem* 269:2790–2795, 1994.

80. Slice LW, Wong HC, Sternini C, et al: The conserved NPXnY motif present in the gastrin releasing peptide receptor is not a general sequestration sequence. *J Biol Chem* 269:21755–21762, 1994.

81. Huang Z, Chen Y, Nissenson RA: The cytoplasmic tail of the G-protein-coupled receptor for parathyroid hormone and parathyroid hormone–related protein contains positive and negative signals for endocytosis. *J Biol Chem* 270:151–156, 1995.

82. Mantyh PW, Allen CJ, Ghilardi JR, et al: Rapid endocytosis of a G protein–coupled receptor: Substance P evoked internalization of its receptor in the rat striatum in vivo. *Proc Natl Acad Sci USA* 92:2622–2626, 1995.

83. Seva C, Dickinson CJ, Yamada T: Growth-promoting effects of glycine-extended progastrin. *Science* 265:410–412, 1994.

84. Fischman AJ, Babich JW, Strauss HW: A ticket to ride: Peptide radiopharmaceuticals. *J Nucl Med* 34:2253–2263, 1993.

85. Reubi JC: The role of peptides and their receptors as tumor markers. *Endocrinol Metab Clin North Am* 22:917–939, 1993.

86. Wiedenmann B, Bader HM, Scherubl H, et al: Gastroenteropancreatic tumor imaging with somatostatin receptor scintigraphy. *Semin Oncol* 21:29–32, 1994.

87. Scherubl H, Bader M, Fett U, et al: Somatostatin-receptor imaging of neuroendocrine gastroenteropancreatic tumors. *Gastroenterology* 105:1705–1709, 1993.

88. Pauwels S, Leners N, Fiasse R, et al: Localization of gastroenteropancreatic neuroendocrine tumors with [111]indium-pentetreotide scintigraphy. *Semin Oncol* 21:15–20, 1994.

89. Sautter-Bihl M-L, Dorr U, Schilling F, et al: Somatostatin receptor imaging: A new horizon in the diagnostic management of neuroblastoma. *Semin Oncol* 21:38–41, 1994.

90. Bong SB, VanderLaan JG, Louwes H, et al: Clinical experience with somatostatin receptor imaging in lymphoma. *Semin Oncol* 21:46–50, 1994.

91. Lip RW, Silly H, Ranner G, et al: Radiolabeled octreotide for the demonstration of somatostatin receptors in malignant lymphoma and lymphadenopathy. *J Nucl Med* 36:13–18, 1995.

92. Dorr U, Sautter-Bihl M-L, Bihl H: The contribution of somatostatin receptor scintigraphy to the diagnosis of recurrent medullary carcinoma of the thyroid. *Semin Oncol* 21:42–45, 1994.

93. Krenning EP, Kwekkeboom DJ, de Jong M, et al: Essentials of peptide receptor scintigraphy with emphasis on the somatostatin analog octreotide. *Semin Oncol* 21:6–14, 1994.

94. Vanhagen PM, Markusse HM, Lamberts SW, et al: Somatostatin receptor imaging. The presence of somatostatin receptors in rheumatoid arthritis. *Arthritis Rheum* 37:1521–1527, 1994.

95. Oyen WJ, Boerman OC, Claessens RA, et al: Is somatostatin receptor scintigraphy suited to detection of acute infectious disease? *Nucl Med Commun* 15:289–293, 1994.

96. Raynor K, Murphy WA, Coy DH, et al: Cloned somatostatin receptors: Identification of subtype-

selective peptides and demonstration of high affinity binding of linear peptides. *Mol Pharmacol* 43:838–844, 1993.

97. Patel YC, Strikant CB: Subtype selectivity of peptide analogs for all five cloned human soma-tostatin receptors (hsstr 1–5). *Endocrinology* 135:2814–2817, 1994.

98. Fitzpatrick VD, Vandlen RL: 6 Agonist selectivity determinants in somatostatin receptor subtypes I and II. *J Biol Chem* 269:24621–24626, 1994.

99. Krenning EP, Kooij PP, Bakker WH, et al: Radiotherapy with a radiolabeled somatostatin ana-logue, [111In-DTPA-D-Phe1]-octreotide. A case history. *Ann N Y Acad Sci* 733:496–506, 1994.

100. Forsell-Aronsson E, Fjalling M, Nilsson O, et al: Indium-111 activity concentration in tissue samples after intravenous injection of indium-111-DTPA-D-Phe-1-octreotide. *J Nucl Med* 36:7–12, 1995.

101. Virgolini I, Raderer M, Kurtaran A, et al: Vasoactive intestinal peptide-receptor imaging for the localization of intestinal adenocarcinomas and endocrine tumors. *N Engl J Med* 331:1116–1121, 1994.

102. Weckbecker G, Raulf F, Stolz B, et al: Somatostatin analogs for diagnosis and treatment of can-cer. *Pharmacol Ther* 60:245–264, 1993.

103. Baldwin GS, Whitehead RH: Gut hormones, growth and malignancy. *Bailleres Clin Endocrinol Metab* 8:185–214, 1994.

104. Shulkes A: Somatostatin: Physiology and clinical applications. *Baillieres Clin Endocrinol Metab* 8:215–236, 1994.

105. Kvols LK, Moertel CG, O'Connell MJ, et al: Treatment of the malignant carcinoid syndrome. *N Engl J Med* 315:663–666, 1986.

106. Arnold R, Frank M, Kajdan U: Management of gastroenteropancreatic endocrine tumors: The place of somatostatin analogues. *Digestion* 55:107–113, 1994.

107. Kubota A, Yamada Y, Kagimoto S, et al: Identification of somatostatin receptor subtypes and an implication for the efficacy of somatostatin analogue SMS 201-995 in treatment of human endo-crine tumors. *J Clin Invest* 93:1321–1325, 1994.

108. Cascinu S, Del Ferro E, Catalano G: A randomised trial of octreotide *vs* best supportive care only in advanced gastrointestinal cancer patients refractory to chemotherapy. *Br J Cancer* 71:97–101, 1995.

109. Logothetis CJ, Hossan EA, Smith TL: SMS 201–995 in the treatment of refractory prostatic car-cinoma. *Anticancer Res* 14:2731–2734, 1994.

110. Rivard N, Lebel D, Laine J, et al: Regulation of pancreatic tyrosine kinase and phosphatase ac-tivities by cholecystokinin and somatostatin. *Am J Physiol* 266:G1130–G1138, 1994.

111. Florio T, Rim C, Hershberger RE, et al: The somatostatin receptor SSTR1 is coupled to phospho-tyrosine phosphatase activity in CHO-K1 cells. *Mol Endocrinol* 8:1289–1297, 1994.

112. Buscail L, Esteve J-P, Saint-Laurent N, et al: Inhibition of cell proliferation by the somatostatin analogue RC-160 is mediated by somatostatin receptor subtypes SSTR2 and SSTR5 through dif-ferent mechanisms. *Proc Natl Acad Sci U S A* 92:1580–1584, 1995.

113. Buscail L, Delesque N, Esteve J-P, et al: Stimulation of tyrosine phosphatase and inhibition of cell proliferation by somatostatin analogues: Mediation by human somatostatin receptor subtypes SSTR1 and SSTR2. *Proc Natl Acad Sci U S A* 91:2315–2319, 1994.

114. Kubota A, Yamada Y, Kagimoto S, et al: Multiple effector coupling of somatostatin receptor sub-type SSTR1. *Biochem Biophys Res Commun* 204:176–186, 1994.

115. Bito H, Mori M, Sakanaka C, et al: Functional coupling of SSTR4, a major hippocampal soma-tostatin receptor, to adenylate cyclase inhibition, arachidonate release and activation of the mitogen-activated protein kinase cascade. *J Biol Chem* 269:12722–12730, 1994.

116. Zeggari M, Esteve J-P, Rauly I, et al: Co-purification of a protein tyrosine phosphatase with acti-vated somatostatin receptors from rat pancreatic acinar membranes. *Biochem J* 303:441–448, 1994.

117. Srikant CB: Cell cycle dependent induction of apoptosis by somatostatin analog SMS 201-995 in AtT-20 mouse pituitary cells. *Biochem Biophys Res Commun* 209:400–406, 1995.

118. Todisco A, Campbell V, Dickinson CJ, et al: Molecular basis for somatostatin action: Inhibition of *c-fos* expression and AP-1 binding: *Am J Physiol* 267:G245–G253, 1994.

119. Reubi JC, Horisberger U, Laissue J: High density of somatostatin receptor in veins surrounding human cancer tissue: Role in tumor-host interaction? *Int J Cancer* 56:681–688, 1994.

120. Reubi JC, Mazzucchelli L, Laissue J: Intestinal vessels express a high density of somatostatin receptors in human inflammatory bowel disease. *Gastroenterology* 106:951–959, 1994.

121. Pinski J, Halmos G, Yano T, et al: Inhibition of growth of MKN45 human gastric-carcinoma xenografts in nude mice by treatment with bombesin/gastrin-releasing-peptide antagonist (RC-3095) and somatostatin analogue RC-160. *Int J Cancer* 57:574–580, 1994.

122. Mantyh PW, Vigna SR, Maggio JE: Receptor involvement in pathology and disease. In Buck SH (ed): The tachykinin receptors. Totowa, NJ, Humana Press, 1994, pp 581–610.

123. Reinshagen M, Patel A, Sottili M, et al: Protective function of extrinsic sensory neurons in acute rabbit experimental colitis. *Gastroenterology* 106:1208–1214, 1994.

124. Mayer EA, Gebhart GF: Basic and clinical aspects of visceral hyperalgesia. *Gastroenterology* 107:271–293, 1994.

125. Gehlert DR: Subtypes of receptors for neuropeptide Y: Implications for the targeting of therapeutics. *Life Sci* 55:551–562, 1994.

126. Dryden S, Frankish H, Wang Q, et al: Neuropeptide Y and energy balance: One way ahead for the treatment of obesity? *Eur J Clin Invest* 24:293–308, 1994.

127. Billington CJ, Briggs JE, Harker S, et al: Neuropeptide Y in hypothalamic paraventricular nucleus: A center coordinating energy metabolism. *Am J Physiol* 266:R1765–R1770, 1994.

128. Zarjevski N, Cusin I, Vettor R, et al: Intracerebroventricular administration of neuropeptide Y to normal rats has divergent effects on glucose utilization by adipose tissue and skeletal muscle. *Diabetes* 43:764–769, 1994.

129. Vettor R, Zarjevski N, Cusin I, et al: Induction and reversibility of an obesity syndrome by intracerebroventricular neuropeptide Y administration to normal rats. *Diabetologia* 37:1202–1208, 1994.

130. Stricker-Krongrad A, Max JP, Musse N, et al: Increased threshold concentrations of neuropeptide Y for a stimulatory effect on food intake in obese Zucker rats—changes in the microstructure of the feeding behavior. *Brain Res* 660:162–166, 1994.

131. Read N, French S, Cunningham K: The role of the gut in regulating food intake in man. *Nutr Rev* 52:1–10, 1994.

132. Lieverse RJ, Jansen JBMJ, Masclee AAM, et al: Satiety effects of cholecystokinin in humans. *Gastroenterology* 106:1451–1454, 1994.

133. Lieverse RJ, Jansen JBMJ, Masclee AAM, et al: Satiety effects of a physiological dose of cholecystokinin in humans. *Gut* 36:176–179, 1995.

CHAPTER 6

Nutrition and Gastroenterology

T.A. Winter, M.D., F.C.P. (S.A.)

Gastrointestinal Clinic, Department of Medicine, University of Cape Town and Groote Schuur Hospital, Cape Town, South Africa

S.J.D. O'Keefe, M.D., M.Sc., F.R.C.P., F.A.C.G.

Professor, Department of Gastroenterology, Groote Schuur Hospital, Cape Town, South Africa

Previously it has been generally perceived that the gut was a simple tube from which food was digested and absorbed and that nutrients were simply sources of energy. Nutritional research, particularly over the past decade, has progressively illustrated the gross oversimplification of this concept. The vital role of the gut as a barrier and immune organ and the novel effects of substrates such as glutamine, arginine, short-chain fatty acids (SCFAs), ω-3 fatty acids, and nucleosides have been clearly shown. The indispensable role of enteral nutrition is also increasingly appreciated, not only in the supportive role of maintenance of the nutritional state but also as primary therapy directed against, or protective of, a number of disease states such as inflammatory bowel disease, cardiovascular disease, and cancer.

GUT FUELS AND NUTRITIONAL PHARMACOLOGY

A variety of nutrients, including glucose, triglycerides, fatty acids, ketone bodies, and amino acids, are provided to intestinal cells by both arterial and luminal supply. The arterial supply does appear to be of greater overall importance because the intermittency of alimentation necessitates an adequate vascular energy supply.[1] In general, substrates absorbed from the intestinal lumen are eventually released into the bloodstream either as the native compound or metabolites and subsequently distributed to the other tissues. On the other hand, utilization of bloodborne nutrients may be associated with extensive metabolism in the intestine. A distinction must be made between "substrate uptake," which refers to the disappearance of the substance from the medium, and "substrate utilization," indicating the amount actually metabolized by the tissue. This difference is often not appreciated, and it may in fact be difficult to distinguish between the two.[2] The heterogeneity of cell types within the gut also makes it difficult to define fuel utilization.

Glutamine

Glutamine is the most abundant free amino acid in the body, with approximately 80% contained in skeletal muscle.[3] It has been shown to be essential for cell proliferation in culture systems[4] and serves as both a fuel and a precursor for purine and pyrimidine biosynthesis. Several studies have shown the importance of glutamine as an energy source for the gut, with the small bowel extracting 20% to 30% of the circulating glutamine in the postabsorptive state. Glutamine released from skeletal muscle forms the preferred fuel for enterocytes[5–7] and can also be used by colonocytes.[8] Glutamine is extensively used by cells of the immune system and also improves glutathione synthesis, an important factor in intracellular antioxidant defense and maintenance of endothelial cell tight-junction integrity.[9] It may therefore play an important, if not indispensable, role in maintenance of the overall efficient functioning of the intestinal mucosa. Furthermore, glutamine utilization by the intestine may spare glucose, allowing absorbed glucose to be transported into the bloodstream and made available for other tissues such as the brain.[1] Glutamine also acts as a transporter of nitrogen and ammonium ion from muscle and gut to the liver and kidney, therefore playing an important role in nitrogen and acid-base balance.[10, 11]

Glutamine is usually classified as a nonessential amino acid because human tissues, particularly skeletal muscle and lung, are able to biosynthesize glutamine from glutamate and branched-chain amino acids. However, studies have now indicated that the capacity of metabolically stressed individuals in producing sufficient endogenous glutamine may be overwhelmed, resulting in deficiency.[12–14] This may result in disruption of the gut barrier and bacterial translocation.[7, 15] Numerous studies have shown that prolonged bowel rest results in gut mucosal atrophy, and because total parenteral nutrition (TPN) solutions do not normally contain glutamine, metabolically stressed individuals receiving TPN may be particularly prone to bacterial translocation and subsequent septic complications.

Babst et al.[16] studied the effects of glutamine supplementation of long-term TPN in healthy rats. Growing rats were fed parenterally for 3 weeks, with or without supplemented glutamine (administered as a 20% solution of dipeptides glycyl-glutamine, and alanyl-glutamine). The TPN solutions were isocaloric, isonitro-genous, and isovolemic, with energy provided by carbohydrates and lipids in a 1:1 ratio. A control group of enterally fed rats was also studied. The effects of these feeding regimens on intracellular and extracellular amino acid patterns, nitrogen balance, serum protein concentrations, as well as growth and morphologic features of liver and small bowel, were analyzed. Glutamine-free TPN resulted in significantly lower intracellular and extracellular glutamine concentrations compared with the enterally fed group. Provision of dipeptides glycyl-glutamine and alanyl-glutamine resulted in a significant increase in intracellular and extracellular concentrations of glutamine. Overall growth rates over the study period were similar in the three groups, but nitrogen balance was significantly better in the glutamine-supplemented group compared with the animals receiving standard TPN (cumulative nitrogen balance 10.59 ± 1.42 vs. 4.18 ± 1.49 g of nitrogen/kg for 20 days). Serum albumin levels remained normal in all groups, and no abnormalities of liver or renal function were detected. Histologic examination revealed mild fatty liver infiltration in the TPN groups, which was not altered by glutamine supplementation. In contrast to several previous studies, neither conventional nor electron microscopy revealed any relevant or consistent alteration to jejunal mucosal architecture induced by TPN or influenced by the provision of glutamine. The authors suggest that provision of 41% of the calories as fat may have antagonized the intestinal atrophy associated with the release of enteroglucagon.[17, 18] Furthermore, in these otherwise healthy animals, endogenous glutamine may be adequate to satisfy the requirements of the intestinal mucosa.

Several studies have illustrated increased intestinal permeability to macromolecules[19, 20] and increased translocation of bacteria[21, 22] in rats receiving TPN. Li et al.[23] recently investigated the role of L-glutamine, supplemented as a 2% solution, in preventing TPN-related increases in intestinal permeability. Eighteen rats were randomly assigned to three groups. The chow group served as a control group and received an infusion of saline solution plus a standard laboratory rat diet. The TPN group received standard TPN, and the Gln group received TPN with 2% of the amino acid content replaced with glutamine. After 7 days of infusion, laparotomies were performed, and 2 mL of a permeability test solution containing 95 mg of lactulose, 38 mg of mannitol, and 1.8 mg of sodium chloride (285 mOsm/L) was injected into a 25-cm segment of isolated jejunum. After 5 hours the urine was collected for analysis of excretion of lactulose and mannitol. The ratio of lactulose to mannitol served an index of intestinal permeability. A segment of the jejunum was also taken for histologic analysis. Results indicated a significant increase in intestinal permeability of the group receiving standard TPN compared with the control group, whereas there was no difference between the control group and those receiving TPN supplemented with glutamine. Mucosal thickness and villus height also decreased significantly in the TPN group but not in the Gln group compared with the controls. However, there did not appear to be a direct correlation between the magnitude of change in permeability and the degree of intestinal atrophy.

These findings support the study by Van der Hulst et al.,[24] who noted increased permeability and decreased villus height in human subjects receiving standard TPN but not in those receiving TPN supplemented with glycyl-L-glutamine. The lack of correlation between changes in permeability and villus macroscopic structure in the Li et al.[23] study suggests that villus atrophy is not the only factor contributing to increased permeability to macromolecules. The authors postulate that glutamine may influence intracellular mediators that enhance tight-junction resistance, possibly by limiting inflammatory events induced by TPN occurring in the intestinal mucosa. In an accompanying editorial, Helton suggests that bacterial chemotactic peptides traversing a permeable mucosa would recruit neutrophils.[9] Activation of the neutrophils and release of oxygen radicals would then further increase permeability. Glutamine may protect against this mechanism by enhancing antioxidant activity.

In another recent study, Tremel et al.[25] investigated the effect of glutamine supplementation (as the dipeptide L-alanine-L-glutamine) on small intestinal absorption in critically ill patients receiving TPN. Twelve intensive care unit patients received isonitrogenous (0.26 g of nitrogen/kg/day) and isocaloric (155 kJ/kg/day) intravenous nutrition over a 9-day period. The control group received a standard amino acid solution (1.5 g of amino acids/kg/day), whereas the study group were supplemented with L-alanine-L-glutamine (300 mg/kg/day). After the period of TPN, small intestinal absorption was assessed by means of a modified D-xylose absorption test. Results showed urinary excretion of D-xylose over 5 hours after a 25-g oral load to be approximately twice as great in the glutamine-supplemented group (7.4 ± 1.1 vs. 3.8 ± 0.9 g, $P < .05$), indicating improved intestinal absorption. Pharmacokinetic evaluation of the serum concentrations of D-xylose showed the control group to have absorption characteristics below accepted normal limits, whereas that of the glutamine-supplemented group was within normal range.

Dose-response studies of supplemented glutamine performed in animals have indicated increased and sustained structural and functional benefits over a wide dose range, with maximal effects achieved when glutamine comprises 33% of the amino acids infused.[26] With a general requirement of approximately 1.5 g of protein/kg of body weight daily, it has been suggested that 0.37 to 0.5 g/kg of this total should be glutamine. This equates to a daily dose of 19 to 35 g of glutamine for patients weighing between 50 and 70 kg.

Glutamine uptake by the intestine has been shown to be decreased during sepsis and endotoxemia apparently as a result of a decrease in the specific activity of mucosal glutaminase and a reduction in the number of active brush-border transporters for glutamine. During septic conditions, this impairment of gut glutamine metabolism may contribute to disruption of the gut mucosal barrier and subsequent bacterial translocation.[27, 28] It has been suggested that provision of glutamine may upregulate both the activity of brush-border glutamine transporters and the activity of intestinal glutaminase, thereby improving gut mucosal metabolism and breaking this vicious circle of events.[11] To investigate the effects of glutamine during endotoxemia, Chen et al.[29] randomized 46 male Wistar rats to receive TPN supplemented with either glutamine or glycine at 2% wt/vol. Endotoxemia was induced by continuous infusion of endotoxin at a rate of 2 mg/kg/daily during the 4-day study period. Although mortality in the two groups was not statistically different (13% in the glutamine group and 22% in the glycine group), the glutamine-supplemented rats had less negative cumulative nitrogen balances (-14.0 ± 132.8 mg vs. -86.8 ± 161.7, $P < .05$) and lower cumulative excretions of urinary 3-methyhistadine (2910 ± 593 vs. 4447 ± 933 nmol, $P < .01$), suggesting inhibition of protein and muscle degradation. Jejunal mucosa glutaminase activity and arterioportal venous blood glutamine concentration differences were significantly higher in the glutamine-supplemented group (15.6 ± 2.3 vs. 11.1 ± 1.9 μmol/g/min, $P < .05$ and 181 ± 52 vs. 147 ± 36 nmol/mL, $P < .05$, respectively). Mucosal weight, villus height, crypt depth, and wall thickness were also significantly greater in the glutamine group, and the arterioportal venous endotoxin difference was less negative (-31 ± 137 vs. -480 ± 672 pg/mL), suggesting that the absorption of endotoxin across the gut was partially reversed.

Arginine is another amino acid that, although classified as nonessential in the diet, is essential for an adequate host response to injury. Dietary arginine supplementation has been associated with improvements in the rates of wound healing, nitrogen balance, and lymphocytic immune responses.[30, 31] The anabolic effects associated with arginine are possibly mediated by the stimulation of secretion of various hormones, including glucagon, insulin, and growth hormone.[32, 33] Arginine is produced in the kidney from citrulline, the most important source of which is the intestine.[34, 35] Citrulline, in turn, is dependent on the metabolism of glutamine.[36, 37] Theoretically, therefore, supplementation with glutamine could lead to increased arginine production by the kidneys. To investigate this possibility, Houdijk et al.[38] randomized rats to receive either a 12.5% glutamine-enriched diet or an isocaloric, isonitrogenous control diet for 14 days. The study showed the glutamine-supplemented group had significantly higher arterial plasma levels of citrulline (30%, $P < .0001$), and arginine (31%, $P < .0005$). Uptake of citrulline and the subsequent production of arginine by the kidneys was also significantly higher in the glutamine-enriched group. The authors suggest that the beneficial effects of glutamine in catabolic states may, at least in part, be related to increased arginine production.

Although much of the work concerning the effects of glutamine has focused on the small intestine, evidence suggests that the proximal colon resembles the ileum in its metabolism of nutrients.[39] However, little is known about the effects of glutamine on colonic mucosa. Scheppach et al.[40] investigated the trophic effects of free glutamine and alanyl-glutamine dipeptide on the human ileum and colon. Biopsy samples from the normal human ileum, proximal colon, and rectosigmoid colon were incubated for 4 hours with glutamine (2 mmol/L), alanyl-glutamine (2 mmol/L), and saline solution (control). Proliferating cells were labeled with bromodeoxiuridine, and uptake was assessed histologically within the whole crypt, as well as for five longitudinal crypt compartments (compartment 1, crypt base; compartment 5, crypt surface). Results showed that both glutamine and alanyl-glutamine dipeptide stimulated crypt cell proliferation in the ileum, as well as in both proximal and distal colon (Fig 1). In the ileal specimens, labeling was greater throughout the entire crypt, whereas in the colonic regions, the trophic effect was confined largely to the basal crypt compartments. In the proximal colon some increase in labeling in compartment 4 might indicate some expansion of the proliferative zone, a feature that has been associated with cancer risk. However, the ϕh value (number of labeled cells in zone 4 and 5 divided by the number of labeled cells in the entire crypt), which indicates an expanded proliferation zone,[41] was unchanged. Thus, glutamine acts as a trophic factor on epithelial cells of the colon, with no evidence of inducing a preneoplastic hyperproliferation. Because the large intestine harbors a far greater number of bacteria than the small bowel, maintenance of an intact mucosal barrier is vital. These trophic effects on the colonic mucosa may therefore have important clinical implications. Whether these effects are specific to glutamine or may be induced by other energy sources such as glucose or short-chain fatty acids needs further investigation.

Hornsby-Lewis et al.[42] investigated the safety and efficacy of L-glutamine when

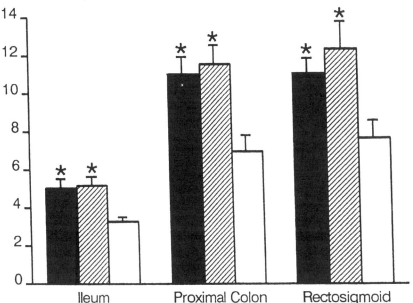

FIGURE 1.

Mean number of cells per crypt column labeled with BrdUrd in biopsy specimens from the human ileum, proximal colon, and rectosigmoid. The biopsy specimens from the three different regions were incubated with 2 mmol of glutamine/L *(solid bars),* 3 mmol of alanyl-glutamine/L *(hatched bars),* or saline solution (control, *clear bars). Asterisks* indicate significantly ($P < .001$) higher cell labeling after glutamine and alanyl-glutamine incubation compared with control conditions. (From Scheppach W, Loges C, Bartram P, et al:*Gastroenterology* 107:429–434, 1994. Used by permission.)

added to the solutions of patients receiving home parenteral nutrition (HPM). Stability studies indicated that the L-glutamine, when mixed by the Pharmix method[43] and kept at 4°C, was stable in solution for at least 22 days. Seven stable patients receiving HPN were given glutamine supplements at a dose of 0.285 g/kg of body weight daily for 4 weeks. The glutamine-containing TPN solutions were prepared weekly. Five of the patients received glutamine-supplemented TPN for the entire 4-week period. Two were discontinued at the end of weeks 2 and 3 because of the development of liver function test abnormalities, with raised liver enzyme levels (particularly aspartate aminotransferase). A third patient was noted to have elevated liver enzyme levels at the end of week 4. The abnormal liver enzyme levels returned to baseline within 2 weeks of discontinuing the glutamine-containing TPN. D-Xylose absorption tests were performed before and after the administration of the glutamine-containing TPN in six of the patients. Baseline D-xylose absorption was markedly abnormal in all patients, but there was no evidence of any improvement after the period of glutamine supplementation. Although the glutamine-containing TPN admixtures were considered stable, the apparent hepatotoxicity of the solutions noted in this study is unexplained and is of concern.

In conclusion, evidence is accumulating that supplementation of TPN with glutamine is of value in the treatment of rats on bowel rest. Studies in patients are less convincing, but such formulations may well prove of benefit to the critically ill on forced bowel rest.

Short-Chain Fatty Acids

Anaerobic bacterial fermentation of nonabsorbed carbohydrate and fiber within the colon results in the production of SCFAs, which have been shown to be important luminal fuel substrates for colonic mucosa. Although enterocytes are able to receive nutrients sufficient for their energy requirements from the bloodstream (glutamine from muscle catabolism and ketone bodies from hepatic ketogenesis), colonocytes are largely dependent on the availability of luminal SCFA, particularly butyrate.[39, 44] During periods of starvation or if the fecal stream is bypassed from the colon, these substrates cannot easily be replaced from endogenous sources. Insufficient mucosal nutrition may subsequently lead to mucosal atrophy, reduced absorption, and inflammation.[45, 46] Ulcerative colitis has been associated with altered fecal concentrations of SCFAs and a decreased ability of the colonic mucosa to metabolize butyrate.[47–49] Furthermore, inhibition of fatty acid metabolism in rats has been shown to cause an acute colitis.[50] Local irrigation with SCFA-containing enemas have been reported to be effective in the management of distal ulcerative colitis, despite the evidence of impaired metabolism.[51–53]

The metabolic effects of SCFAs on the colon are summarized in Figure 2. The two, three-, and four-carbon fatty acids (acetate, propionate, and butyrate) are important respiratory fuels for colonocytes and are found in the colonic lumen in a

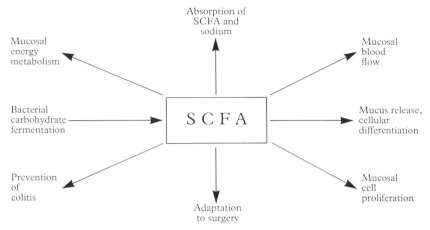

FIGURE 2.
Effects of short-chain fatty acids *(SCFAs)* on colonic morphology and function (facts and hypotheses). (From Scheppach W: *Gut* 35(suppl 1):S35–S38, 1994. Used by permission.)

molar ratio of about 60:20:20, with a total concentration of between 60 and 150 mmol/L.[54, 55] Kinetic studies have shown that colonic epithelial cells utilize SCFAs in a preferential order of butyrate > propionate > acetate,[56] with butyrate providing about 60% to 70% of the colon's energy requirements.[57, 58] These SCFAs are trophic to the intestinal mucosa.[59–61] They also stimulate sodium and water absorption,[62, 63] enhance mucosal blood flow,[64, 65] and have been shown to stimulate ileocolonic motility[66, 67] and mucus release. Although SCFAs stimulate normal colonic cell proliferation, butyrate in particular has been shown to slow proliferation and promote the expression of phenotypic markers of differentiation in colon cancer cells cultured in vitro.[68, 69] Consequently, they may provide protection against the development of malignancy.[70]

Although SCFAs from the lumen have a direct effect on colonocytes, an indirect stimulatory effect on the jejunal epithelium has been reported.[71, 72] To investigate whether these effects are mediated by the autonomic nervous system, enterotrophic hormones, or both, Frankel et al.[73] studied 60 male Sprague-Dawley rats who had undergone cecal isolation. An infusion catheter was placed into the proximal cecum, a distal cecocutaneous stoma was formed, and intestinal continuity was restored with ileocolonic anastomosis. The rats then either underwent cecal denervation or remained normally innervated and received intracecal infusions of either SCFAs (150 mmol/L of acetate, 30 mmol/L of propionate, 90 mmol/L of butyrate), saline solution, or no infusion for 10 days. Twenty-four additional rats underwent cecectomy, ileocolonic anastomosis, and placement of a proximal colonic infusion catheter. These rats were also assigned to receive either SCFAs, saline solution, or no infusion. After the period of infusion, the rats were killed, and jejunal and colonic samples were taken for histologic and biochemical analyses. In the innervated rats, cecal infusion of SCFAs significantly ($P < .05$) increased jejunal DNA, villous height, surface area, crypt depth, and gastrin, whereas in the denervated animals, there was no significant change. There was no evidence of trophic effects to the colon in either of these two groups. However, direct intracolonic infusions of SCFAs increased ($P < .05$) colonic mucosal DNA and crypt depth. These results indicate that in rats, the trophic effects of SCFAs on the jejunum are, at least in part, mediated by the autonomic nervous system and are associated with increased tissue levels of gastrin. However, the colon appears to be dependent on direct contact with luminal SCFAs. This finding is supported by the study of Koruda et al.,[74] who noted that intravenous supplementation with SCFAs prevented TPN-associated atrophy of the jejunal but not of the colonic mucosa. Stein et al.[75] have also recently reported improved mucosal protein synthesis in the jejunum but not in the colon after the addition of butyrate to TPN in rats.

The integrity of colonic epithelium depends on the ability of the cells to adhere to each other and to the basement membrane. Colonic epithelium is, however, in a dynamic state. The cells must also be able to loosen such adhesion to allow cell migration from the crypt base to the surface, with subsequent loss to the lumen. Urokinase (u-PA) is a neutral protease, the major physiologic substrate of which is plasminogen, from which plasmin, another neutral protease, is produced.[76] Substrates for plasmin include major constituents of basement membranes such as laminin, fibronectin, and proteoglycans. Urokinase also digests fibronectin directly.[77] Colonic epithelium secretes u-PA and has u-PA associated with its plasma membrane.[78]

Urokinase activity may therefore directly modulate epithelial cell adhesion and play an integral part in the physiologic mechanisms that allow migration of cells within the crypts. Plasmin is also an important activator of the cytokine transforming growth factor–β (TGF-β),[79] the putative functions of which include control of intestinal epithelial proliferation, differentiation, and restitution.[80, 81] Therefore the production and control of u-PA may have particular relevance to the normal functioning of colonic epithelium. Furthermore, increased mucosal u-PA activity has been reported in colitis,[82, 83] a state where disturbed cell adhesion, increased permeability, elevated cell turnover, and ulceration are characteristic.

In view of the importance of SCFAs in colonic metabolism and function, Gibson et al.[84] investigated the effects of butyrate on secretion of u-PA by human colonic epithelium. Colonic crypt cells were isolated from surgically resected colons from two groups of patients. The first group (10 patients) had undergone colectomy for nonneoplastic conditions (diverticular disease, recurrent sigmoid volvulus, unexplained lower gastrointestinal bleeding), and the second group (10 patients) had undergone colectomy for carcinoma of the colon. The cell suspensions were then cultured with or without the addition of sodium butyrate (0.001–4.0 mmol/L). After 24 hours of incubation, the cells were harvested and u-PA content measured in supernatants and cell homogenates. Results indicated that sodium butyrate caused a concentration-dependent inhibition of both secreted and cell-associated u-PA content. In contrast, addition of acetate or propionate to the culture medium had minimal effects. Butyrate was also shown to stimulate the secretion of the u-PA inhibitor, plasminogen activator inhibitor 1 by $25\% \pm 7\%$ ($P < .02$). The magnitude of the inhibitory effect of butyrate on u-PA secretion was significantly greater in colonic crypt cells from cancer-bearing colon (62% ± 2%) than normal colons (39% ± 7%; P = .02). This difference probably reflects the diffuse abnormalities previously observed in colonic epithelium distant from large bowel cancers.[85–87]

These effects on u-PA secretion may explain some of the beneficial effects of butyrate on the colon. Mucosal inflammation develops in a SCFA-deficient luminal environment, as in segments of colon from which the fecal stream has been diverted. This "diversion colitis" has been shown to resolve after instillation of SCFAs,[88] possibly by blocking the passage of macromolecules into the mucosa. Inhibition of u-PA may also explain the link between butyrate and intestinal permeability, as well as the beneficial effects of SCFA enemas in the treatment of distal ulcerative colitis.[51–53]

The increased osmotic load of SCFAs produced from malabsorbed carbohydrate in small intestinal disease was thought to contribute to the diarrheal fluid losses in these conditions. However, recent evidence suggests that they do, in fact, play an important role in stimulating colonic fluid and electrolyte absorption, thereby compensating for small intestinal malabsorption.[89] Short-chain fatty acids are important regulators of colonic sodium, and thereby fluid, transport, and stimulate sodium absorption, by enhancing Na^+-H^+ exchange.[90, 91] Absorption of Na^+ and SCFAs are coupled, and therefore regulation of transcellular active Na^+ transport may play an important part in colonic SCFA conservation. However, the identification of the putative transporter for specific SCFAs remains to be determined.

Butzner et al.[92] investigated the effects of infective enterocolitic disease on SCFA and SCFA-stimulated Na^+ absorption. Rabbits were infected with the enteric pathogen *Yersinia enterocolitica,* which is known to result in injury to the entire small bowel, cecum, and proximal colon. This results in malabsorption and increased manifestation of fermentable carbohydrate to the proximal colon. After 6 days, luminal SCFA concentrations were measured and Na^+ and SCFA (propionate) transport assessed in the proximal colon using an Ussing chamber technique. In a control group of noninfected rabbits, butyrate and propionate were shown to stimulate Na^+ absorption, and the absorption of both Na^+ and propionate was blocked by the Na^+-H^+ inhibitor amiloride. In the infected group, increased luminal content of SCFAs was confirmed. However, both butyrate and propionate failed to stimulate colonic Na^+ absorption, and propionate absorption was inhibited. These results indicate that not only does infective enteric disease result in an increased osmotic load to the colon due to malabsorption of carbohydrate and inhibition of SCFA absorption, but it also impairs SCFA-stimulated Na^+ absorption. Consequently, it seems unlikely that SCFA therapy will be of use in diarrheal states of infective etiology.

Starvation and severe malnutrition have been associated with diarrhea, particularly when one is attempting to refeed such individuals. A number of studies have indicated that complete luminal starvation for 2 to 5 days prevented ion absorption in the colon.[93–95] Although a relationship between diminished luminal SCFAs and diarrhea in malnourished patients has not been established, it is empirically thought to exist,[96] and provision of fermentable fiber to refeeding regimens and oral rehydration solutions has been suggested (Fig 3).[97, 98] However, severely malnourished patients may be prone to other physiologic derangements that may further complicate refeeding strategies. Small intestinal hypersecretion of fluid has been documented in rats,[99, 100] and we[101] have demonstrated significant impairment in the production of digestive enzymes in human subjects. In these individuals, a period of feeding with predigested (semielemental) formulas or even parenteral nutrition may be useful or possibly essential in breaking the vicious circle of malnutrition, malabsorption, and diarrhea.

ω-3 Fatty Acids

Dietary fats are directly involved in the production of eicosanoids and as such are important mediators of the inflammatory and immune responses. Linoleic acid, an n-6 fatty acid found in animal and vegetable oils, is a precursor for arachidonic

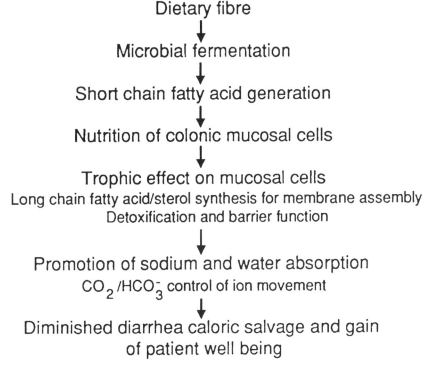

Dietary fibre
↓
Microbial fermentation
↓
Short chain fatty acid generation
↓
Nutrition of colonic mucosal cells
↓
Trophic effect on mucosal cells
Long chain fatty acid/sterol synthesis for membrane assembly
Detoxification and barrier function
↓
Promotion of sodium and water absorption
CO_2/HCO_3^- control of ion movement
↓
Diminished diarrhea caloric salvage and gain
of patient well being

FIGURE 3.
Sequence of functional events established by experimentation that occur in colonocytes and the colon when exposed to SCFAs derived from the fermentation of dietary fiber. Breakdown of the sequence occurs under severe starvation conditions or inhibition of bacterial fermentation. (From Roediger WEW: *JPEN J Parenter Enteral Nutr* 18:4–8, 1994. Used by permission.)

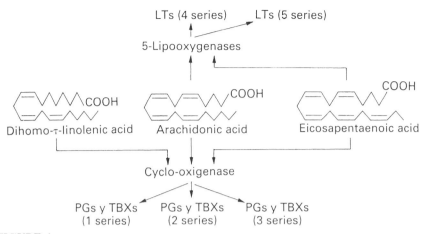

FIGURE 4.
Eicosanoid (prostaglandin *[PG]*, thromboxane *[TBX]*, and leukotriene *[LT]* synthesis from long-chain n-6 and n-3 polyunsaturated fatty acids. (From Fernandes-Bañares F, Cabre E, González-Huix F, et al: *Gut* 35(suppl 1):S55–S59, 1994. Used by permission.)

acid synthesis. Prostaglandins of the 2 series and leukotrienes of the 4 series are then produced by the actions of cyclo-oxygenase and lipoxygenase on arachidonic acid, respectively (Fig 4). The products prostaglandin E_2 (PGE_2) and thromboxane A_2 are powerful mediators of inflammation and cellular proliferation. Prostaglandin E_2 in particular has been shown to exert a proliferative effect on colonic mucosa,[102] and increased mucosal levels have been found in colonic cancer tissues.[103, 104]

Such n-3 fatty acids as eicosapentaenoic acid and docosahexaenoic acid, found in fish oils, compete with arachidonic acid, with the subsequent production of prostaglandins of the 3 series and leukotrienes of the 5 series. These are less inflammatory and are associated with altered cytokine function with suppression of the production of interleukin-1 and tumor necrosis factor.[105] As detailed in earlier chapters in *Current Gastroenterology,* fish oil n-3 fatty acids may play an important role in a number of clinical conditions. Diets high in fish oil have been associated with a decreased risk of cancer in general and colon cancer in particular.[108–112] Fish oils have also been found useful in the management of inflammatory conditions such as ulcerative colitis.[113–116]

Anti et al.[117] attempted to determine the optimal dose of fish oil required to reduce the cytokinetic anomalies associated with the rectal mucosa in patients with sporadic colonic adenomas. Sixty patients with adenomas were randomized to receive 2.5, 5.1, or 7.7 g of fish oil daily or placebo for 30 days. The fish oil was administered as capsules, each containing 455 mg of eicosapenaenoic acid, 395 mg of docosahexaenoic acid, and 0.3 mg of α-tocopheral alcohol (as an antioxidant). The placebo capsules contained a blend of n-6 fatty acids (25% saturated, 65% monounsaturated, and 10% polyunsaturated). Rectal epithelial proliferation was assessed before and after the study period by means of autoradiographic measurement of the uptake of [³H]thymidine into biopsy specimens. In addition, to evaluate persistence of the effect during long-term administration, 15 patients received 2.5 g of fish oil daily for 6 months, and proliferative parameters were assessed before, during, and after the dietary period.

Mucosal eicosapentaenoic and docosahexanoic acid levels increased, and arachidonic acid levels decreased in all patients who received the fish oil supplementation. This was associated with a significant reduction in the rectal proliferation indices in all groups receiving fish oil, with the reduction confined to patients shown to have abnormal baseline patterns. The degree of suppression was similar in the three fish oil groups, and the effects were shown to persist during the long-term, low-dose treatment. There were no significant side effects. This study indicates that low-dose n-3 fatty acid supplementation, administered in capsule form, is well tolerated and is associated with sustained normalization of the rectal proliferation patterns. Assuming that the changes in the rectal mucosa are representative of the rest of the colon, this may reflect a reduction in cancer risk.

Polyunsaturated fatty acids influence the immune system, with both n-3 and n-6 fatty acids reported to have immunosuppressive effects.[118, 119] Grimm et al.[120] investigated the in vivo immunoregulatory influence of various ratios of n-3 to n-6 fatty acids in lipid emulsions administered to a rat heart transplant model. Twenty percent emulsions of safflower oil (n-3:n-6 = 1:370), fish oil (n-3:n-6 = 7.6:1), soybean oil (n-3:n-6 = 1:6.5), and a mixture of safflower oil and fish oil (n-3:n-6 = 1:2.1) were continuously infused at a rate of 9 g of fat/kg of body weight/daily from time of transplantation until complete rejection. Another group of rats received a continuous infusion of saline solution and served as non-oil-treated controls. The non-oil-treated controls and those receiving the balanced mixture of fish and safflower oil rejected their allografts around day 7 (7.8 ± 0.3, and 6.7 ± 0.56 days, respectively). However, infusion of safflower oil, soybean oil, and fish oil prolonged graft survival to 13.3 ± 1.0 days, 10.4 ± 0.7 days, and 12.3 ± 0.4 days, respectively. Soybean oil caused significantly weaker immunosuppression than safflower oil or fish oil.

These results indicate that the ratio of n-3 to n-6 fatty acids influence the immunosuppressive effects of fat emulsions. Safflower oil (n-3:n-6 = 1:370) and fish oil (n-3:n-6 = 7.6:1) were equally immunosuppressive. Soybean oil, with a more balanced n-3 to n-6 ratio (1:6.5), was significantly less immunosuppressive, and the balanced mixture of safflower oil and fish oil had no suppressive effect. The authors[121, 122] comment that although n=6 eicosanoids have a net rejection effect, PGE_2 has been reported to inhibit the cell-mediated response. Predominance of n-6 fatty acids has been shown to increase the production of PGE_2 and decrease that of thromboxane A_2 from rat macrophages.[123] A selective increase in PGE_2 production may therefore explain the prolonged graft survival in the safflower-treated group.

Whereas the immunosuppressive properties of n-6 fatty acids are evident only when there is a marked imbalance in the n-6:n-3 ratio, a moderate surplus of n-3 fatty acids appears sufficient to reveal the effect. This probably reflects the preferential synthesis of n-3-derived eicosanoids, which have a net immunosuppressive effect.

SHORT BOWEL SYNDROME

The mechanism of adaptation to small intestinal resection has continued to intrigue investigators. In addition to the role played by the amino acid glutamine reviewed earlier, SCFAs may also influence the process of adaptation. It is common knowledge to those involved in the management of patients with severe short bowel syndrome and particularly those requiring HPN that the nutritional management of patients with retained colons is far easier than those with jejunostomies. The explanation probably involves the capacity of colon bacteria to salvage maldigested nutrients. Maldigested carbohydrate arriving in the colon is metabolized by bacteria to produce hydrogen and SCFAs. One of the SCFAs, butyrate, is the preferred metabolic substrate for colonic cells and maintains epithelial health. In addition, SCFAs are absorbed and may provide up to 10% of energy requirements in normal individuals. However, with the increased malabsorption of food and particularly carbohydrate, SCFA production can reach levels where it may provide a major energy source for the body. Furthermore, the uptake of SCFAs facilitates the absorption of salt and water, thereby reducing diarrhea. Recent studies also suggest that the absorbed SCFAs can act distally and influence the proliferation of small intestinal mucosa, enhancing the adaptation process.

To investigate this question further, Aghdassi et al.[124] studied four groups of adult Wistar rats. Two of the groups underwent 80% resection of the small intestine, and the other two had simple transections. All rats were fed a liquid diet by gastrostomy for 16 days. Half of the rats with resection and half with transection were also given metronidazole at a dose of 30 mg/kg daily. At day 16 they were weighed and then killed. Resected rats not receiving metronidazole had significantly greater weight gain, carcass protein, nitrogen balance, and higher mucosal dry weight, protein, and DNA content compared with the same measurements in resected rats receiving metronidazole. On the other hand, the addition of metronidazole to the rats with simple transection had no significant effect on these parameters. The authors therefore concluded that although the suppression of colonic fermentation in intact rats had little effect on body composition, the suppression of colon metabolism in rats with massive small bowel resection significantly impaired the adaptive response and nutritional recovery. In other words, the absorptive function of the colon becomes significant only when there is a loss of small intestinal absorptive capacity. That the changes were linked to the production of SCFAs was supported by the finding of reduced SCFAs in the cecum of resected rats receiving metronidazole. The question remains whether the improvement in nutrition is simply related to increased energy absorption in the form of SCFAs or is caused indirectly by stimulation of intestinal adaptation by SCFAs.

The production of intestinal growth factors has also been linked to the process of intestinal adaptation. In a study by O'Loughlin et al.,[125] 4-week-old New Zealand white rabbits were divided into two groups, one being subjected to 60% proximal jejunectomy and the other a sham operative procedure. Mucosal adaptation was studied 10 and 21 days after surgery. In a second series of experiments, animals with similar resections received oral epidermal growth factor (EGF) for 5 days, and the effect on adaptation was assessed 10 days after surgery. After the animals were killed, the ileum was resected, with samples being taken for epithelial transport studies (using Ussing chambers) and for the measurement of brush-border disaccharidase levels. The results demonstrated that simple transection produced a hyperplastic response in the mucosa observed at day 10 but not at day 21. In those who, in addition, had jejunal resection, there was an observed increase in disaccharidase activity but a decrease in 3-*O*-methyl-D-glucose transport. Mucosal hyperplasia was noted at both time periods, indicating that intestinal digestive and absorptive function do not always parallel mucosal hyperplasia. In comparison, the resected animals receiving EGF treatment were shown to have a threefold to fourfold increase in glucose transport and fluorescein binding but no specific effect on digestive enzymes. The authors concluded that EGF may have a therapeutic role in the management of short bowel syndrome by increasing the absorptive capacity of the otherwise hyperplastic mucosa. This is theoretically possible because EGF is a remarkably stable peptide that can be taken orally because it is resistant to gastric and intestinal digestion. Resistance to digestion is essential for its action because unlike other growth factors, it is not expressed throughout the gastrointestinal tract but is released into salivary, duodenal, and pancreatic secretions. However, it must be remembered that the turnover in the intestinal mucosa is finely regulated by the balance between stimulatory and inhibitory mediators, and the pharmacologic application of one factor might result in unexpected side effects.

One example of such side effects from the therapeutic use of regulatory peptides was described by O'Keefe et al.[126] Recent studies have shown that the long-acting somatostatin analogue octreotide can reduce the fluid and electrolyte requirements of patients with permanent end-jejunostomies receiving HPN.[127] The effect, however, was variable; some patients responded dramatically, with a reduction of stomal volumes from more than 10 L daily to less than 5 L daily, whereas others experienced only a 20% reduction. The mechanism of action appears to include reductions in levels of gastric acid, pancreatic enzyme, and intestinal fluid secretion, together with increased absorption due to suppressed intestinal motility. Although digestive enzyme secretion is reduced, the contact time between food, enzymes, and the absorptive surface is increased, permitting greater absorption in the remnant small intestine.

Unfortunately, octreotide has an overall inhibitory effect on most gastrointestinal processes and may therefore interfere with the normal process of intestinal adaptation. A further study in such patients measured amino acid metabolism, pancreatic enzyme synthesis, and mucosal protein turnover by primed continuous infusion of carbon-14-label leucine tracer.[126] Results confirmed that octreotide therapy improved fluid and electrolyte balance but also suppressed gut hormone (insulin, gastrin, glucagon, and peptide yy) levels in the bloodstream. More important, the uptake of amino acids into pancreatic enzyme and mucosal proteins was reduced, with decreased villous growth rates, and there was an increase in amino acid oxidative losses (Fig 5). Consequently, the concomitant use of octreotide with HPN may interfere with the utilization of infused nutrients and suppress splanchnic protein synthesis rates and the process of intestinal adaptation. Other studies have demonstrated the suppressive effect of somatostatin on splanchnic blood flow and gut immunity, and therefore treated patients may be at increased risk of bacterial translocation.[126] This may be of importance in view of the increased risk of such patients to catheter-related sepsis.[128] In addition, increased expression of somatostatin receptors has been noted in neoplastic diseases, granulomatous diseases such as tuberculosis, lymphadenopathies, and in human inflammatory bowel disease.[129] Somatostatin analogues are also expensive. Consequently, their use should be restricted to situations where definite cost benefit can be proved.

Oral Rehydration Solutions

Two recent studies deserve comment. One of the major advances in gastroenterology worldwide has been the development of simple oral rehydration solutions (ORSs). This led to the development of the so-called World Health Organization

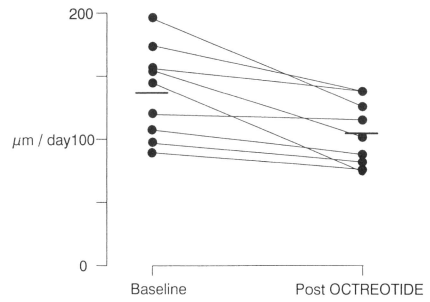

FIGURE 5.
Individual changes in villus growth rates calculated from isotope incorporation and morphologic measurements in patients before and after 10-day octreotide treatment showing significant ($P < .05$) suppression. (From O'Keefe SJ, Haymond MW, Bennett WM, et al: *Gastroenterology* 107:379–388, 1994. Used by permission.)

oral rehydration solution with an osmolarity of 311 mOsm/L and a glucose concentration of 2%. The mechanism of ORSs exploits the capacity of the enterocyte to passively transport water with the active transport of glucose and salt to maintain osmolarity. More recently, ORSs have been modified to contain higher quantities of carbohydrate in the form of glucose polymers to improve not only hydration but also energy absorption.[130] Argenzio et al.[131] have applied similar logic to the development of solutions containing amino acids, which are also actively transported. In a series of experiments on ileal mucosa obtained from newborn piglets infected with cryptosporidi, they measured mucosal sodium absorption by Ussing chamber technique. Although the results demonstrated that glucose and glutamine induced equivalent increases in sodium absorption in noninfected animals, those with infections showed a far greater sodium absorption enhancement with glutamine. In addition, glutamine was oxidized to carbon dioxide at rates three times those of glucose. These effects of glutamine were shown to be inhibited by PGE_2 and enhanced by indomethacin, indicating that the glutamine-stimulated sodium absorption was mediated by a prostaglandin-sensitive Na^+-H^+ exchange mechanism. They concluded that glutamine may be superior to glucose for use in oral rehydration solutions. Following on the same line of logic, one might expect a wide variety of nutrients that have active transport mechanisms to be useful in facilitating the absorption of water across the mucosa. Perhaps the answer is simply to give patients with diarrhea, and normal digestive capacity, normal food!

SUMMARY

Nutritional research continues to focus on the novel effects of the various gut fuels. The plethora of studies concerning the use of glutamine in animal models have certainly produced interesting results, but its role in clinical practice in human subjects still remains to be determined. The relevance of SCFAs, produced by bacterial fermentation to human colonic metabolism is more established, and the findings of recent studies are likely to contribute significantly to our understanding of the pathophysiology of intestinal disease. It is also anticipated that dietary variations, with subsequent differences in availability and metabolism of SCFAs, will, at least in part, explain population differences in the prevalence of colonic diseases such as inflammatory bowel disease and cancer. We can now await the results of larger-scale clinical trials to determine whether specific dietary factors can influence specific disease processes and therefore find a role in the primary management of sick patients.

REFERENCES

1. Newsholme EA, Carrie A-L: Quantitative aspects of glucose and glutamine metabolism by intestinal cells. *Gut* 35(suppl 1):S13–S17, 1994.
2. Newsholme EA, Crabtree B, Newsholme P: Use of enzyme activities as indicators of maximum rates of fuel utilization. *Ciba Found Symp* 73:245–258, 1980.

3. Bergstroem J, Fuerst P, Noree LO, et al: Intracellular free amino acid concentration in human muscle tissue. *J Appl Physiol* 36:693–397, 1974.

4. Eagle H, Oyama VI, Levy M, et al: The growth response of mammalian cells in tissue culture to L-glutamine and L-glutamic acid. *J Biol Chem* 218:607–616, 1956.

5. Windmueller HG, Spaeth AE: Respiratory fuels and nitrogen metabolism in vivo in small intestine of fed rats: Quantitative importance of glutamine, glutamate and aspratate. *J Biol Chem* 255:107–112, 1980.

6. Souba WW, Smith RJ, Wilmore DW: Glutamine metabolism by the intestinal tract. *J Parenter Nutr* 9:608–617, 1985.

7. Souba WW: Glutamine: A key substrate for the splanchnic bed. *Annu Rev Nutr* 11:283–308, 1991.

8. Ardawi MSM, Newsholm EA: Fuel metabolism in colonocytes of the rat. *Biochem J* 231:713–719, 1985.

9. Helton WS: The pathophysiologic significance of alterations in intestinal permeability induced by total parenteral nutrition and glutamine. *JPEN J Parenter Enteral Nutr* 18:289–290, 1994.

10. Welbourne TC: Interorgan glutamine flow in metabolic acidosis. *Am J Physiol* 253:F1069–F1076, 1987.

11. Souba WW, Klimberg VS, Plumley DA, et al: The role of glutamine in maintaining a healthy gut and supporting the metabolic response to injury and infection. *J Surg Res* 48:393–391, 1990.

12. Lacey JM, Wilmore DW: Is glutamine a conditionally essential amino acid? *Nutr Rev* 48:297–309, 1990.

13. Vinnars E, Bergstroem J, Fuerst P: Influence of the postoperative state on the intracellular free amino acids in human muscle tissue. *Ann Surg* 182:665–671, 1975.

14. Souba WW: The gut as a nitrogen-processing organ in the metabolic response to critical illness. *Nutr Supp Serv* 8:15–22, 1988.

15. O'Dwyer ST, Smith RJ, Hwang TL, et al: Maintenance of the small bowel mucosa with glutamine-enriched parenteral nutrition. *JPEN J Parenter Enteral Nutr* 13:579–585, 1989.

16. Babst R, Horig H, Stehle P, et al: Glutamine peptide-supplemented long-term total parenteral nutrition: Effects on intracellular and extracellular amino acid patterns, nitrogen economy, and tissue morphology in growing rats. *JPEN J Parenter Enteral Nutr* 17:566–574, 1993.

17. Christiansen J, Bech A, Fahrenkrug J, et al: Fat-induced jejunal inhibition of gastric acid secretion and release of pancreatic glucagon, enteroglucagon, gastric inhibitory polypeptide, and vasoactive intestinal polypeptide in man. *Scand J Gastroenterol* 14:161–166, 1979.

18. Bloom SR, Polak JM: The hormonal pattern of intestinal adaption. A major role for enteroglucagon. *Scand J Gastroenterol* 74S:93–103, 1982.

19. Illig KA, Ryan CK, Sax HC, et al: Total parenteral nutrition-induced changes in gut mucosal function: Atrophy alone is not the issue. *Surgery* 112:631–637, 1992.

20. Helton S, Smith R, Hong R, et al: Are intestinal permeability, bacterial translocation, and intestinal atrophy during TPN and enteral feeding related? *JPEN J Parenter Enteral Nutr* 15(suppl):17, 1991.

21. Alverdy JC, Aoys E, Moss GS: Total parenteral nutrition promotes bacterial translocation from the gut. *Surgery* 104:185–190, 1988.

22. Helton WS, Garcia R: Oral prostaglandin E2 prevents gut atrophy during intravenous feeding but not bacterial translocation. *Arch Surg* 128:178–184, 1993.

23. Li J, Langkamp-Henken B, Suzuki K, et al: Glutamine prevents parenteral nutrition–induced increases in intestinal permeability. *JPEN J Parenter Enteral Nutr* 18:303–307, 1994.

24. Van der Hulst RWJ, Von Meyenfeldt MF, Arends JW, et al: Glutamine and the preservation of gut integrity. *Lancet* 341:1363–1365, 1993.

25. Tremel H, Kienle B, Weilemann LS, et al: Glutamine dipeptide-supplemented parenteral nutrition maintains intestinal function in the critically ill. *Gastroenterology* 107:1595–1601, 1994.

26. Wilmore DW: Glutamine and the gut. *Gastroenterology* 107:1885–1886, 1994.

27. Souba WW, Herskowitz K, Klimberg VS, et al: The effects of sepsis and endotoxemia on gut glutamine metabolism. *Ann Surg* 211:543–549, 1990.

28. Salloum RM, Copeland EM, Souba WW: Brush border transport of glutamine and other substrates during sepsis and endotoxemia. *Ann Surg* 213:401–410, 1991.

29. Chen K, Okuma T, Okumura K, et al: Glutamine-supplemented parenteral nutrition improves gut mucosal integrity and function in endotoxemic rats. *JPEN J Parenter Enteral Nutr* 18:167–171, 1994.

30. Barbul A, Lazarou SA, Efron DT, et al: Arginine enhances wound healing and lymphocytic immune responses in humans. *Surgery* 108:331–336, 1990.

31. Seifter E, Rettura G, Barbul A, et al: Arginine: An essential amino acid for injured rats. *Surgery* 48:224–230, 1978.

32. Merimee TJ, Lillicrap DA, Rabinowitz D: Effect of arginine on serum levels of human growth hormone. *Lancet* 2:668–670, 1965.

33. Palmer JP, Walter RM, Ensinck JW: Arginine-stimulated acute phase response of insulin and glucagon secretion. *Diabetes* 24:735–740, 1975.

34. Dhanakoti SN, Brosman JT, Hertzberg GR, et al: Renal arginine synthesis: Studies *in vivo* and *in vitro*. *Am J Physiol* 259:E437–E442, 1990.

35. Windmueller HG, Spaeth AE: Source and fate of circulating citrulline. *Am J Physiol* 241:E473–E480, 1981.

36. Windmueller HG, Spaeth AE: Respiratory fuels and nitrogen metabolism *in vivo* in small intestine of fed rats. *J Biol Chem* 253:69–76, 1978.

37. Windmueller HG, Spaeth AE: Intestinal metabolism of glutamine and glutamate from the lumen as compared to glutamine from blood. *Arch Biochem Biophys* 171:662–672, 1975.

38. Houdijk APJ, van Leeuwen PAM, Teerlink TT, et al: Glutamine-enriched enteral diet increases renal arginine production. *JPEN J Parenter Enteral Nutr* 18:422–426, 1994.

39. Roediger WEW: Role of anaerobic bacteria in the metabolic welfare of the colonic muscosa in man. *Gut* 21:793–798, 1980.

40. Scheppach W, Loges C, Bartram P, et al: Effect of free glutamine and alanyl-glutamine dipeptide on mucosal proliferation of the human ileum and colon. *Gastroenterology* 107:429–434, 1994.

41. Lipkin M, Blattner WE, Fraumeni JF, et al: Tritiated thymidine (φp, φh) labeling distribution as a marker for hereditary predisposition to colon cancer. *Cancer Res* 43:1899–1904, 1983.

42. Hornsby-Lewis L, Shike M, Brown P, et al: L-Glutamine supplementation in home parenteral nutrition patients: Stability, safety, and effects on intestinal absorption. *JPEN J Parenter Enteral Nutr* 18:268–273, 1994.

43. *Caremark Procedures Manual.* Totowa, NJ, Caremark International, 1992.

44. Souba WW, Herskowitz, Austgen TR, et al: Glutamine nutrition: Theoretical considerations and therapeutic impact. *JPEN J Parenter Enteral Nutr* 14:237–243, 1990.

45. Roediger WEW: The starved colon—diminished mucosal nutrition, diminished absorption, and colitis. *Dis Colon Rectum* 33:858–862, 1990.

46. Scheppach W: Effects of short chain fatty acids on gut morphology and function. *Gut* 35(suppl 1):S35–S38, 1994.

47. Vernia P, et al: Organic anions and the diarrhoea of inflammatory bowel disease. *Dig Dis Sci* 33:1353–1358, 1988.

48. Chapman MAS, et al: Failure of colonic mucosa to oxidize butyrate in ulcerative colitis [abstract]. *Gut* 33(suppl 2):T158, 1992.

49. Roediger WEW: The colonic epithelium in ulcerative colitis: An energy deficient disease? *Lancet* 2:712–715, 1980.

50. Roediger WEW, Nance S: Metabolic induction of experimental ulcerative colitis by inhibition of fatty acid oxidation. *Br J Exp Pathol* 67:773–782, 1986.

51. Bruer RI, Buto SK, Christ ML, et al: Rectal irrigation with short-chain fatty acids for distal ulcerative colitis. Preliminary report. *Dig Dis Sci* 36:185–187, 1991.

52. Senagore AJ, Mackeigan JM, Scheider M, et al: Short-chain fatty acid enemas: A cost-effective alternative in the treatment of nonspecific proctosigmoiditis. *Dis Colon Rectum* 35:923–927, 1992.

53. Scheppach W, Sommer H, Kirchner T, et al: Effect of butyrate enemas on the colonic mucosa in distal ulcerative colitis. *Gastroenterology* 103:51–56, 1992.

54. Mortensen PB, Hove H, Clausen MR, et al: Fermentation to short-chain fatty acids and lactate in human faecal batch cultures. Intra- and inter-individual variations versus variations caused by changes in fermented saccharides. *Scand J Gastroenterol* 26:1285–1294, 1991.

55. Rubinstein R, Howard AV, Wrong OM: In vivo dialysis of faeces as a method of stool analysis: IV. The organic anion component. *Clin Sci* 37:549–564, 1969.

56. Clausen MR, Mortensen PB: Kinetic studies on the metabolism of short-chain fatty acids and glucose by isolated rat colonocytes. *Gastroenterology* 106:423–432, 1994.

57. Bergman EN: Energy conditions of volatile fatty acids from the gastrointestinal tract in various species. *Physiol Res* 70:567–590, 1990.

58. Rowe WA, Bayless TM: Colonic short-chain fatty acids: Fuel from the lumen? *Gastroenterology* 103:336–338, 1992.

59. Sakata T: Stimulatory effect of short chain fatty acids on epithelial cell proliferation in the rat intestine: A possible explanation for the trophic effects of fermentable fibre, gut microbes, and luminal trophic effects. *Br J Nutr* 58:95–103, 1987.

60. Kripke SA, Fox AD, Berman JM, et al: Stimulation of intestinal mucosal growth with intracolonic infusion of short chain fatty acids. *JPEN J Parenter Enteral Nutr* 13:109–116, 1989.

61. Scheppach W, Bartram P, Richter A, et al: Effect of short-chain fatty acids on the human colonic mucosa in vitro. *JPEN J Parenter Enteral Nutr* 16:43–48, 1992.

62. Roediger WEW, Moore A: The effect of short-chain fatty acids on sodium absorption in the human colon perfused through the vascular bed. *Dig Dis Sci* 26:100–106, 1981.

63. Ruppin H, Bar-Meir S, Soergel KH, et al: Absorption of short-chain fatty acids by the colon. *Gastroenterology* 78:1500–1507, 1980.

64. Kvietys PR, Granger DN: Effect of volatile fatty acids on blood flow and oxygen uptake by the dog colon. *Gastroenterology* 80:962–969, 1981.

65. Mortensen FV, Nielsen H, Mulvany MJ, et al: Short chain fatty acids dilate isolated human colonic resistance arteries. *Gut* 31:1391–1394, 1990.

66. Kamath PS, Phillips SF, Zinsmeister AR: Short-chain fatty acids stimulate ileal motility in humans. *Gastroenterology* 95:1496–1502, 1988.

67. Yajima T: Contractile effects of short-chain fatty acids on the isolated colon of the rat. *J Physiol* 368:667–678, 1985.

68. Whitehead RH, Young GP, Bhathal PS: Effects of short chain fatty acids on a new human colon carcinoma line (LIM 1215). *Gut* 27:1457–1463, 1986.

69. Kim YS, Tsao D, Siddiqui B: Effects of sodium butyrate and dimethylsulfoxide on biochemical properties of human cancer cells. *Cancer* 45:1185–1192, 1980.

70. McIntyre A, Gibson PR, Young GP: Butyrate production from dietary fibre and protection against large bowel cancer in a rat model. *Gut* 34:386–391, 1993.

71. Kripke SA, Fox AD, Berman JM, et al: Stimulation of intestinal mucosal growth with intracolonic infusion of short-chain fatty acids. *JPEN J Parenter Enteral Nutr* 13:185–187, 1989.

72. Sakata T: Stimulatory effect of short-chain fatty acids on epithelial cell proliferation in the rat intestine: A possible explanation of trophic effects of fermentable fibre, gut microbes and luminal trophic factors. *Br J Nutr* 58:95–103, 1987.

73. Frankel WL, Zhang W, Singh A, et al: Mediation of the trophic effects of short-chain fatty acids on rat jejunum and colon. *Gastroenterology* 106:375–380, 1994.

74. Koruda MJ, Rolandelli RH, Settle RG, et al: Effect of parenteral nutrition supplemented with short-chain fatty acids on adaption to massive small bowel resection. *Gastroenterology* 95:715–720, 1988.

75. Stein TP, Yoshida S, Schluter MD, et al: Comparison of intravenous nutrients on gut mucosal synthesis. *JPEN J Parenter Enteral Nutr* 18:447–452, 1994.

76. Blasi F: Surface receptors for urokinase plasminogen activator. *Fibrinolysis* 2:73–84, 1988.

77. Gold LI, Schwimmer R, Quigley JP: Human plasma fibronectin as a substrate for human urokinase. *Biochem J* 262:529–534, 1989.

78. Gibson PR, van der Pol E, Doe WF: Cell associated urokinase activity and colonic epithelial cells in health and disease. *Gut* 32:191–195, 1991.

79. Lyons RM, Gentry LE, Purcio AF, et al: Mechanism of activation of latent recombinant transforming growth factor β_1 by plasmin. *J Cell Biol* 110:1361–1367, 1990.

80. Koyama S, Podolsky DK: Effects of growth factors on an intestinal epithelial line: Transforming growth factors **A** and **B** in rat intestinal epithelial cells. *J Clin Invest* 83:1768–1773, 1989.

81. Ciacci C, Lind SE, Podolsky DK: Transforming growth factor B regulation of migration in wounded rat intestinal epithelial monolayers. *Gastroenterology* 105:93–101, 1993.

82. Elliott R, Stevens RW, Doe WF: Expression of urokinase-type plasminogen activator in the mucosal lesions of inflammatory bowel disease. *J Gastroenterol Hepatol* 2:517–523, 1987.

83. De Bruin PAF, Crama-Bohbouth G, Verspaget HW, et al: Plasminogen activators in the intestine of patients with inflammatory bowel disease. *Thromb Haemost* 60:262–266, 1986.

84. Gibson PR, Rosella O, Rosella G, et al: Butyrate is a potent inhibitor of urokinase secretion by normal colonic epithelium in vitro. *Gastroenterology* 107:410–419, 1994.

85. Gibson PR, Folino M, Rosello O, et al: Neoplasia and hyperplasia of large bowel: Focal lesions in an abnormal epithelium. *Gastroenterology* 103:1452–1459, 1992.

86. Terpstra OT, Van Blankenstein M, Dees J, et al: Abnormal pattern of cell proliferation in the entire colonic mucosa of patients with colon adenoma or cancer. *Gastroenterology* 93:704–708, 1987.

87. Wilson RG, Smith AN, Bird CC: Immunohistochemical detection of abnormal cell proliferation in colonic mucosa of subjects with polyps. *J Clin Pathol* 43:744–747, 1990.

88. Harig JM, Soegel KH, Komorowski RA, et al: Treatment of diversion colitis with short-chain fatty acid irrigation. *N Engl J Med* 320:23–28, 1989.

89. Ramakrishna BS, Roediger WEW: Bacterial short chain fatty acids: Their role in gastrointestinal disease. *Dig Dis Sci* 8:337–345, 1990.

90. Binder HJ, Mehta P: Short-chain fatty acids stimulate active sodium and chloride absorption in the rat distal colon. *Gastroenterology* 96:989–996, 1989.

91. Sellin JH, De Soignie R: Short-chain fatty acid absorption in rabbit colon *In vitro*. *Gastroenterology* 99:676–683, 1990.

92. Butzner JD, Meddings JB, Dalal V: Inhibition of short-chain fatty acid absorption and Na^+ absorption during acute colitis in the rabbit. *Gastroenterology* 106:1190–1198, 1994.

93. Roediger WE, Rae DA: Trophic effect of short chain fatty acids on the mucosal handling of ions by the defunctioned colon. *Br J Surg* 69:23–25, 1982.

94. Nzegwu H, Young A, Levin RJ: Effects of starvation and refeeding on electrogenic transport in rat colon: A model for famine diarrhoea [abstract]. *Gut* 28:A1395–A1396, 1987.

95. Levin RJ, Nzegwu HC, Young A: Proximal colon secretion in fed and starved rats [abstract]. *J Physiol* 396:33P, 1988.

96. Roediger WE: Famine, fibre, fatty acids, and failed colonic absorption: Does fibre fermentation ameliorate diarrhoea? *JPEN J Parenter Enteral Nutr* 18:4–8, 1994.

97. Carpenter CCJ, Greenough WB, Pierce NF: Oral-rehydration therapy: The role of polymeric substrates. *N Engl J Med* 319:1346–1348, 1988.

98. Cereal-based oral rehydration solutions: Bridging the gap between fluid and food [editorial]. *Lancet* 339:219–220, 1992.

99. Young A, Levin RJ: Intestinal hypersecretion of the refed starved rat: A model for alimentary diarrhoea. *Gut* 33:1050–1056, 1992.

100. Young A, Pereira MMC, Warren MA, et al: Hypersecretion associated with the action of *Escherichia coli* enterotoxin on the jejunum and ileum from starved and chronically undernourished rats. *Med Sci Res* 16:573–575, 1988.

101. Winter TA, Ogden JM, Lemmer ER, et al: The vicious circle of malnutrition, maldigestion and malabsorption: Response to specialized refeeding [abstract]. *Nutrition* 10:489, 1994.

102. Tutton PJM, Barkla DH: Influence of prostaglandin analogs on epithelial cell proliferation and xenograft growth. *Br J Cancer* 41:47–51, 1980.

103. Minoura T, Takata T, Sakaguchi M, et al: Effect of dietary eicosapentaenoic acid on azoxymethane-induced colon carcinogenesis. *Cancer Res* 48:4790–4794, 1988.

104. Bennett A, Del Tacca M, Stamford IF, et al: Prostaglandins from tumors of human large bowel. *Br J Cancer* 35:881–884, 1977.

105. Endres S, Ghorbani R, Kelley VE, et al: The effect of dietary supplementation with n-3 polyunsaturated fatty acids on the synthesis of interleukin-1 and tumor necrosis factor by mononuclear cells. *N Engl J Med* 320:265–271, 1989.

106. Winter TA, O'Keefe SJD: Nutrition and gastroenterology. In Gitnick G (ed): *Current Gastroenterology.* St Louis, Mosby, vol 14, 1994.

107. Winter TA, O'Keefe SJD: Nutrition and gastroenterology. In Gitnick G (ed): *Current Gastroenterology.* St Louis, Mosby, vol 15, 1995.

108. Blot WJ, Lanier A, Fraumeni JF, et al: Cancer mortality among Alaskan natives, 1960–69. *J Natl Cancer Inst* 55:547–554, 1975.

109. Bang HO, Dyerberg J, Hjorne N: The composition of food consumed by Greenland Eskimos. *Acta Med Scand* 200:69–73, 1976.

110. Anti M, Marra G, Armelao F, et al: Effect of ω-3 fatty acids on rectal proliferation in subjects at risk for colon cancer. *Gastroenterology* 103:883–891, 1992.

111. Wargovich MJ: Fish oil and colon cancer. *Gastroenterology* 103:1096–1101, 1992.

112. Bartram HP, Gostner A, Scheppach W, et al: Effect of fish oil on rectal cell proliferation, mucosal fatty acids, and prostaglandin E$_2$ release in healthy subjects. *Gastroenterology* 105:1317–1322, 1993.

113. Silk DB: Medical management of severe inflammatory disease of the rectum: Nutritional aspects. *Baillière's Clin Gastroenterol* 6:27–41, 1992.

114. Aslan A, Triadafilopoulos G: Fish oil fatty acid supplementation in active ulcerative colitis: A double-blind, crossover study. *Am J Gastroenterol* 87:432–437, 1992.

115. Stenson WF, Cort D, Rodgers J, et al: Dietary supplementation with fish oil in ulcerative colitis. *Ann Intern Med* 116:609–614, 1992.

116. Hawthorn AB, Daneschmend TK, Hawkey CJ, et al: Treatment of ulcerative colitis with fish oil supplementation: A prospective 12 month randomized trial. *Gut* 33:922–928, 1992.

117. Anti M, Armelao F, Marra G, et al: Effects of different doses of fish oil on rectal cell proliferation in patients with sporadic colonic adenomas. *Gastroenterology* 107:1709–1718, 1994.

118. Perez RV, Waymack JP, Munda R, et al: The effect of donor specific transfusions and dietary fatty acids on rat cardiac allograft survival. *J Surg Res* 32:335–340, 1987.

119. Otto DA, Kahn DR, Hamm MW, et al: Improved survival of heterotrophic cardiac allografts in rats with dietary n-3 polyunsaturated fatty acids. *Transplantation* 50:193–198, 1990.

120. Grimm H, Tibel A, Norrlind B, et al: Immunoregulation by parenteral lipids: Impact of the n-3 to n-6 fatty acid ratio. *JPEN J Parenter Enteral Nutr* 18:417–421, 1994.

121. Goodwin JS, Webb DR: Regulation of the immune response by prostaglandins. *Clin Immunol Immunopathol* 15:106–111, 1980.

122. Kunkel SL, Chensue SW, Phan SH: Prostaglandins as endogenous mediators of interleukin 1 production. *J Immunol* 136:186–192, 1986.

123. Chouaib S, Chatenoud L, Klatzman D, et al: The mechanisms of inhibition of human IL-2 production: II. PGE_2 induction of suppressor T-lymphocytes. *J Immunol* 132:1851–1857, 1984.

124. Aghdassi E, Plapler H, Kurian R, et al: Colonic fermentation and nutritional recovery in rats with massive small bowel resection. *Gastroenterology* 107:637–642, 1994.

125. O'Loughlin E, Winter M, Shun A, et al: Structural and functional adaptation following jejunal resection in rabbits: Effect of epidermal growth factor. *Gastroenterology* 107:87–93, 1994.

126. O'Keefe SJ, Haymond MW, Bennett WM, et al: Long-acting somatostatin analogue therapy and protein metabolism in patients with jejunostomies. *Gastroenterology* 107:379–388, 1994.

127. O'Keefe SJ, Petersen ME, Fleming CR: Octreotide as an adjunct to home parenteral nutrition in the management of permanent end-jejunostomy syndrome. *JPEN J Parenter Enteral Nutr* 18:26–34, 1994.

128. O'Keefe SJ, Burnes JU, Thompson RL: Recurrent sepsis in home parenteral nutrition patients: An analysis of risk factors. *JPEN J Parenter Enteral Nutr* 18:256–263, 1994.

129. Reubi JC, Mazzucchelli L, Laissue JA: Intestinal vessels express a high density of somatostatin receptors in human inflammatory bowel disease. *Gastroenterology* 106:951–959, 1994.

130. Zheng BY, Khin-Maung-U, Lu RB, et al: Absorption of glucose polymers from rice in oral rehydration solutions by rat small intestine. *Gastroenterology* 104:81–85, 1993.

131. Argenzio RA, Rhoades JM, Armstrong M, et al: Glutamine stimulates prostaglandin-sensitive Na^+-H^+ exchange in experimental porcine cryptosporidiosis. *Gastroenterology* 106:1418–1428, 1994.

CHAPTER 7

Abdominal Imaging

Sharon S. Burton, M.D.
Associate Professor of Radiology, Chief, Division of Gastrointestinal Radiology, University of Florida College of Medicine, Gainesville, Florida

Patricia L. Abbitt, M.D.
Associate Professor of Radiology, Chief, Division of Ultrasound, University of Florida College of Medicine, Gainesville, Florida

Gladys M. Torres, M.D.
Associate Professor of Radiology, University of Florida College of Medicine, Gainesville, Florida

Joseph Cernigliaro, M.D.
Clinical Fellow of Radiology, Division of Body Imaging, University of Florida College of Medicine, Gainesville, Florida

Pablo R. Ros, M.D.
Professor and Associate Chairman of Radiology, Chief, Division of Body Imaging and Magnetic Resonance Imaging, University of Florida College of Medicine, Gainesville, Florida

Abdominal imaging is a dynamic field that continues to evolve as new diagnostic and therapeutic approaches are developed and validated. This chapter will summarize current approaches to the diagnosis of selected gastrointestinal (GI) tract diseases using plain radiography, barium studies, sonography, computed tomography (CT), and magnetic resonance imaging (MRI). An update on percutaneous interventional techniques used for diagnosis and treatment is also provided.

Current Gastroenterology®, vol. 16
© 1996, Mosby–Year Book, Inc.

PLAIN FILMS

Abdominal radiographs are a useful screening tool in patients with signs and symptoms of bowel obstruction. Recent proposals for improving plain film diagnosis include (1) use of LaPlace's law in suspected colonic obstruction, (2) appropriate interpretation of differential air fluid levels in small bowel dilation, and (3) recognition of radiographic signs of colonic obstruction due to traumatic diaphragmatic hernia.

Wittenberg[1] demonstrated pitfalls in the diagnosis of colonic obstruction and use of LaPlace's law as a diagnostic tool (Fig 1). His patient had gas in the rectum and no fecal retention proximal to a near complete obstruction in the rectum. Wittenberg[1] proposes the use of LaPlace's law as a more reliable criterion for colonic obstruction.[2]

According to this law of physics, when a patent tube is subjected to constant intraluminal pressure, the part of the tube with the greatest diameter will be under the greatest tension. In the colon, the cecum has the largest diameter and should be at least as dilated, if not more dilated, than the rest of the colon in the presence of

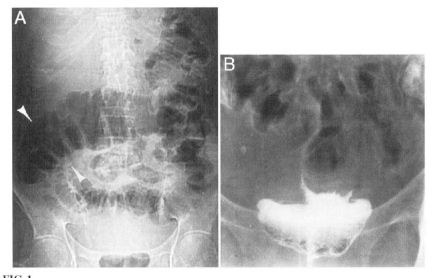

FIG 1.
Distal colonic obstruction in a 60-year-old woman with history of gastric adenocarcinoma. **A,** digital radiograph of abdomen immediately before computed tomography (CT). Gas is seen in the rectum. The proximal colon is dilated, and the maximum diameter of cecum *(arrowheads)* is greater than that of all other segments of colon. With CT, maximum colonic distension was confirmed to be at level of ileocecal valve consistent with LaPlace's law. No colonic fluid and a paucity of feces were seen. **B,** barium enema shows tapered total retrograde obstruction of rectum. Laparotomy revealed a large obstructing pelvic mass and other intraperitoneal metastases from gastric adenocarcinoma. (From Wittenberg J: *AJR* 161:443–444, 1993. Used by permission.)

obstruction. If the entire colon is dilated and the cecum is not, mechanical obstruction is unlikely.

Differentiating mechanical obstruction from adynamic ileus may require additional films.[1] A left decubitus film is recommended for assessment of the descending colon[3] and a prone film for suspected rectosigmoid obstruction. If air or fluid do not extend past the site of colonic dilation on these views, distal mechanical obstruction must be excluded by contrast enema. This combination of plain film techniques will improve accuracy of diagnosis of colonic obstruction.

Harlow et al.[4] investigated the significance of differential air fluid levels in patients with small bowel dilation. They reviewed in retrospect abdominal films from patients with 62 episodes of small bowel obstruction and 38 episodes of adynamic obstruction. Differential air-fluid levels were defined as air-fluid interfaces seen on horizontal beam films (erect or decubitus) at different heights within the same loop of bowel. The vertical separation between fluid levels within the same loop was measured in millimeters. Differential air-fluid levels were seen in 32 of 62 cases of obstruction (52%) and in 11 of 38 episodes of adynamic ileus (29%). The sensitivity for detection of mechanical obstruction was only 52%, and specificity was 71%. Differential air-fluid levels measuring 20 mm high or greater were moderately suggestive of mechanical obstruction, because they rarely occurred to this degree in adynamic ileus.

Colonic obstruction due to traumatic diaphragmatic hernia is a rare occurrence that may follow blunt or penetrating trauma to the upper half of the abdomen or the chest. Cruz and Minagi[4a] reported radiographic findings in four patients with obstruction after stab injury to the left upper quadrant. Patients had abdominal pain. The mean time interval since stab injury was 70 days, with a range from 4 to 150 days. Initial chest radiographs in all patients showed abnormalities of the left hemidiaphragm, including elevation, loss of definition of the diaphragm, pleural effusion (two cases), and small cystic lucencies above the diaphragmatic contour (one case). Initial abdominal films showed mild dilation of the colon proximal to the splenic flexure in two patients. Progressive colonic dilation proximal to the splenic flexure was seen on serial films in three patients. Contrast enema showed colonic obstruction at the splenic flexure level in three patients. At surgery, all patients showed colonic obstruction due to herniation of colon, omentum, or both through a traumatic diaphragmatic defect. This unusual cause of colonic obstruction must be considered in patients with abdominal pain and prior history of injury to the upper half of the abdomen.

BARIUM STUDIES

Topics of interest regarding barium studies of the GI tract include (1) gastric cancer detection using double-contrast barium examinations, (2) natural history of fundic gland polyposis, and (3) serial changes in intestinal Behçet's disease (BD).

Accuracy of radiographic diagnosis of gastric cancer using single-contrast barium studies is limited. The average reported sensitivity of cancer detection using single-contrast technique is 75%.[5] Double-contrast barium examinations provide improved distension and mucosal detail that improves detection of smaller, more subtle lesions, including early gastric cancer.[6]

At the Hospital of the University of Pennsylvania, a retrospective study was done to assess the sensitivity of double-contrast barium studies for detection of gastric carcinoma. In 80 patients with pathologically proven gastric carcinoma, the lesion was visible on radiographs in all cases. One patient's ulcerative lesion was missed on a prior barium examination 2 years before, and therefore double-contrast barium studies detected 79 of 80 gastric carcinomas (99%). Malignant neoplasms were diagnosed or suspected in 77 of 80 patients (96%) undergoing barium studies. Two or three patients who were diagnosed as having benign disease had gastric outlet obstruction. The presence of retained fluid and food material in patients with outlet obstruction was the most important pitfall for radiographic diagnosis of gastric cancer.

The radiographic appearances of gastric cancer are shown in Figure 2. The lesion was predominantly polypoid in 59%, had an infiltrative or scirrhous pattern in 31% (see Figure 2, A), and showed an ulcerative pattern in 10% of patients (see Figure 2, B). Early gastric cancer was found in 5 of 50 patients undergoing surgery. The early cancers were polypoid or plaquelike lesions (see Figure 2, C) in four patients and ulcerative in one patient. Gastric cancer was located in the cardia or fundus in 38 patients (48%), the body in 16 patients (20%), and antrum in 21 patients (26%).

The number of false-positive barium studies that could have led to unnecessary referral for endoscopy was also investigated.[5] Over a 1-year period, 54 of 1,546 patients (3.5%) undergoing double-contrast barium studies were referred for endoscopy because of radiographic findings that were equivocal or suggestive of malignancy (ulcers, thickened folds or nodular mucosa, and gastric narrowing). Ten of 54 patients referred (19%) proved to have gastric cancer, and 3 had large ulcerated masses that were presumed to be malignant. In 19 patients who had endoscopy showing no malignancy, other diagnoses included *Helicobactor pylori* gastritis in 8 patients, nonspecific gastritis in 5 patients, hyperplastic polyps in 3 patients, and normal findings in 3 patients.

In summary, these studies indicate that the double-contrast barium examination of the stomach provides a sensitive screening tool for gastric cancer without leading to a high number of unnecessary referrals for endoscopy. The increasing frequency of cancers in the upper half of the stomach, 48% in this series, makes use of double-contrast methods even more important. Lesions in the fundus and cardia may be missed on single-contrast barium examinations because it is not possible to compress the stomach behind the rib cage or achieve full distension with barium alone. Optimal double-contrast technique will be required to maintain a high level of sensitivity for detection of gastric cancer in clinical practice.

Fundic gland polyposis (FGP) is a non-neoplastic condition initially described

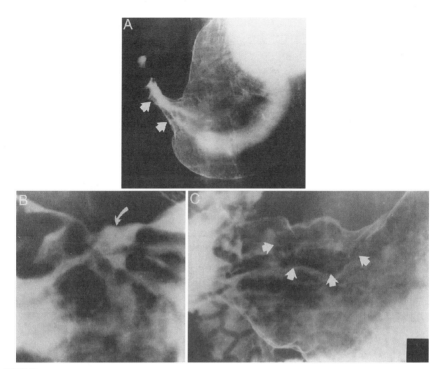

FIG 2.
Radiographic features of gastric carcinoma. **A,** scirrhous carcinoma of gastric antrum. Radiograph from double-contrast barium study shows irregular narrowing of distal part of antrum *(arrows)* from infiltrative/scirrhous carcinoma. **B,** malignant gastric ulcer. Prone compression view from double-contrast barium study shows a meniscoid ulcer *(arrow)* on lesser curvature of gastric antrum. Intraluminal projection of ulcer and nodular, clubbed appearance of folds radiating to edge of ulcer crater are characteristic findings of a malignant ulcer. **C,** early gastric cancer. Radiograph from double-contrast barium study shows a 3-cm plaquelike lesion *(arrows)* straddling lesser curvature of gastric antrum. Examination of biopsy specimens and brushings from follow-up endoscopy showed no evidence of tumor. However, examination of biopsy specimens from a second endoscopic examination confirmed the presence of malignant tumor. Early gastric cancer was found at surgery. (From Low VHS: *AJR* 162:329–334, 1994. Used by permission.)

in patients with familial adenomatosis coli (FAC), but it can occur in patients without FAC.[7] The natural history of FGP was evaluated in 31 patients who were followed with endoscopy and radiography over a period of 1 to 13 years. Of 25 women and 6 men, ranging in age from 32 to 73 years, none had evidence of a polyposis syndrome. Double-contrast barium studies and endoscopy showed fundic gland polyps as smooth, round, protrusions less than 9 mm and located in the fundus and body of the stomach (Fig 3, A). Histology revealed hyperplasia of the fundic glands with cystic dilation (Fig. 3, B). In 8 of 11 patients with a solitary lesion, the polyp was completely resected at the time of diagnosis, and no further polyps developed.

Seven of 20 patients with multiple polyps on initial diagnosis showed a change in the number of polyps over time. The pattern of change included complete resolution of polyps, transient disappearance followed by recurrence of numerous polyps, or simple increase in number over time. In 16 patients, no visible changes were seen in the number of polyps over time. The reasons for regression and recurrence of polyps and the pathogenesis of this benign condition remain unknown.

In a similar study, Iida et al.[8] investigated the natural history of intestinal BD. Behçet's disease is characterized by aphthous stomatitis, genital ulcers, and ocular inflammation. It may affect multiple organ systems, including the intestinal tract, where it results in deep ulcers that may perforate, requiring surgical resection. Seven patients with intestinal BD who did not require surgery were followed with serial barium studies for an average of 4.5 years. Abdominal symptoms included pain, diarrhea, and bloody stools. Five patients had initial barium studies showing deep ulcers in the terminal ileum or ileocecal region (Fig 4, A–C). Follow-up examinations in four patients showed healing or improvement in ulcers after treatment, but the lesions recurred. The colon was the only site affected in two patients who had numerous aphthoid ulcerations and shallow longitudinal ulcers (Fig 4, D). Treat-

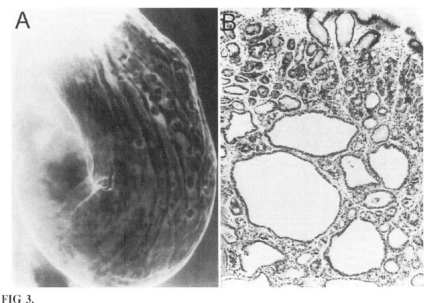

FIG 3.
Fundic gland polyposis. **A,** this female patient was diagnosed with fundus gland polyposis (FGP) at age 32 and showed spontaneous disappearance of polyps on radiographic and endoscopic examination at age 35. This gastric radiograph obtained 12.9 years (age 45) after initial examination shows reappearance of FGP, with a remarkable increase in the number of polyps (≥ 100). **B,** micrograph of biopsy specimen taken from gastric polyps shows simple hyperplasia of normal fundic glands with microcysts (hematoxylin-eosin stain; original magnification ×140). (From Hizawa K: *Radiology* 189:429–432, 1993. Used by permission.)

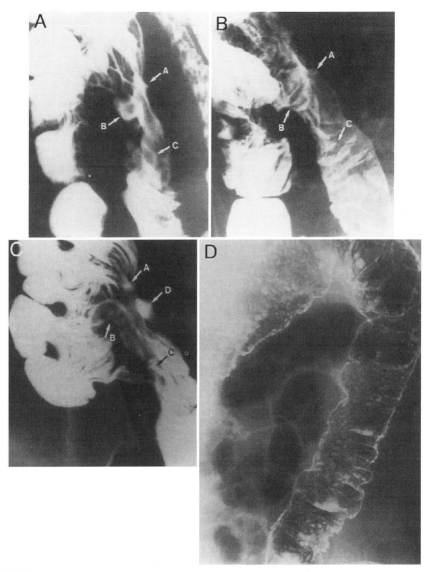

FIG 4.
Serial changes in intestinal Behçet's disease. **A,** inital radiograph with compression reveals three deep ulcers in the terminal ileum *(arrows A–C).* **B,** follow-up radiograph obtained 5 months after the initial examination shows three ulcers that are almost healed *(arrows A–C).* **C,** follow-up radiograph obtained 2 years 7 months after the initial examination shows an open ulcer *(arrow A),* two healed ulcers *(arrows B* and *C),* and a newly developed ulcer *(arrow D).* **D,** double-contrast radiograph of the colon in another patient shows innumerable aphthoid ulcers and loss of haustration in the left side of the colon. (From Iida M: *Radiology* 188:65–69, 1993. Used by permission.)

ment with sulfasalazine and total parenteral nutrition resulted in transient healing of colonic ulcers, followed by recurrence.

The differential diagnosis of intestinal BD includes other forms of inflammatory bowel disease. The ileocecal distribution of intestinal BD and tendency to wax and wane with treatment resemble Crohn's disease. Typically the ulcers in BD tend to be larger, rounder, and deeper than those seen in Crohn's disease. Other features commonly seen in Crohn's disease, such as longitudinal ulcers, cobblestoning, and stricture formation, are not usually present in BD. Colonic involvement with BD may mimic ulcerative colitis, except that the ulcerations of BD tend to occur in a background of normal mucosa instead of the diffuse mucosal inflammation found in ulcerative colitis. Identification of other clinical features of BD may be required to differentiate these inflammatory diseases of the GI tract.

Ultrasonography

Topics of interest in ultrasonography this past year dealt with ways to improve the sonographic diagnosis of commonly encountered conditions, including (1) appendicitis, (2) hemangioma of the liver, and (3) portal vein thrombosis.

Appendicitis is the most common cause of an intra-abdominal nontraumatic emergency requiring surgical intervention. The diagnosis may be readily apparent in the typical patient, but 30% to 45% of patients may have an atypical manifestation, resulting in clinical uncertainty. Interest has been keen in the technique of graded compression ultrasonography for the diagnosis of appendicitis since it was first described by Puylaert[9] in 1986. Numerous articles in the radiologic literature have studied the use of this technique and its effectiveness in diagnosing acute appendicitis.

In a 1994 commentary by Puylaert[9] himself, he describes the effect that the use of graded compression has had on our understanding of the natural history of appendicitis since the inception of the technique. In patients with appendicitis, approximately 10% to 15% may show an "abortive" course, with resolution of symptoms early in the disease. This improvement in clinical appendicitis occurs as serial ultrasonography studies show a gradual decrease in appendiceal diameter and inflammation. The sonographic resolution usually lags behind the clinical improvement. This has confirmed what surgeons had believed: Appendicitis can resolve at an early stage.

Balthazar et al.[10] at New York University–Tisch Medical Center prospectively compared the accuracy of CT and ultrasonography in 100 consecutive patients with suspected appendicitis. The CT diagnosis of appendicitis was based on the presence of an abnormal appendix or pericecal inflammation or abscess associated with an appendicolith (Fig 5). Computed tomography had a higher sensitivity than ultrasonography (96% vs. 76%), a higher accuracy (94% vs. 83%), and a higher negative predictive value (95% vs. 76%). The degree and extent of inflammation was

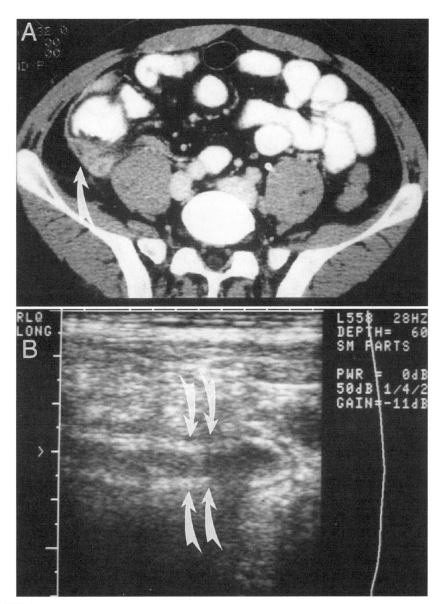

FIG 5.
Acute appendicitis. Both CT and ultrasonography yielded true-positive results. **A,** CT shows a thick-walled appendix and inflammation posterior to the cecum *(arrow)*. **B,** ultrasonography demonstrated the thickened and distended appendix *(arrows)*. (From Balthazar EJ: *Radiology* 190:31–35, 1994. Used by permission.)

better evaluated with CT than ultrasonography. Unrelated conditions responsible for the patient's symptoms were more often explained by CT than ultrasonography. Although CT was superior to sonography in detecting appendicitis in their hospital, Balthazar et al.[10] recommended the use of sonography as the initial test for patients with suspected appendicitis, especially children, young women, and women in the first trimester of pregnancy, because of the lower cost, ready availability, lack of ionizing radiation, and high positive predictive value. Computed tomography scanning was recommended for obese patients or children with suboptimal or nonspecific sonography.

Jeffrey et al.[11] reviewed the sonographic features diagnostic of acute appendicitis and pitfalls leading to a false-negative diagnosis of appendicitis by sonography.

The sonographic diagnosis of appendicitis can be made with confidence if the appendix is noncompressible and measures 7 mm or greater in anteroposterior dimension. The recognition of an appendicolith in a patient with right lower quadrant pain is also considered positive for appendicitis.

Pitfalls leading to a false-negative diagnosis of appendicitis sonographically include appendicitis confined to the tip of the appendix, retrocecal appendicitis, an already perforated or gangrenous appendix, or a gas-filled appendix. The diagnosis of appendicitis may be made inappropriately when the appendicitis is resolving and could be managed without surgery (Fig 6), when a dilated fallopian tube or muscle fibers of the psoas muscle are mistaken for the appendix, or when a patient has periappendicitis from surrounding inflammation in conditions such as Crohn's disease.

Quillin and Siegel[12] described the use of color Doppler in 100 children with suspected appendicitis and determined that hypervascularity in the appendiceal wall or within a right lower quadrant mass suggested appendicitis but could not definitely distinguish a normal from an abnormal appendix. Color Doppler sonography did not increase the sensitivity of detecting appendicitis when compared with gray-scale ultrasonography alone.

Two key articles in the sonographic literature highlighted the hepatic hemangioma, a common benign liver mass sometimes confused with a more ominous diagnosis. Hemangiomas are often discovered by ultrasonography, and CT and follow-up studies at 4 to 6 months are often suggested to confirm their stable appearance. Mungovan et al.[13] followed 21 patients with biopsy-proven hemangiomas for 5 to 84 months to see if change in size occurred commonly. The hemangiomas ranged from 1.5 to 3.5 cm. Ninety percent showed no change on follow-up scans. The study's conclusion was that the size of hemangiomas of the liver are usually stable, and if growth is identified, prompt reassessment of the lesion must be considered.

Moody and Wilson[14] from Toronto described a commonly identified sonographic pattern for an "atypical" hepatic hemangioma. The typical hepatic hemangioma is seen sonographically as a well-circumscribed highly echogenic mass, often in the subcapsular region, sometimes with enhancement posterior to it. The authors studied 29 patients with atypical hemangiomas having echogenic borders with an in-

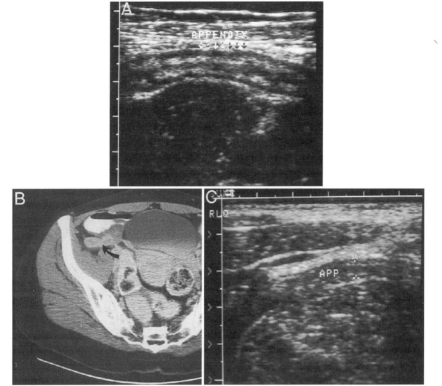

FIG 6.
Resolving appendicitis. **A,** sonogram shows an enlarged appendix measuring 9 mm in anteroposterior diameter, consistent with appendicitis. **B,** CT scan confirmed appendicitis. Note the thick-walled, enlarged appendix. **C,** follow-up sonogram 2 weeks later with resolution of symptoms showed a normal-sized appendix. (From Jeffrey RB: *AJR* 162:55–59, 1994. Used by permission.)

ternal echo pattern that was at least partially hypoechoic. This particular pattern should increase the suspicion of a hepatic hemangioma and led to the rapid performance of a confirmatory study, often the nuclear medicine–tagged red blood cell study.

Multiple articles appeared regarding the evaluation of the portal vein and its splanchnic tributaries, as well as evaluations focused on the transjugular intrahepatic portosystemic shunt (TIPS) in patients with portal hypertension.

Parvey et al.[15] reviewed portal vein thrombosis and its imaging features. Associated conditions such as cirrhosis, abdominal malignancy, or inflammation, as well as myeloproliferative conditions, may be present. Portal vein thrombosis may complicate TIPS placement or liver transplantation. Imaging findings on sonography, CT, MRI, and angiography were reviewed.

Dodd and Carr[16] performed percutaneous biopsy of portal vein thrombus in 19 patients with portal vein thrombosis and known cirrhosis. Thirteen of the patients had hepatocellular carcinoma (HCC). Biopsy of the portal vein thrombus was undertaken to facilitate staging of patients with HCC (Fig 7). Malignant hepatocytes were obtained in 12 patients; benign thrombi were obtained in two. This was confirmed by surgical resection or clinical course, suggesting that biopsy of portal vein thrombosis can be a safe and effective way to stage patients with HCC and portal vein involvement.

Petit et al.[17] sought to determine the frequency of splenic vein thrombosis after splenectomy. In a group of 183 consecutive patients undergoing splenectomy, 119 underwent postoperative ultrasound or CT. Splenic vein thrombosis was detected in 13 patients in the first 2 weeks after surgery. Of the 13 patients, 12 had splenectomy for hematologic disorders and 1 patient had it for traumatic injury. The authors conclude that splenic vein thrombosis occurs in at least 7% of patients after splenectomy. Routine sonographic studies should be performed after splenectomy so that anticoagulant therapy may be instituted early and appropriately if splenic vein thrombosis occurs.

Ultrasonography remains a first-line imaging modality for commonly seen conditions in the abdomen: appendicitis, hepatic hemangioma, and portal vein thrombosis related to cirrhosis or HCC.

COMPUTED TOMOGRAPHY

Topics of current interest in CT include (1) two-phase dynamic incremental CT for detection of small HCCs, (2) use of CT in the evaluation of inflammatory diseases of the colon, and (3) efficacy of CT in distinguishing small bowel obstruction from other causes of bowel dilation.

Patients with a history of chronic hepatitis and cirrhosis have an increased incidence of HCC, and early detection is an important factor in their prognosis.[18] Most HCCs are hypervascular, and examination with CT should focus on the arterial phase of enhancement. Well-differentiated HCCs are small and tend to be hypovascular; their detection requires scanning during the parenchymal phase of enhancement.[19] Newer CT scanners have shorter scanning times and interscan delays, and the use of a power injector allows imaging of the liver during the arterial phase.[18]

FIG 7.
Ultrasound-guided biopsy of portal vein thrombus. **A,** diagram of sonographically guided biopsy technique allows precise placement of needle in portal vein thrombus. **B,** the echogenic needle tip *(arrows)* is in the center of the portal vein thrombus. **C,** diagram of biopsy of portal vein thrombus shows maximal needle excursion during biopsy. The tip of the needle is kept within the lumen of the portal vein. (From Dodd GD: *AJR* 161:229–233, 1993. Used by permission.)

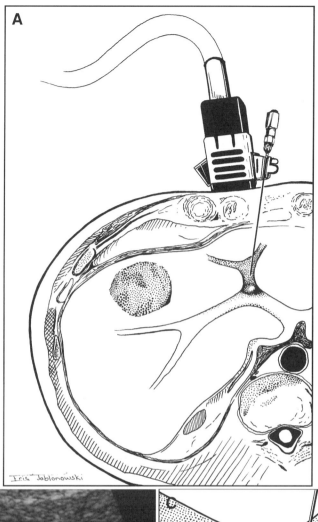

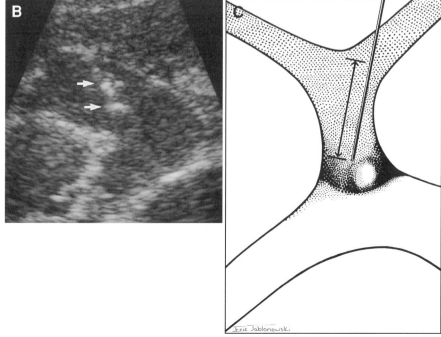

Ohashi et al.[18] compared several imaging techniques in a study of 184 patients with chronic liver disease. Two-phase (early-vascular and parenchymal) dynamic incremental CT of the entire liver was performed and compared with ultrasound and CT after intra-arterial injection of iodized oil. The HCC detection rate was 92% with dynamic incremental CT, 69% with ultrasound, and 81% with iodized oil–enhanced CT. These results indicate that two-phase dynamic incremental CT is suitable for routine examinations for the early detection of small HCCs (Figs 8–10).[18]

The features of colitis on CT scans are generally nonspecific. Philpotts et al.[20] retrospectively reviewed the CT scans of 117 patients with documented colitis and colon wall thickening to determinate if CT can help to differentiate among the various infectious and inflammatory causes of colitis. The parameters evaluated were mural thickness and homogeneity, presence of pneumatosis, distribution of disease, mesenteric and small bowel disease, and extracolonic findings.

Although considerable overlap of mural thickness was observed, the mean thickness in Crohn's colitis was greater than in ulcerative colitis. The majority of the patients with Crohn's colitis showed homogeneous attenuation of the bowel wall (70%). In contrast, 70% of patients with ulcerative colitis and infectious colitis had

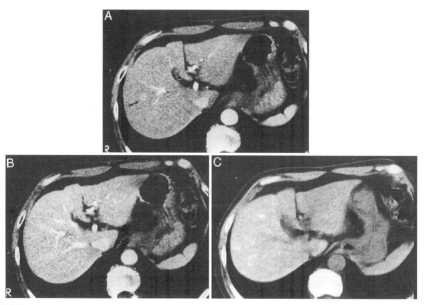

FIG 8.
Well differentiated hepatocellular carcinoma (HCC). **A,** CT scan from the first series of dynamic incremental CT shows a slightly high-attenuating, 9-mm lesion *(arrow).* **B,** CT scan from the second series of dynamic incremental CT, obtained in the same plane as **A,** shows equivocal findings. **C,** iodized oil–enhanced CT scan obtained in the same plane shows no accumulation of iodized oil in the same lesion. At resection, the lesion was confirmed to be a well-differentiated HCC. (From Ohashi I: *Radiology* 189:851–855, 1993. Used by permission.)

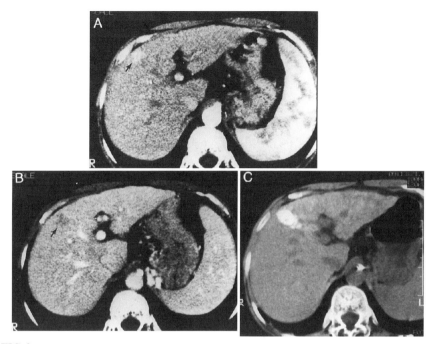

FIG 9.
Hypervascular HCC. **A,** CT scan from the first series of incremental CT shows a high-attenuation 22-mm lesion *(arrow).* **B,** CT scan from the second series shows the same lesion but with low attenuation *(arrow).* **C,** iodized oil–enhanced CT shows a high-attenuation lesion accumulating iodized oil. The lesion shows the typical pattern of a hypervascular HCC. (From Ohashi I: *Radiology* 189:851–855, 1993. Used by permission.)

heterogeneous wall attenuation. The heterogeneity of the wall in patients with ulcerative colitis is caused primarily by submucosal fat and in patients with infectious colitis is caused by mural water attenuation. Submucosal fat was seen only in chronic and subacute colitides.[20]

Pneumatosis is a feature associated with ischemia or infarction of the bowel wall,[21] although it has been described in cases of severe ulcerative colitis. Fibrofatty mesenteric proliferation surrounding the involved colon is typical of Crohn's colitis. Small bowel involvement is most common with Crohn's disease, although it has been seen in about 4% of patients with ulcerative colitis. The presence of abscess is virtually diagnostic of Crohn's colitis (Fig 11). Ascites was present in cases of acute colitides, particularly pseudomembranous, ischemic, and infectious colitides.[20] In summary, although the CT features of colitis are nonspecific, several findings can be helpful in suggesting a specific diagnosis.[20]

Small bowel obstruction is a common clinical entity associated with signs and symptoms that can be similar to other intra-abdominal disorders. The radiologic work-up of patients with suspected small bowel obstruction starts with a plain film. Many times it is difficult to differentiate mechanical obstruction from ileus.[21] The objective of a study performed at Harvard Medical School was to evaluate the efficacy of CT in distinguishing small bowel obstruction from other causes of bowel dilation. The presence of continuous small bowel dilation, prestenotic dilation, and a transition zone correlated with the presence of small bowel obstruction. Identification of these CT features will help differentiate patients who have small bowel obstruction from patients with nonobstructive bowel dilation.[22] Computed tomography also provides information about the specific causes and location of the obstruction.[23]

In patients with partial small bowel obstruction and colonic obstruction with predominant small bowel dilation, GI contrast studies still play an important diagnostic role. These examinations, combined with the clinical findings, have more impact than CT on the therapeutic decisions made in these patients.[23]

MAGNETIC RESONANCE IMAGING

Applications of MRI to the GI tract have progressed with regard to (1) faster MRI techniques to suppress motion and shorten examination time, (2) clinical tri-

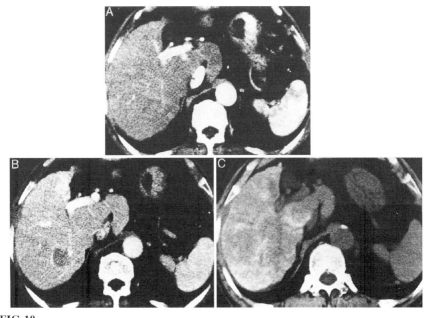

FIG 10.
Hypovascular HCC. **A,** CT scan from the first series of dynamic CT shows no areas of high attenuation. **B,** CT scan from the second series, obtained in the same plane as **A,** shows a low-attenuation lesion in the right lobe. **C,** iodized oil–enhanced CT scan shows no accumulation of oil in the lesion, which was considered to be hypovascular. Findings of a subsequent tissue-core biopsy confirmed this lesion to be a well-differentiated HCC. (From Ohashi I: *Radiology* 189:851–855, 1993. Used by permission.)

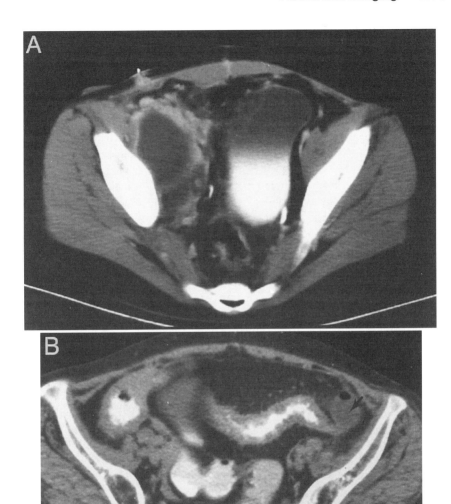

FIG 11.
Abscess in two patients with Crohn's colitis. **A,** contrast-enhanced CT scan demonstrates a large fluid collection that replaces a portion of the right iliopsoas muscle in a 17-year-old man. **B,** a small air-containing fluid collection *(arrow)* is identified adjacent to a segment of thickened sigmoid colon on this contrast-enhanced CT scan in a 52-year-old woman. (From Philpott LE: *Radiology* 190:445–449, 1994. Used by permission.)

als for the first Food and Drug Administration (FDA)–approved oral contrast agent for MRI, and (3) MR capabilities for evaluation of gastric malignancies, perianal fistulas, and rectal neoplasms. Of particular interest for gastroenterologists is the initial description of a new MR technique, MR cholangiography.

Regarding faster MRI techniques for the abdomen, a paper published by a group[24] at Thomas Jefferson University Hospital in Philadelphia is worth mentioning. In this paper, 48 patients with known or suspected liver disease were imaged using two MR sequences: T_2-weighted conventional spin-echo and T_2-weighted fast spin-echo sequences. Different parameters were compared, including signal intensity, ratios of signal to noise, and signal difference to noise for the spleen, pancreas, muscle, fat, normal liver, and liver tumors. The majority of malignant liver lesions showed lower signal intensity ratios on the fast spin-echo sequences compared with the conventional spin-echo sequences. Other significant differences were found with hemangiomas and other benign liver tumors (Fig 12). The authors conclude that the use of fast spin-echo sequences may be less suitable for the depiction of malignant liver lesions. However, fast spin-echo sequences may improve the distinction of benign lesions (hemangioma) compared with conventional spin-echo images. The practical impact of these findings is that the heralded fast-spin echo sequences, which reduce imaging time by 50%, may not be the most sensitive method for detection of malignant liver lesions.

During the last year, the first FDA-approved oral contrast agent specifically designed for MRI was released.[25] This agent, known commercially as Imagent GI, is known generically as perflubron and consists of perfluorooctyl bromide. Perflubron is a clear, inert liquid that contains no hydrogen atoms and therefore generates no signal and is black by MRI. The MRI characteristics of perflubron are unlike those of any other agent, and its physical and chemical characteristics are also unique. Its low surface tension, high specific gravity, and immiscibility with water allow perflubron to move rapidly through the bowel while remaining as a tight bolus. Regardless of the bowel content, this is accomplished without either dilution or concentration of the agent.

The results of the phase 3 clinical trial using perflubron as a contrast oral agent for MRI were reported by Mattrey et al.,[25] including researchers from the University of California at San Diego, Stanford University, and Nice, France. They reported their results in 127 subjects who were imaged before and after oral administration of perflubron. Perflubron increased the bowel darkening in more than 92% of subjects in all pulsing sequences and field strengths used. Definition of the left lobe of the liver and body and tail of the pancreas was improved in 67%, 29%, and 42% of the subjects, respectively. Other abdominal organs, such as the uterus and bladder, were improved in their definition in 80% and 76%, respectively. In 69% of the subjects, abnormal tissues were more conspicuous after the use of perflubron. There were no image artifacts or side effects attributed to the perflubron used. The images performed with the use of perflubron (Fig 13) demonstrate the favorable effects produced by this contrast. Perflubron is a safe contrast agent with high efficacy in demonstrating the GI tract, abdominal organs surrounded by the GI tract, and abdominal abnormalities by MRI.

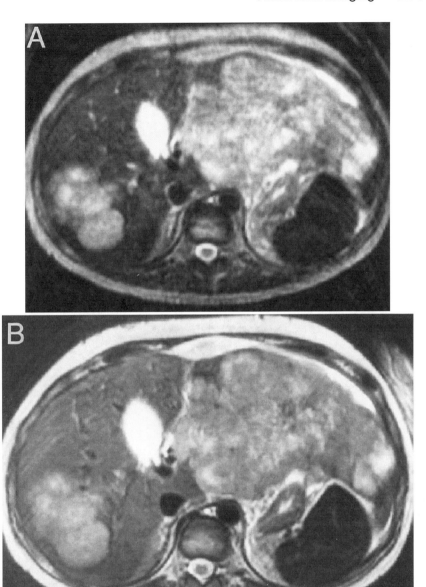

FIG 12.
Tissue contrast comparison on spin-echo and fast spin-echo images. Spin-echo (**A**) and fast spin-echo (**B**) images in a patient with hepatic metastases show generally similar tissue contrast. However, the signal intensity ratio and signal difference to noise ratio are lower for the metastases on the fast spin-echo image. Note that although there is increased motion artifact in **A,** the signal intensity of the large metastases in the right lobe is higher in **A** compared with **B.** (From Outwater EK: *Radiology* 190:425–429, 1994. Used by permission.)

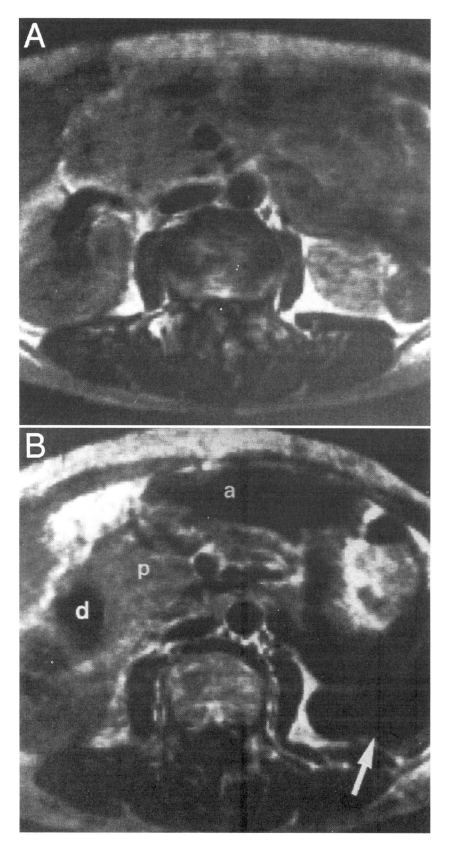

The utility of high–field strength MRI for evaluation of gastric anatomy was reported by Korean researchers who used a 4.7-tesla superconducting MR unit to study the stomach in vitro.[26] Nine specimens with gastric cancer and 29 normal stomachs were imaged using a 4.7-tesla magnet and compared with pathologic specimens. The mucosa, submucosa, and muscularis propria were clearly identified with MRI. The submucosa of the fresh specimens had the lowest signal intensity. There was no statistical correlation between the signal intensity and the duration of fixation of the specimens. Tumor invasion was detected in seven of eight specimens with mucosal invasion and in all patients with submucosal invasion. This work shows that in vitro MRI can demonstrate the three layers of the stomach wall, detect gastric cancer, and measure the depth of invasion. The detailed demonstration of the gastric wall layers with in vitro MRI raises the potential for in vivo application of this technique. Evaluation of the stomach may also be improved with the use of GI agents such as perflubron.

Another application of MRI to the GI tract is the study of perianal fistulas. A group of Norwegian investigators[27] described MRI using a saline solution as a contrast agent to diagnose perianal fistula disease. They studied 16 consecutive patients who had a clinical history of perianal fistulous tracts. The patients were imaged before and after the instillation of saline solution into the fistula tracts. Fistula tracts, fluid cavities, and secondary fibrotic tracts were identified easily. The extent of fistulas and fluid collections was better delineated on contrast-enhanced examinations than on noncontrast examinations because of the expansion of the collapsed portions of the fistulous tracts after saline solution administration. T_2-weighted images were the most sensitive sequence for depicting these abnormalities. With its multiplanar capabilities, MRI may become the best method to visualize fistulous tracts and their relationship to normal anatomic structures in patients with complex fistulas. The use of a contrast agent, such as saline solution, may help in patients who have sparse secretion to better identify the fistula (Fig 14).

Of all regions of the GI tract, MRI of rectal cancer has received the greatest research interest to date. Another key paper appeared last year indicating the potential for the use of MRI in rectal tumor staging using an endorectal coil.[28] Thirty-six patients with rectal tumors underwent MRI with an endorectal surface coil. In all cases, MR images were compared and correlated with specimens from the resected tumors. With endorectal MRI, the rectal wall layers were reliably demonstrated. Tumor staging by MRI agreed with pathologic findings in 81% of cases. Retrospectively, the integrity of the rectal wall layers at the lesion center was found

FIG 13.
Efficacy of oral perflubron as a contrast agent. T_1-weighted magnetic resonance (MR) images obtained at the level of the head of the pancreas in a 65-year-old woman with a pancreatic mass before (**A**) and after (**B**) ingestion of perflubron. In **B**, filling of the duodenum (*d*) and antrum (*a*) improves the definition of the enlarged head of the pancreas (*p*). Also note the darkened jejunal loops (*arrow* in **B**). (From Mattrey RF: *Radiology* 191:841–848, 1994. Used by permission.)

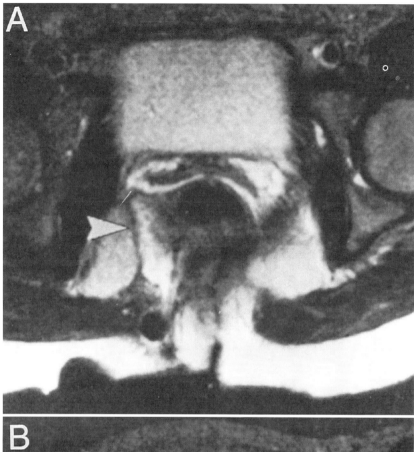

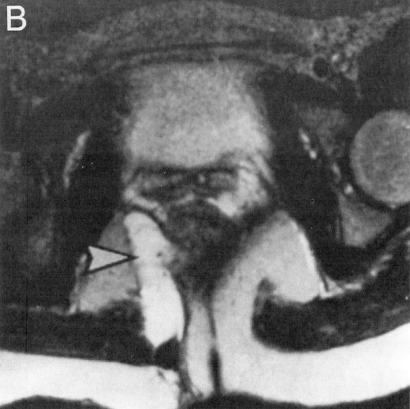

to be an accurate criterion for interpreting the local extent of the lesions. Lymph nodes as small as 2 mm were demonstrated. Although sensitive for demonstrating perirectal adenopathy, MRI had a specificity of only 82% for N1 disease. It can be concluded that the use of an endorectal surface coil is a promising method to stage rectal lesions preoperatively. This method demonstrates the multiple layers of the rectum and potential invasion in patients with rectal cancer (Fig 15).

A final area of interest for the gastroenterologist is the initial description of MR cholangiography. A group[29] of researchers, including radiologists, gastroenterologists, and surgeons from the Middlesex Hospital in London, reported their experience in 40 patients with obstructive jaundice. In all patients, three-dimensional MR cholangiography was performed and compared with conventional cholangiography. Magnetic resonance cholangiography correlated very well with conventional cholangiography, demonstrating the level of obstruction or absence of obstruction accurately in 36 of 40 patients with MR cholangiography and in 37 of 39 patients with conventional cholangiography. The peripheral biliary tree was shown more completely with MR cholangiography than with endoscopic retrograde cholangiography in all patients undergoing diagnostic studies with both modalities. Magnetic resonance cholangiography is a noninvasive technique that shows particular promise for the assessment of patients with complex strictures in whom conventional cholangiography carries a higher risk of sepsis. This may be helpful in planning the optimal drainage route before intervention. Magnetic resonance cholangiography and MR pancreatography may play an important role in patients who have had upper GI surgery and in situations where a noninvasive scanning method is desired to study the biliary tree (Fig 16).

INTERVENTIONAL PROCEDURES

Interesting topics pertaining to intervention in the GI tract are (1) percutaneous removal of "dropped" gallstones after laparoscopic cholecystectomy, (2) a coaxial system for the decompression of colonic pseudo-obstruction, (3) percutaneous drainage and sclerosis of symptomatic hepatic cysts, (4) the utilization of portal vein embolization for left hepatic lobe hypertrophy before surgery, (5) percutaneous hot saline solution injection therapy of hepatic tumors, and (6) hepatic arterial injury after TIPS.

With the increasing popularity of laparoscopic cholecystectomy, the report of per-

---

FIG 14.
Magnetic resonance imaging (MRI) of perianal fistulous tract. Before (**A**) and after (**B**) saline solution instillation. In **A** the fistula is seen collapsed, whereas in **B** the fluid cavity is seen expanded. An area of communication between the cavity and rectal lumen is suspected (*arrowheads*). (From Myhr GE: *Radiology* 191:545–549, 1994. Used by permission.)

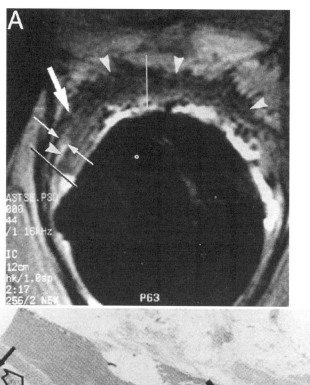

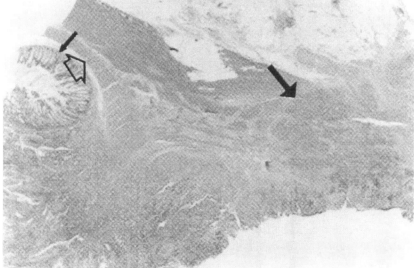

FIG 15.
Endorectal surface core imaging in rectal cancer. **A,** axial T_2-weighted fast spin-echo image demonstrates mucosal thickening of the rectal cancer *(arrowheads)* that is seen completely disrupting the submucosa *(small arrows)* and the muscularis propria *(large arrow).* This indicates a stage T3 lesion. **B,** pathologic section obtained from the area between the lines shown at **A.** As in MRI, the tumor invades completely through the muscularis propria *(large solid arrow).* The border of mucosa and submucosa *(small solid arrow)* and the border of submucosa and muscularis propria *(open arrow)* in the adjacent and involved rectal wall are identified. (From Schnall MD: *Radiology* 190:709–714, 1994. Used by permission.)

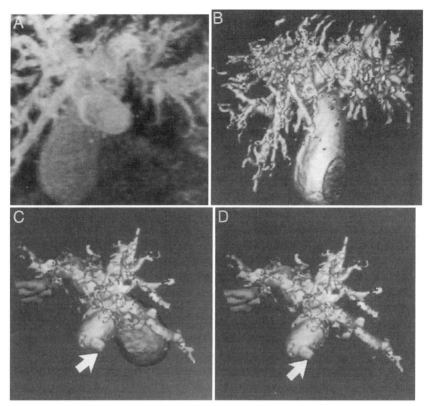

FIG 16.
Magnetic resonance cholangiography in a 42-year-old woman with jaundice. **A,** on MR cholangiography of the complete data set, it is difficult to appreciate the level of obstruction because of overlying peripheral ducts and the gallbladder. **B–D,** after transfer of the complete data set to a three-dimensional work station, the image is rotated and pruned of the peripheral branches, as well as the gallbladder **(D),** revealing the point of obstruction in the common bile duct *(arrows).* (From Hall-Craggs MA, Allen CM, Owens CM, et al: *Radiology* 189:423–427, 1993. Used by permission.)

cutaneous removal of "dropped" gallstones is timely.[30] Most patients with spilled bile and stones suffer no adverse consequences. However, spillage of infected bile and stones can lead to abscess formation. Percutaneous stone removal can be performed after abscess drainage using a basket device (Fig 17). Stones greater than 1 cm in diameter require fragmentation before removal. This percutaneous technique for stone removal can spare the patient further surgical intervention.

Colonic pseudo-obstruction can be very uncomfortable and, on occasion, dangerous to the patient. A paper from Madigan Army Medical Center reports preliminary results with decompression of colonic pseudo-obstruction and related entities using a tricomponent coaxial system (TAS).[31] In four patients, a 20 Fr Madigan-DC catheter was placed in the transverse or ascending colon as necessary to allow for adequate decompression (Fig 18). The catheters were left in from 6 hours to 4 days. Tube placement was achieved in 20 to 90 minutes, and there were no complications. No problems maintaining tube patency occurred because of the multiple large side holes in the catheter. This technique does not require air insufflation, which can further distend a dilated colon. This may provide an advantage over colonoscopic

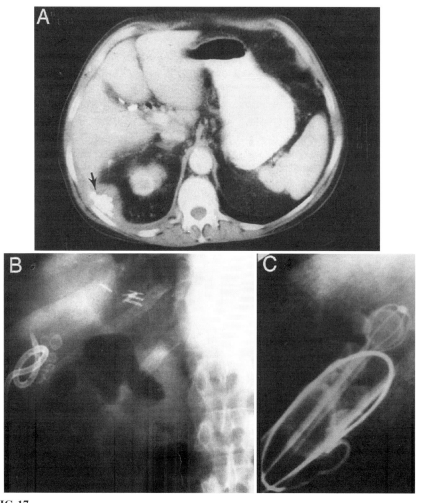

FIG 17.
Percutaneous removal of "dropped" gallstone after laparoscopic cholecystectomy. **A,** CT examination obtained 2 months after laparoscopic cholecystectomy shows multiple small stones *(arrows)* in an abscess cavity. **B,** radiograph after drainage of abscess shows the 12 Fr pigtail catheter adjacent to the gallstones. **C,** spot radiograph obtained during initial stone extraction shows an 8-mm calculus trapped in the Burhenne basket. The basket was introduced via a 30 Fr sheath. A guidewire is coiled within the abscess cavity as a safety wire. (From Trerotola SO: *Radiology* 188:419–421, 1993. Used by permission.)

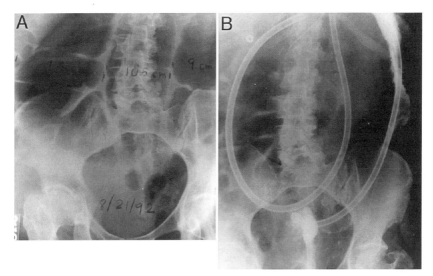

FIG 18.
Fluoroscopic decompression of colonic pseudo-obstruction. **A,** radiograph of the abdomen of a 64-year-old woman with metastatic breast cancer and acute colonic pseudo-obstruction. **B,** after placement of the 20 Fr catheter using the tricomponent coaxial system, the dilated colonic loops are decompressed. (From Bender GN: *Radiology* 188:395–398, 1993. Used by permission.)

decompression. Use of this technique in the treatment of chronic pseudo-obstruction is not recommended currently because the risk of colonic wall erosion and perforation from a chronically indwelling 20 Fr polyurethane catheter is unknown.

Hepatic cysts are a developmental anomaly that can cause symptoms of pain, early satiety secondary to gastric or duodenal compression, edema secondary to vena cava compression, biliary dilation due to extrahepatic ductal compression, and portal hypertension secondary to compression of the portal vein. vanSonnenberg et al.[32] described their experience with percutaneous drainage and sclerosis of 24 symptomatic hepatic cysts. Twenty-two-gauge needles were used for initial localization and aspiration, followed by trocar insertion of a 7 to 12 Fr catheter via CT or ultrasound guidance. The cysts were drained and a fluoroscopic sinogram was performed to evaluate for biliary communication. No communications were found, although one cyst had peritoneal spill precluding sclerosis at that time. Before sclerosis, 10 to 15 mL of 1% lidocaine was instilled into the cyst and left for 5 to 10 minutes. Although no controlled study proves superiority, the sclerosant of choice was alcohol. On occasion, tetracycline or doxycycline was used. Patients returned every 1 to 2 days for assessment of catheter drainage and cyst reaccumulation. If drainage was more than 10 to 15 mL, resclerosis was performed. Most cysts were treated in three or fewer sessions. In this series of patients, the long-term improvement rate was 88%. Significant complications occurred on three occasions. Two were large right pleural effusions/hemothorax, and one was a case of secondary cyst infection. Several patients experienced pain on alcohol instillation. The authors[32] conclude that percutaneous drainage and sclerosis of hepatic cysts should prove effective in the majority of cases. Likely nonresponders to this form of therapy include patients with nondominant cysts, multiple small cysts, and cystic neoplasms.

Patients with unresectable liver metastases from colorectal carcinoma have a dismal prognosis. On the other hand, patients who are able to undergo curative resection have a 30% 5-year survival.[33] Removal of more than 65% of the adult liver increases the risks of postoperative hepatic failure. Certain patients can undergo safe resection if the future remaining liver is allowed to hypertrophy[34] before surgery. de Baere et al.[34] describe the use of right portal vein embolization to induce preoperative hypertrophy of the left lobe to maximize hepatic function after surgical resection of the liver. The authors describe the subxiphoid placement of a 5 Fr needle catheter into the right portal vein and subsequent embolization with gelatin sponges or N-butyl-2-cyanoacrylate. No significant complications occurred in the 10 patients studied. On average, portal vein embolization produced a 64% hypertrophy of the left lobe after 4 to 5 weeks. Nine of the 10 patients were able to undergo liver resection without postoperative liver failure. The tenth patient was not resected because of the interval discovery of lung metastases. This technique should be considered in patients who may not otherwise be considered operative candidates.

In volume 15 of *Current Gastroenterology,* the technique of percutaneous ethanol injection therapy of HCCs was described. Recently Honda et al.[35] described their experience in 20 patients using percutaneous hot saline solution injection therapy for hepatic tumors. Patients with HCC measuring less than 3 cm in diameter were studied. Saline solution was heated to the hottest temperature possible. With local anesthetic (1% lidocaine) used for analgesia, 10 to 20 mL of the hot saline solution was injected into the lesion until the patients complained of intense pain. The authors report that saline solution has significantly decreased toxicity when compared with alcohol because there is no risk of acute ethanol poisoning. This limits complications in case of intraperitoneal or intrapleural spills. In addition, favorable results in treating larger (~3 cm) tumors were obtained in two to three treatment sessions on average with hot saline solution injection compared with seven to nine sessions with alcohol because of the fact that larger amounts of saline solution can be injected in one session. The decreased number of treatment sessions should decrease the risks of arterioportal shunts and bile duct injury, which are known complications of percutaneous hepatic therapy.[36] This technique has promise as an alternative form of therapy for relatively small HCCs.

Transjugular intrahepatic portosystemic shunts continue to be performed as an effective treatment for portal hypertension and variceal hemorrhage. Previously reported complications have included fever, self-limited peritoneal hemorrhage, myocardial infarction, transient hemobilia, and transient renal failure.[37–39] Haskal et al.[40] describe two cases of hepatic arterial injury, a newly reported complication of TIPS. In both cases, inadvertent injury to branches of the right hepatic artery occurred during attempts to puncture the portal vein. In one case, the injury resulted in right hepatic arterial occlusion and irreversible hepatic failure. In the second patient, the injury led to intraperitoneal bleeding, and embolization could not be performed because of celiac acis occlusion. Despite surgical repair, the patient died of multiorgan failure. Although TIPS remains a good alternative to surgical shunts and an excellent bridge to liver transplantation, one must be prepared for intraprocedural or postprocedural complications.

SUMMARY

We reviewed highlights from the current literature on abdominal imaging and interventional techniques. Criteria for plain film diagnosis of bowel obstruction are expanded and clarified. The double-contrast barium study is shown to be a sensitive technique for detecting gastric cancer, and serial changes in fundic gland polyposis and intestinal Behçet's disease were described.

In cross-sectional imaging, we discussed the role of sonography for diagnosis of appendicitis, hepatic hemangioma, and portal vein pathologic conditions, including a technique for ultrasound-guided needle biopsy of portal vein thrombus. Technical advances in CT that allow rapid, dual-phase imaging of the liver during arterial and portal venous phases of enhancement were illustrated. This has been helpful in detection of HCCs and other liver neoplasms. Computed tomography features of inflammatory colitis and criteria that differentiate small bowel obstruction and adynamic ileus were also discussed.

Advances in abdominal MRI include release of the first approved enteric contrast agent, use of saline solution for perianal fistula evaluation, and endorectal coils for preoperative staging in patients with rectal carcinoma. The first results on MR cholangiography were presented. Innovations in interventional procedures in the abdomen include percutaneous removal of dropped gallstones, decompression of colonic pseudo-obstruction, and various therapies for benign and malignant liver disease.

Continued research in abdominal imaging and interventional techniques will further improve the diagnosis and management of patients with diseases of the GI tract.

REFERENCES

1. Wittenberg J: The diagnosis of colonic obstruction on plain abdominal radiographs: Start with the cecum, leave the rectum to last. *AJR* 161:443–444, 1993.
2. Baker SR: Plain film radiology of the intestines and appendix. In *The Abdominal Plain Film.* Norwalk, Conn, Appleton & Lange, pp 155–241, 1990.
3. Laufer I: The left lateral view in the plain-film assessment of abdominal distension. *Radiology* 119:265–266, 1976.
4. Harlow CL, Stears RLG, Zeligman BE, et al: Diagnosis of bowel obstruction on plain abdominal radiographs: Significance of air-fluid levels at different heights in the same loop of bowel. *AJR* 161:291–295, 1993.

4a. Cruz CJ, Minagi H: Large bowel obstruction resulting from traumatic diaphragmatic hernia: Imaging findings in four cases. *AJR* 162:843–845, 1994.

5. Low VHS, Levine MS, Rubesin SE, et al: Diagnosis of gastric carcinoma: Sensitivity of double-contrast barium studies. *AJR* 162:329–334, 1994.

6. Murayama M: Early diagnosis of gastric cancer. In Laufer I, Levine MS (eds): *Double Contrast Radiology,* ed 2. Philadelphia, WB Saunders, 1992, pp 495–532.

7. Hizawa K, Iida M, Matsumoto T, et al: Natural history of fundic gland polyposis without familial adenomatosis coli: Follow-up observations in 31 patients. *Radiology* 189:429–432, 1993.

8. Iida M, Kobayashi H, Matsumoto T, et al: Intestinal Behçet disease: Serial changes at radiography. *Radiology* 188:65–69, 1993.

9. Puylaert JBCM: When in doubt, sound it out. *Radiology* 191:320–321, 1994.

10. Balthazar EJ, Birnbaum BA, Yee J, et al: Acute appendicitis: CT and US correlation in 100 patients. *Radiology* 190:31–35, 1994.

11. Jeffrey RB, Jain KA, Ngheim HV: Sonographic diagnosis of acute appendicitis: Interpretive pitfalls. *AJR* 162:55–59, 1994.

12. Quillin SP, Siegel MJ: Appendicitis: Efficacy of color Doppler sonography. *Radiology* 191:557–560, 1994.

13. Mungovan JA, Cronan JJ, Vacarro J: Hepatic cavernous hemangiomas: Lack of enlargement over time. *Radiology* 191:111–113, 1994.

14. Moody AR, Wilson SR: Atypical hepatic hemangioma: A suggestive sonographic morphology. *Radiology* 188:413–417, 1993.

15. Parvey HR, Raval B, Sandler CM: Portal vein thrombosis: Imaging findings. *AJR* 162:77–81, 1994.

16. Dodd GD, Carr BI: Percutaneous biopsy of portal vein thrombus: A new staging technique for hepatocellular carcinoma. *AJR* 161:229–233, 1993.

17. Petit P, Bret PM, Atri M, et al: Splenic vein thrombosis after splenectomy: Frequency and role of imaging. *Radiology* 190:65–68, 1994.

18. Ohashi I, Hanafusa K, Yoshida T: Small hepatocellular carcinomas: Two-phase dynamic incremental CT in detection and evaluation. *Radiology* 189:851–855, 1993.

19. Yoshimatsu S, Inoue Y, Ibukuro K, et al: Hypovascular hepatocellular carcinoma undetected at angiography and CT with iodized oil. *Radiology* 171:343–347, 1989.

20. Philpotts LE, Heiken JP, Wescott MA, et al: Colitis: Use of CT findings in differential diagnosis. *Radiology* 190:445–449, 1994.

21. Smerud MJ, Johnson CD, Stephens DH: Diagnosis of bowel infarction: A comparison of plain film and CT scans in 23 cases. *AJR* 154:99–103, 1990.

22. Gazelle GS, Goldberg MA, Wittenberg J, et al: Efficacy of CT in distinguishing small bowel obstruction from other causes of small bowel dilation. *AJR* 162:43–47, 1994.

23. Frager D, Medwid SW, Baer JW, et al: CT of small bowel obstruction: Value in establishing the diagnosis and determining the degree and cause. *AJR* 162:37–41, 1994.

24. Outwater EK, Mitchell DG, Vinitski S: Abdominal MR imaging: Evaluation of a fast spin-echo sequence. *Radiology* 190:425–429, 1994.

25. Mattrey RF, Trambert MA, Brown JJ, et al: Perflubron as an oral contrast agent for MR imaging: Results of a phase III clinical trial. *Radiology* 191:841–848, 1994.

26. Auh YH, Lim T-H, Lee DH, et al: In vitro MR imaging of the resected stomach with a 4.7-T superconducting magnet. *Radiology* 191:129–134, 1994.

27. Myhr GE, Myrvold HE, Nilsen G, et al: Perianal fistulas: Use of MR imaging for diagnosis. *Radiology* 191:545–549, 1994.

28. Schnall MD, Furth EE, Rosato EF, et al: Rectal tumor stage: Correlation of endorectal MR imaging and pathologic findings. *Radiology* 190:709–714, 1994.

29. Hall-Craggs MA, Allen CM, Owens CM, et al: MR cholangiography: Clinical evaluation in 40 cases. *Radiology* 189:423–427, 1993.

30. Trerotola SO, Lillemoe KD, Malloy PC, et al: Percutaneous removal of "dropped" gallstones after laparoscopic cholecystectomy. *Radiology* 188:419–421, 1993.

31. Bender GN, Do-Dai DD, Briggs LM, et al: Colonic pseudo-obstruction: Decompression with tri-component coaxial system under fluoroscopic guidance. *Radiology* 188:395–398, 1993.

32. vanSonnenberg E, Wroblicka JT, D'Agostino HB, et al: Symptomatic hepatic cysts: Percutaneous drainage and sclerosis. *Radiology* 190:387–392, 1994.

33. Fortner JG, Silva JS, Golbey RB, et al: Multivariate analysis of a personal series of 247 consecutive patients with liver metastases from colorectal cancer: I. Treatment by hepatic resection. *Ann Surg* 199:306–316, 1984.

34. de Baere T, Roche A, Vavasseur D, et al: Portal vein embolization: Utility for inducing left hepatic lobe hypertrophy before surgery. *Radiology* 188:73–77, 1993.

35. Honda N, Guo Q, Uchida H, et al: Percutaneous hot saline injection therapy for hepatic tumors: An alternative to percutaneous ethanol injection therapy. *Radiology* 190:53–57, 1994.

36. Sheu JC, Sung J-L, Huang G-T, et al: Intratumor injection of absolute ethanol under ultrasound guidance for the treatment of small hepatocellular carcinoma. *Hepatogastroenterology* 34:255–261, 1987.

37. LaBerge JM, Ring EJ, Gordon RL, et al: Creation of transjugular intrahepatic portosystemic shunts with the wallstent endoprosthesis: Results in 100 patients. *Radiology* 187:413–420, 1993.

38. Noeldge G, Haag K, Sellinger M, et al: Treatment of portal hypertension with the transjugular intrahepatic portosystemic shunt: Follow-up studies in 92 patients [abstract]. *Radiology* 185(P):179, 1992.

39. Zemel G, Katzen BT, Becker GJ, et al: Percutaneous transjugular portosystemic shunt. *JAMA* 266:390–393, 1991.

40. Haskal Z, Pentecost MJ, Rubin RA, et al: Hepatic arterial injury after transjugular intrahepatic portosystemic shunt placement: Report of two cases. *Radiology* 188:85–88, 1993.

CHAPTER 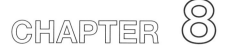 8

Gastrointestinal Endoscopy

Barry De Gregorio, M.D.

Division of Gastroenterology, Oregon Health Sciences University, Portland, Oregon

M. Brian Fennerty, M.D.

Division of Gastroenterology, Oregon Health Sciences University, Portland, Oregon

Gastrointestinal endoscopy remains a crucial diagnostic and therapeutic procedure in the management of gastrointestinal diseases. Previously inaccessible organs are now routinely investigated endoscopically. Endoscopy continues to evolve at a furious pace as technology expands. This chapter deals with recent developments in endoscopic techniques, outcomes, and equipment.

GENERAL ISSUES

Sedation

Efforts continue to ensure that upper gastrointestinal endoscopy is performed efficiently, competently, and safely. Although diagnostic upper endoscopy is generally safe, complications do occur and are generally cardiopulmonary in origin. Cardiopulmonary events are believed to be related to arterial oxygen desaturation secondary to the anesthesia (conscious sedation) used during these procedures. Some authors have advocated performing routine diagnostic upper endoscopy without sedation to avoid sedation-related risks. Iwao et al. studied oxygenation by pulse oximetry in 120 patients undergoing nonsedated diagnostic upper endoscopies.[1] They found that 44% of their patients experienced some degree of oxygen desaturation. In most cases oxygen desaturation was mild (in 35% of the patients, O_2 saturation was between 90% and 94%), but 11 patients (9%) experienced "severe" desaturation defined as 89% or lower. Age, gender, smoking, hemoglobin level, body mass index, and duration of the procedure did not predict the occurrence of desaturation. In a second study, Iwao et al. compared oxygen saturation during nonsedated diagnostic upper endoscopy in 80 patients with cirrhosis and 80 controls.[2] Although baseline oxygen saturation was lower in the cirrhotic group than controls, during endoscopy desaturation levels were similar for both groups. Significant hypoxia was found in 28 (35%) with cirrhosis vs. 29 (36%) of the controls. Mild hypoxia (90% to 95%) was seen in 21 cirrhotics vs. 22 controls, and severe hypoxia (<90%) was seen in 7 patients in both groups. Analysis of variance failed to show a correlation between the degree of desaturation and the extent of liver disease. They concluded that patients with cirrhosis undergoing nonsedated upper endoscopy were not at any increased risk for oxygen desaturation. These two studies suggest that patients undergoing nonsedated examinations are still at risk for significant arterial oxygen desaturation. These data indicate that desaturation may be related to events other than anesthesia and monitoring for cardiopulmonary compromise is necessary even when sedation is not given. Therefore, cardiopulmonary risk may not be decreased by avoiding sedation.

Sedation use during colonoscopy is similarly controversial, with some suggesting that in expert hands the majority of patients do not require sedation for reasonably comfortable completion of the examination. However, traditional use of intravenous opiates and benzodiazepines is the norm but leads to increased postprocedural recovery time and may increase the risk of cardiopulmonary complications. Previous studies of various opiates and benzodiazepines have failed to show an advantage in efficacy or safety of a particular agent. Saunders et al. in a double-blind, randomized placebo-controlled study compared the efficacy of a patient-administered inhaled nitrous oxide/oxygen mixture vs. conventional conscious sedation (benzodiazepine/opiate) in patients undergoing colonoscopy.[3] Both agents were more effective than placebo, and there was no statistically significant difference in the number of pain episodes, need for additional sedation, and patient pain scores. Oxygen desaturation was not observed in the nitrous oxide/oxygen group but was seen in six patients in the benzodiazepine group. Postprocedural recovery was shorter in the nitrous oxide/oxygen group. Alternative methods of sedation may be as effective as traditional means, but any advantage in complication rate and clinical outcomes has yet to be proved.

Antibiotic Prophylaxis and Infectious Issues

Various guidelines and recommendations for the use of prophylactic antibiotics in patients undergoing gastrointestinal endoscopic procedures are available. In an effort to clarify who is at risk for infectious complications during endoscopy, Zuckerman et al. prospectively evaluated 486 patients undergoing 507 procedures.[4] Former and current American Heart Association and American Society of Gastrointestinal Endoscopy guidelines were used. A decision regarding antibiotic prophylaxis was deemed necessary in 15% of the patients. Depending on which guideline was used, between 1% and 3% of the patients were candidates for antibiotics. Cardiac conditions were the most commonly encountered (10% of all patients), and mitral valve prolapse was the most common cardiac lesion.

Mogadam et al.[5] reviewed all endoscopic outpatient procedures for compliance with published prophylaxis guidelines. They found that only 10% of board-certified gastroenterologists in northern Virginia and Washington, DC, used antibiotic prophylaxis according to guidelines. Antibiotics were given more frequently than guidelines would suggest, and in some cases antibiotics were not given even though they were recommended. The risk of native valve bacterial endocarditis following endoscopic gastrointestinal procedures is rare (1 in 5 to 10 million procedures). Whether prophylaxis with antimicrobials is effective in preventing endocarditis is unproved, and these data suggest that endoscopists do not comply with published guidelines. This may not be appropriate inasmuch as the cost of prophylaxis is high yet efficacy is unproved.

Prevention of Disease Transmission/Acquired Immunodeficiency Syndrome

The gastrointestinal manifestations of human immunodeficiency virus (HIV) infection/acquired immunodeficiency syndrome (AIDS) are numerous, and as a result gastroenterologists' consultative and endoscopic skills are frequently requested to aid in the diagnosis and treatment of these patients. In 1987, Raufman and

TABLE 1.
Frequency That Protective Attire Is Worn During Endoscopy*

Attire	Patients in General, n (%)	HIV-Positive or AIDS Patients, n (%)
Gowns/scrub suits	91 (75)	121 (99)
Disposable	43 (35)	82 (67)
Waterproof	38 (31)	64 (52)
Gloves	120 (98)†	120 (98)†
Two or more pairs	19 (16)	68 (56)
Surgical masks	25 (20)	109 (89)
Surgical caps	6 (5)	45 (37)
Eye protectors	54 (44)	110 (90)
Shoe protectors	6 (5)	33 (27)

*From Shapiro M, Brandt LJ: *Gastrointest Endosc* 40:477–480, 1994. Used by permission.
†The remaining responses were left blank.

Strauss[6] concluded that anxiety among gastroenterologists and endoscopy personnel regarding the transmission of HIV has resulted in inefficient, costly practices. Shapiro and Brandt[7] resurveyed 200 gastroenterology program directors and found that although perception of the transmission risk had not changed, the level of concern was relatively low and endoscopy personnel were less reluctant to become involved in the care of HIV-infected patients. It was found, however, that endoscopy personnel used protective equipment two to seven times more often when the patient had known HIV disease (Table 1). Despite employment of universal blood and body fluid precautions, it seems that many endoscopists use less protection with assumed non–HIV-infected patients, especially regarding face mask and eye protection. Other infectious disease risks, e.g., hepatitis C, in addition to HIV make more compulsive use of blood/body fluid precautions an area requiring attention.

Training

Competence and adequate training in gastrointestinal endoscopy continue to be major topics of interest among gastroenterology fellowship program directors and the gastroenterology societies. Adequate, well-supervised training with quantifiable measures of technical and cognitive competency is essential for developing the expertise necessary to perform complete, safe examinations. Undetected or unrecognized pathology can be particularly devastating and is a major reason for emphasis on comprehensive training for all those who perform endoscopic procedures. The number of endoscopic examinations leading to technical and cognitive competence is unknown and results in problems in establishing minimally accepted standards. Church prospectively studied completion rates and reasons for examination failure in 2,907 patients undergoing colonoscopy.[8] The overall rate for reading the cecum for all colonoscopies was 93.6%. When adjusted for poor preparation, significant colonic disease, tortuosity, or patient discomfort, the adjusted completion rate was 98.8%. Completion rates were lower in women and in patients younger than 20 or older than 80 years of age. Additionally, patients in intensive care units and women post-hysterectomy had lower completion rates. Completion rate differences disappeared except for female sex and post-hysterectomy when adjusted completion rates were used. Adjusted completion rates may be a better reflection of technical competence and may allow for a quantitative means of establishing procedural standards.

Some endoscopists suggest that terminal ileum intubation should be attempted at every colonoscopy, whereas others attempt intubation only when the clinical setting dictates (e.g., inflammatory bowel disease, ileal tissue sampling, radiographic abnormalities on barium studies, etc.). However, the success of terminal ileum intubation is unknown, as are the time and the experience necessary for successful intubation. Kundrotas et al.[9] successfully intubated the terminal ileum in 213 of 270 patients (79%) in a mean time of 3.4 minutes (range, 30 seconds to 10 minutes). There was no statistically significant difference between success rates among various training levels, and the yield of finding significant pathology was low (4 cases with abnormal endoscopic findings and only 1 of those 4 with histologic abnormalities). Ileoscopy is a necessary skill for endoscopists but requires training to gain proficiency. These data suggest that the yield of pathology does not justify "routine" ileoscopy during colonoscopy.

Endoscopic Biopsy/Lesion Size

Documentation of *Helicobacter pylori* infection is frequently sought during clinical evaluation of dyspeptic patients. Newer methods of detection including noninvasive methods such as urea breath testing or office-based serology are evolving and soon to be available. There continues, however, to be discrepancies between the yield of *H. pylori* by various testing methods (breath test, polymerase chain reaction [PCR], serology) and by gastric biopsy. Many experts believe that the location of the gastric biopsy is important in determining whether *H. pylori* will be detected. Genta and Graham[10] reported the results of 89 patients with known *H. pylori* infection who underwent histologic "mapping" of the stomach by endoscopic biopsy to determine which anatomic site gave the highest diagnostic yield. This study supports the dogma that antral biopsies give the highest diagnostic yield. In patients with *H. pylori* (demonstrated on any histologic specimen), the antral lesser curve at or near the incisura had the highest yield (no false-negatives). Surprisingly, corpus biopsies had greater than 90% accuracy. Although bacterial distribution throughout the stomach was nearly uniform, the inflammatory response was greatest in the antrum. This study emphasizes the importance of endoscopic targeting of biopsies to maximize the diagnostic of *H. pylori* and/or associated inflammation.

Gastrointestinal endoscopy is a valuable tool in establishing specific pathologic diagnoses, and tissue sampling is integral to the successful completion of this goal. Reusable biopsy forceps have been the usual method for obtaining tissue samples in most endoscopy units, but recently disposable biopsy forceps have been introduced in an attempt to minimize the transmission of infection as well as the mechanical problems encountered with reusable forceps. Yang et al.[11] prospectively compared various forceps for performance and adequecy of specimen acquisition. Jumbo forceps, regardless of the type, provided specimen sizes that were twice as large as regular forceps (Fig 1). Regular disposable forceps provided histologic specimen depths comparable to those of jumbo forceps. Regular reusable biopsy forceps yielded specimens with the smallest overall volume and depth. Yang et al. recommend using jumbo biopsy forceps of either type whenever possible to ensure optimal tissue volume for histologic evaluation.

Biopsy of submucosal gastrointestinal lesions with conventional biopsy forceps frequently yields little diagnostic information because these forceps sample only the superficial mucosal tissue. Karita and Tada[12] described the use of a combined strip biopsy and bite biopsy technique to obtain a histologic diagnosis in patients with submucosal gastrointestinal tumors. After puncturing the mucosa overlying the

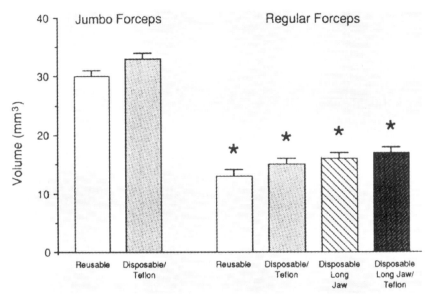

FIG 1.
Mean volumes obtained by the various forceps. The jumbo forceps obtained biopsy specimens twice the size of those obtained with regular forceps. *$P < 0.05$, significantly different from jumbo size. (From Yang R, Naritoku W, Laine L: *Gastrointest Endosc* 40:671–674, 1994. Used by permission.)

submucosal lesion, 2 to 3 mm of normal saline is injected. A snare is placed over the elevated tissue, which is held in place by special grasping forceps. A blended cutting and coagulation current is then used for resection. Bite biopsy forceps are then inserted into the mucosal defect created by the strip biopsy and a tissue specimen is obtained from the base of the defect. Nine of 11 tissue specimens gave a pathologic diagnosis, and there were no major complications. This technique appears to be useful in the diagnosis of submucosal lesions. The safety of this technique, however, remains to be demonstrated. Additionally, comparison to needle aspiration cytology directed endoscopically or by endoscopic ultrasound (EUS) requires study.

Biopsy forceps are also used by clinicians as a reference when measuring the size of a lesion, although this technique has never been validated. Yet accurate lesion measurement is important in the design and performance of clinical trials. A specific example would include estimates of the malignant potential of colonic neoplastic polyps based on polyp size. Margulies et al.[13] evaluated how accurately endoscopists estimate the size of objects at endoscopy when open biopsy forceps are used as the reference. Measurements were performed by gastroenterology attending physicians, fellows, and medical residents who used various-sized objects in a latex colon model viewed through a video colonoscope with and without the aid of open biopsy forceps. Mean estimates of size were consistently lower for all groups, and the use of open forceps did not improve accuracy. There was no difference in performance based on endoscopic experience. This study confirmed earlier studies concluding that endoscopists consistently underestimate the size of lesions observed endoscopically. Vakil et al.[14] believe that some of the difficulty in endoscopic measurements may be related to distortion of images because of the wide-angle lenses employed in current video endoscopes. His group has developed a computer program to correct distortion of the wide-angle lens. They compared the open-biopsy forceps reference technique for estimation of lesion size with a new image processing technique. Both techniques were tested in both an in vitro and in vivo system. With the in vitro ulcer model, the open-biopsy forceps technique underestimated lesion size by 41.8% ± 23.3%. When the new image processing technique was used to correct distortion, the estimate error was reduced to 1.8% ± 2.2% (P < .05) (Fig 2). In vivo testing revealed similar decreases in underestimation error, from 26.5% ± 5.7% to 2.8% ± 3.2% (P < .05). Technological advances in imaging will likely result in far greater accuracy in estimating lesion size.

Dilation

Balloon dilation for ulcer-induced pyloric strictures causing gastric outlet obstruction provides a viable endoscopic alternative to surgical treatment. DiSario et

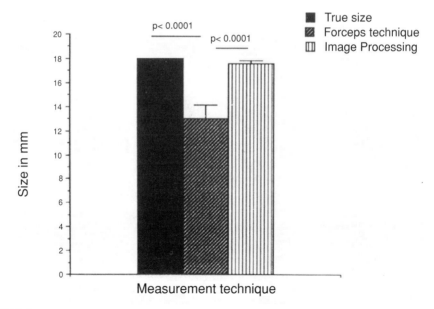

FIG 2.
Data indicating that comparisons to forceps uniformly underestimate the size of a lesion and this error is largely corrected through image processing. (From Vakil N, Smith W, Bourgeois K, et al: *Gastrointest Endosc* 40:178–183, 1994. Used by permission.)

al.[15] reported the largest series to date of the success of endoscopic balloon dilation for gastric outlet obstruction. Thirty patients with an average of 6 months of obstructive symptoms underwent treatment with through-the-scope (TTS) dilation using balloons measuring between 6 and 18 mm (median, 15 mm). Twenty-four patients (80%) achieved sustained symptom relief: 17 with a single procedure and 7 requiring multiple sessions. Four patients (13%) failed dilation and 2 (6.7%) suffered perforation (both with 18-mm balloons). Endoscopic balloon dilation is a proven technique for the treatment of gastric outlet obstruction secondary to stricturing from peptic ulcer disease and, if successful, may obviate the need for surgery. Perforation can occur and appears to be related to balloon size.

GASTROINTESTINAL BLEEDING

Peptic Ulcer Disease

Ulcer rebleeding risk is based in part on endoscopic appearance of the ulcer. Appropriate management of the bleeding ulcer hinges on the correct identification of various endoscopic stigmata, including active bleeding, visible vessels, adherent clots, and black/red spots in the ulcer base. Endoscopic ulcer features, just as ulcer size and polyp size, are subject to observer variation in interpretation. Laine et al.[16] assessed the interobserver agreement among endoscopists asked to label certain characteristic endoscopic features of bleeding ulcers before and after a short teaching session. Two hundred two endoscopists attending the 1992 American College of Gastroenterology Post-graduate Course answered questions regarding endoscopic pictures of ulcer stigmata before and after a teaching session. The proportion of correct identification increased with years of endoscopic experience and plateaued at 6 years beyond training. Endoscopists who performed five or fewer procedures per month had fewer correct responses. Teaching sessions benefited trainees (15% increase in correct answers) to a greater extent than it did physicians with 0 to 20 years' experience (8% increase) or greater than 20 years' experience (3%). Agreement on various ulcer stigmata ranged between 35% and 91%. Endoscopists disagreed on labeling of ulcer features greater than 25% of the time and more frequently with "more difficult" stigmata. These data indicate that significant variation exists among endoscopists' interpretation of ulcer stigmata and that development of a more accurate and reproducible measure of stigmata is necessary to facilitate optimal patient care.

The natural history of a bleeding peptic ulcer is presumed to follow an endoscopically identifiable progression. Our understanding of the natural history of ulcer stigmata was further advanced by Yang et al.,[17] who studied 85 patients with recent ulcer hemorrhage with repeated endoscopy at 2-day intervals. Visible vessels took 4.1 ± 2.1 days to disappear as compared with adherent clot and black/red spot stigmata, which took 2.4 ± 0.8 and 2.4 ± 1.3 days to disappear, respectively ($P < .05$). Bleeding did not recur after the stigmata resolved, and the time to resolution was not affected by age, sex, smoking, a history of peptic ulcer disease, ulcer location, severity of bleeding, comorbidities, or endoscopic therapy. Interestingly, most stigmata evolve through phases, but visible vessels occasionally disappear without going through other various stages.

Healing of gastroduodenal ulceration may depend somewhat on adequate mucosal blood flow; however, measurement of mucosal blood flow has been technically difficult. Leung et al.[18] used the technique of endoscopic reflectance spectrophotometry to measure the index of oxygen saturation (IOS) in 97 consecutive patients with bleeding duodenal ulcers. The IOS correlates reasonably well with mucosal blood flow. Those ulcers that healed had ulcer margins that exhibited increased IOS. This provocative work suggests that other measurable factors, in addition to stigmata of recent hemorrhage, may aid in assessing ulcer prognosis. The clinical impact of this endoscopic technique remains unclear.

Injection of a bleeding peptic ulcer is effective in controlling the bleeding in most cases. However, consensus on which injected agent is most effective at controlling bleeding is lacking. The mechanism of hemostasis following injection therapy also remains controversial, i.e., whether hemostasis is related to the pharmacologic effects of a particular agent or simply a local tamponade effect. Lai et al.[19] in a randomized, double-blind study compared endoscopic injection treatment with equal volumes of epinephrine (1 : 10,000) or distilled water in patients with bleeding ulcers. Twenty-five of 27 patients in the epinephrine group and 22 of 25 patients in the distilled water group achieved initial hemostasis ($P > .05$). There were no serious complications in either group. These investigators concluded that local tamponade of bleeding peptic ulcers with distilled water is as effective and safe as epinephrine injection. Berg et al.[20] performed a prospective, randomized pilot study of fibrin glue vs. polidocanol injection in the treatment of bleeding gastrointestinal ulcers. Thirty-eight patients were treated with fibrin glue injections and 41 with polidocanol. Recurrent bleeding was seen in 5 patients in the fibrin glue group and 10 patients in the polidocanol group. They concluded that fibrin glue injection is an effective method for treating bleeding gastroduodenal ulcers and is worth further investigation. These studies indicate that the specific injectate may be less important than previously believed and the mechanism may not be related to a "sclerosant" effect. The cheapest, safest, and most effective injection agent has not yet been determined.

Variceal Bleeding

Variceal hemorrhage is the most frequent cause of massive upper gastrointestinal bleeding. The mainstay of endoscopic management has been injection sclerotherapy using a variety of sclerosants. Sclerotherapy is effective in eradicating varices in a compliant population over numerous endoscopic sessions and results in less rebleeding and improved survival if eradication is achieved. Sclerotherapy is not without significant morbidity, including ulceration, bleeding, and stricture formation. Whether sclerotherapy is also associated with an increase in infectious complications is debated. Bac et al.[21] recorded the incidence of bacterial peritonitis within 2 weeks of variceal sclerotherapy in 216 patients undergoing 1,092 sclerotherapy sessions. Bacterial peritonitis developed in 60 patients at a mean time from variceal sclerotherapy to diagnosis of 3.5 days. The risk of bacterial peritonitis developing after emergency sclerotherapy was 3.0% as compared with a 0.5% risk of peritonitis with elective sclerotherapy ($P = .019$). Gut-derived gram-negative microorganisms were the most common bacteria cultured from the ascites. Bac and associates concluded that the risk of bacterial peritonitis is determined mainly by factors associated with variceal bleeding and not the sclerotherapy itself. Additionally, it was concluded that routine antibiotic prophylaxis before variceal sclerotherapy is not indicated.

Capitalizing on a ligation technique used to treat hemorrhoids, band ligation has been shown to eradicate varices. In this technique, small O-rings are applied with an endoscope tip attachment device. Studies by Stiegman (1992), Laine (1993), and Hashizume (1993) have all found that variceal ligation was as effective as sclerotherapy in eradicating varices and that it was associated with significantly fewer complications. Berner et al.[22] conducted a prospective, randomized comparison of sclerotherapy and ligation to study the short-term effect of these procedures on pulmonary and coagulation function, esophageal motility, gastroesophageal reflux, and bacteremia. They concluded that neither sclerotherapy nor ligation produced clinically significant changes in pulmonary function, coagulation parameters, or bacteremia. However, sclerotherapy was associated with significantly greater esophageal dysmotility and worsening gastroesophageal reflux. Whether these findings are clinically significant requires further study.

ESOPHAGEAL DISORDERS

Esophageal Cancer

The overall prognosis for esophageal cancer continues to be poor, with a 5-year survival rate of less than 10%. Few patients can be cured surgically, so palliation of dysphagia and maintenance of nutrition are the major therapeutic goals. The use of rigid esophageal endoprostheses to alleviate dysphagia has been proved effective but is limited by significant morbidity. Whether location of the tumor affected the morbidity of endoprosthesis placement was unknown. Spinelli[23] reviewed 76 patients with distal-third esophageal cancer (43 patients) or gastric cardia cancer (33 patients) who received esophageal endoprostheses for the palliation of malignant dysphagia. Atkinson, Celestin, and Wilson-Cook endoprostheses were used.

Forty patients (56%) had improvement in dysphagia allowing them to eat semi-solid or solid food. Twenty-five (35%) could only swallow liquids, and 6 (8%) were unimproved. They found that the combined early and late complication rate was 22%. When compared with endoprostheses placed in the upper and middle thirds of the esophagus (previous studies from this group), patients with distal esophageal and gastric cardiac lesions had higher complication rates, less improvement in dysphagia, and overall shorter survival.

Self-expanding, metallic stents have shown great promise in efficacy and safety in palliating esophageal carcinoma with apparently less morbidity than rigid endoprostheses. Various stent designs are being introduced that are easier to place than rigid endoprostheses; however, data from randomized control trials are lacking. Raijman et al.[24] reported their experience with a new Nitinol self-expanding stent in 14 patients with nonoperable esophageal carcinoma (Fig 3). Morbidity was minimal and efficacy was impressive. Ell et al.[25] compared the efficacy of coated (5 patients) with uncoated (26 patients) self-expanding metallic stents; all stents were placed successful and improvement in dysphagia was seen in 21 of 31 patients within 48 hours. Acute problems noted in the first week following placement included stent migration, insufficient expansion of the stent, placement-related epigastric and chest pain, and pouch formation at the superior margin of the stent. Major complications during the follow-up period included stent migration, stent obstruction caused by tumor overgrowth/ingrowth, and food impaction (35%). Problems of tumor overgrowth were successfully remedied with placement of a second stent or tumor tissue ablation by electrocoagulation.

Although placement of self-expanding, metallic stents is less difficult and less

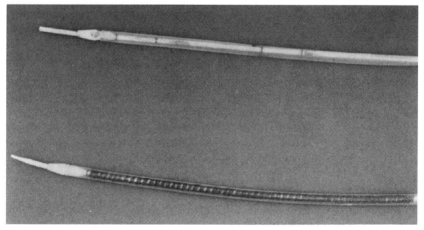

FIG 3.
Nitinol stent delivery system (*below*) and stabilizer *(above)* showing the compressed nature (8 mm) of this system. (From Raijman I, Walden D, Kortan P, et al: *Gastrointest Endosc* 40:614–615, 1994. Used by permission.)

traumatic than placement of rigid stents, accurate placement can be challenging and is essential for successful palliation of dysphagia. Raijman et al.[26] reported a clever and simple method for marking tumor margins that uses Hypaque contrast injections (Fig 4). Injections were made intramucosally at the proximal and distal margins of the tumor mass with a standard sclerotherapy needle. Three to 4 mm of diatrizoate (Hypaque 50%) was used at each injection site to confirm tumor margins fluoroscopically. This is a worthwhile technique for aiding in the accuracy of stent placement without significantly lengthening the time of the procedure.

Esophageal stents are but one method of palliation for malignant obstruction

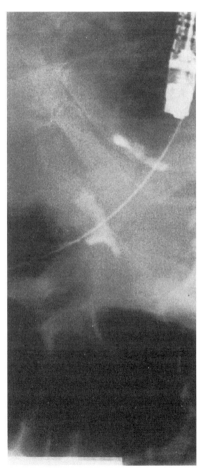

FIG 4.
Fluoroscopic view of contrast demonstrating both the proximal and distal tumor margins. (From Raijman I, Kortan P, Haber GB, et al: *Gastrointest Endosc* 40:222–224, 1994. Used by permission.)

caused by esophageal carcinoma. Other modalities, including endoscopic dilation, BICAP, and laser photocoagulation, have also been shown to be effective. Injection of ethanol into an obstructive tumor mass is another method that has previously been described. Chung et al.[27] treated 36 patients with inoperable esophageal or gastric cardia carcinoma by the intralesional injection of absolute ethanol. A sclerotherapy needle was used to deliver 0.5- to 1-cc increments of 100% ethanol with a mean volume per session of 7.8 cc. Complications included mediastinitis (1 patient) and tracheoesophageal fistula (2 patients). The mean dysphagia grade improved from 2.7 to 1.4 following treatment ($P < .001$). Dysphagia grade improvement appears better following stent placement, but the low cost and technical simplicity of ethanol injection, especially with bulky, exophytic lesions, make this technique a treatment option in selected situations.

Endoscopic ultrasonography is a new gastrointestinal diagnostic technique that has shown particular promise in the staging of gastrointestinal malignancies; EUS more accurately determines the depth of tumor invasion and identifies lymph node involvement. Superficial esophageal carcinoma is curable in many instances, but accurate preoperative staging is essential. Yoshikane et al.[28] used EUS to stage suspected superficial esophageal carcinoma and compared the ultrasonographic findings with histopathologic findings. Nine patients with mucosal carcinomas and 19 patients with submucosal lesions were evaluated with EUS for depth of invasion and lymph node metastases. Endoscopic ultrasound had accuracy rates for identifying the depth of invasion of 67% for mucosal lesions and 79% for submucosal lesions. The accuracy rate for identifying lymph node involvement was 72%, with a sensitivity and specificity of 58% and 85%, respectively. Endoscopic ultrasonography may be an important tool for better differentiating superficial esophageal carcinomas from more advanced lesions so that appropriate therapy can be applied.

Achalasia

Achalasia is characterized by the inability of the lower esophageal sphincter to relax in response to normal physiologic stimuli (swallows). Achalasia has traditionally been treated by balloon dilatation and/or surgical myotomy (Heller myotomy), with drug therapy reserved for mild cases or those patients who are poor candidates for more definitive treatment. A retrospective review of the University of Alabama, Birmingham Medical Center experience in treating achalasia was reported by Abid et al.[29] They compared those patients treated with balloon dilatation (36 patients) with those treated with Heller myotomies (19 patients). The severity of dysphagia, regurgitation, heartburn, and chest pain were assessed before and after treatment for both groups, and all showed significant improvement ($P < .01$). Heartburn was more frequently observed in the myotomy group. In this study the outcome was equal in those treated by balloon dilation and those treated by myotomy, which confirms previous investigations; thus balloon dilation remains a viable treatment option.

SCREENING AND SURVEILLANCE

Colorectal Neoplasia

The success of any screening program depends largely on the majority of patients participating and compliance. To ensure better compliance, screening examinations must be tolerable to the patient with minimal discomfort. The value of screening for colorectal neoplasia by flexible sigmoidoscopy and/or fecal occult blood testing seems to be established. One method of improving patient acceptance of sigmoidoscopy screening may be to simplify the bowel preparation while maintaining the quality of the preparation to optimize the value of the examination. The use of hypertonic phosphate enemas before examination has been standard practice, but clear consensus does not exist for how to best prepare the distal end of the colon for sigmoidoscope examination. Preston et al.[30] prospectively compared three preparation regimens—one enema 1 hour before examination, two enemas 1 hour before examination, or two enemas given 3 and 1 hour before sigmoidoscopy—to determine which regimen provided the optimal preparation. There was no statistical difference among the various regimens, with adequate or excellent colon preparation achieved in 80% of the patients. Preston et al. suggest that one hypertonic phosphate enema 1 hour before flexible sigmoidoscopy will provide for a high-quality examination and will be better tolerated by patients.

Patients at higher risk for colorectal carcinoma stand to benefit most from screening efforts. Although women with a history of breast, endometrial, or ovarian cancer have been considered to be at higher risk for the development of colorectal carcinoma, debate continues as to how important this association is. A recent meta-analysis by Schoen et al.[31] found that the age-adjusted relative risks for the development of colorectal cancer after breast, endometrial, or ovarian cancer were 1.1, 1.4, and 1.6, respectively. Ultimately, the degree of increased risk is small, and a consensus opinion regarding the screening modality, e.g., colonoscopy vs. sigmoidoscopy, in these patients is lacking.

Polyps greater than 1 cm in size carry an increased malignant potential, but it is unclear how great the malignant potential is in a patient with diminutive polyps (less than 0.5 cm) of the distal and of the colon. Zarchy and Ershoff[32] prospectively studied 226 patients who had benign neoplasms on flexible sigmoidoscopy and also underwent follow-up colonoscopy to determine what findings on flexible sigmoidoscopy predicted other advanced lesions (i.e., adenoma greater than 1 cm, villous or severe dysplasia on histology) on colonoscopy. Twenty-four percent of the patients with distal adenomas had other adenomas found on colonoscopy, but only 6% had advanced lesions and none had carcinoma. However, if an advanced lesion was found on flexible sigmoidoscopy, there was a greater than 10% chance of finding a similar advanced lesion on colonoscopy.

Endoscopic differentiation of hyperplastic and adenomatous polyps is unreliable and as a result requires biopsy for histologic confirmation. Bertoni et al.[33] prospectively evaluated the predictive value of the "disappearing phenomenon" (a diminutive rectal polyp's disappearance following maximal air insufflation during endoscopy) of diminutive polyps in the distal 20 cm of the colon as a means of differentiating neoplastic from non-neoplastic polyps. Two hundred eighteen polyps in 90 patients were identified, and complete disappearance of 93 (43%) was noted. Disappearance was significantly more prevalent with polyps in the middle and lower regions of the rectum ($P < .05$) and with smaller, paler, smooth-surfaced polyps ($P < .001$). Multiple logistic regression analysis also suggested that disappearance was the strongest predictor of nonadenomatous polyps ($P < .001$). However, the technique was not uniformly accurate and thus biopsy-documented histology is still required.

Krevsky and Fisher[34] raised the question of whether or not the recent American Cancer Society screening guideline modification that eliminated repeat flexible sigmoidoscopy 1 year after the initial screening would result in a missed opportunity to identify clinically significant colorectal neoplasia. Repeat flexible sigmoidoscopies were performed on 81 patients 1 year after the initial screening of 202 patients. Thirty-two percent of the patients had polyps identified at the index flexible sigmoidoscopy. On repeat examination, 5 patients (6%) had polyps and 2 of the 5 were under 50 years old. Although it appears that neoplastic polyps can be identified at short intervals after previous screening examinations, the clinical importance appears to be minimal and the cost high. Therefore, less frequent screening intervals appear justified.

Adding to our uncertainty about screening intervals and targeted populations was a study by Squillace et al.[35] that suggested that a normal colonoscopic examination in patients with no history of colonic polyps who are 50 years or older does not predict a polyp-free status for life. It was hypothesized that patients who had no previous neoplastic polyps at an index colonoscopic examination may represent a low-risk population and may not require further screening examinations. However, this study found that the incidence of adenomatous polyps in 29 patients between 50 and 70 years old who had had normal colonoscopic results at least 5 years previously was 41.4%.

These data indicate that 1-year follow-up examinations result in a low yield of new or undetected polyps. However, the lack of finding polyps on flexible sigmoidoscopy or colonoscopy does not preclude further neoplasia formation (i.e., identifies a low-risk group), and a continued screening program for colorectal neoplasia appears necessary.

Barrett's Esophagus

The increased risk of esophageal adenocarcinoma in patients with Barrett's esophagus is the justification for endoscopic surveillance in these patients. An assumption of such a program is that surveillance leads to the diagnosis of either high-grade dysplasia or earlier-stage cancer and results in improved survival. Provenzale et al.[36] used a decision analysis computer model to assess the efficacy and cost-effectiveness of various Barrett's esophagus surveillance strategies. Twelve strategies were examined: (1) no surveillance, esophagectomy performed only for cancer on biopsy; (2) no surveillance, esophagectomy for high-grade dysplasia; (3 to 7) surveillance at intervals from 1 to 5 years with esophagectomy for cancer; and (8 to 12) surveillance at intervals from 1 to 5 years with esophagectomy for high-grade dysplasia. Life expectancy, quality-adjusted life expectancy, and cost-effectiveness were determined for each strategy. Annual surveillance with esophagectomy for high-grade dysplasia would prevent more cancers and is the most effective strategy if life expectancy were the only criteria. When quality-adjusted life expectancy is considered, surveillance every 2 to 3 years is the most favorable strategy. Surveillance at 5-year intervals is the most cost-effective while still providing increased life expectancy. This model required many assumptions, some of which are subject to debate. Thus the clinical applicability of this model is questionable but suggests that as more outcomes data become available, recommended surveillance intervals may change. It also remains to be proved whether surveillance in patients with Barrett's esophagus results in a decrease in mortality.

Consistently reproducible endoscopic examination is critical to meaningful surveillance of Barrett's esophagus. Hiatal hernias, interobserver bias, and short-segment Barrett's esophagus cause inconsistencies in diagnosing Barrett's esophagus as well as accurately measuring Barrett's esophagus more commonly than is often appreciated. Kim et al.[37] reported the results of the endoscopic findings in 192 patients with gastroesophageal reflux disease and found 116 patients meeting for diagnostic criteria for Barrett's esophagus. Endoscopies were repeated at 6 weeks, with 10% having a greater than 4-cm change in length of the previously measured Barrett's esophagus and 20% having specialized columnar epithelium demonstrated at only one of the two endoscopies. Overall, there was an change in the diagnosis in 18% of patients. These inconsistencies in the ability to detect and measure Barrett's esophagus underscore the difficulties in studying the lesion.

The use of other endoscopic techniques may aid in the diagnosis of Barrett's esophagus. Stevens et al.[38] reported a technique of combined Lugol's iodine and indigo carmine dye spraying with magnification endoscopy to identify Barrett's epithelium. This technique appeared especially helpful in identifying short-segment Barrett's esophagus. Endoscopic ultrasonography has become the gold standard for staging esophageal malignancy, but its role in dysplasia/carcinoma surveillance in Barrett's esophagus is unproved. Falk et al. demonstrated that EUS cannot reliably differentiate benign from dysplastic or malignant Barrett's esophagus.[39] Therefore, the gold standard of increased risk of malignancy in Barrett's esophagus remains histologic demonstration of high-grade dysplasia.

COLONOSCOPY

Polypectomy

The National Polyp Study (1993) confirmed what had long been assumed; removal of adenomatous polyps significantly reduces a patient's risk for the development of colorectal carcinoma. Polypectomy has generally been performed with standard-sized snares and/or hot biopsy forceps. However, these larger snares are at times cumbersome, especially when dealing with diminutive polyps. Removal of diminutive polyps can be achieved efficiently, safely, and quickly with the use of tiny oval and hexagonal snares.[40] McAfee et al. removed 183 diminutive polyps from 90 patients with a success rate of 93% (88% of the polyps recovered). The only complication was one major hemorrhage in a patient in whom a polypectomy was performed without cautery. The use of tiny snares appears to enhance the endoscopist's ability to quickly and efficiently remove diminutive polyps. Whether cautery or a cold snare is the preferable technique requires further study.

Hot biopsy forceps are sometimes used to remove small polyps because of their ease of use. However, concerns over colonic perforation and delayed hemorrhage, especially in the right colon, have tempered enthusiasm for the use of these instruments. Additionally, many polyps can be difficult to approach with this technique. In an effort to decrease bleeding risk and improve efficacy, newer polypectomy devices have been evaluated. A bipolar polypectomy device was evaluated by McNally et al.[41] The device has four small teeth that are used to hook into the polyp tissue and then draw the tissue into a cutting cup. A total of 52 polyps were removed from 39 patients with this technique. The device is technically difficult to use but has the advantages of minimizing the amount of current needed for polypectomy and reducing thermal scatter to surrounding tissues, and theoretically it should decrease the risk of serious complications such as perforation and delayed hemorrhage. Its clinical utility remains uncertain and requires further study.

Aspirin and other nonsteroidal anti-inflammatory drugs (NSAIDs) cause platelet dysfunction by direct inhibition of the cyclooxygenase pathway. Nonsteroidal anti-inflammatory drugs are thought to increase the risk of bleeding after endoscopic biopsy or polypectomy if the use of such medications is not discontinued before the procedure and for a variable time after. This assumption has not been validated in prospective trials. Shiffman et al.[42] studied 694 patients who had undergone upper gastrointestinal endoscopy or colonoscopy with biopsy or polypectomy; 320 of these patients had recently consumed NSAIDs. Postprocedure bleeding was assessed by questionaires and telephone follow-up. Thirty-two patients (4.6%) reported bleeding. Twenty patients who had taken NSAIDs (20/320, 6.3%) had minor, self-limiting, clinically insignificant bleeding as opposed to 8 patients who did not take NSAIDs (8/374, 2.1%, P = .009). Two patients in each group had major bleeding. This report suggests that although the incidence of minor bleeding increased with NSAID use, the risk of major bleeding is low. Because bleeding risk with polypectomy is low (1% to 2%), a large trial will be necessary to show significantly decreased major bleeding by discontinuing NSAID use. Even though such a trial may never be performed, it still appears prudent to discontinue NSAID use before endoscopy and after polypectomy or biopsy.

Hemorrhoid Treatment

Hemorrhoidal disease is extremely common in the United States and although rarely fatal, hemorrhoids can cause a significant amount of morbidity for patients. Various treatment modalities have been developed for symptomatic internal hemorrhoids and include rubber band ligation, Nd-YAG laser treatment, sclerotherapy, infrared coagulation, bipolar coagulation, and dc coagulation. Randal et al.[43] conducted the first prospective, randomized study comparing bipolar and dc electrocoagulation for the treatment of bleeding internal hemorrhoids (Figs 5 and 6). Fifty patients were randomized to bipolar coagulation treatment and 50 to dc coagulation. All patients had chronic blood loss from internal hemorrhoids and had received previous medical and/or surgical treatment for hemorrhoids. Hemorrhoids were graded on a scale of 1 to 4 at each treatment session. At the initial evaluation, 98% of the study patients had grade 2 or 3 hemorrhoids, 2% had grade 1, and none had grade 4. The dc hemorrhoidal probe was placed 1 cm or more above the den-

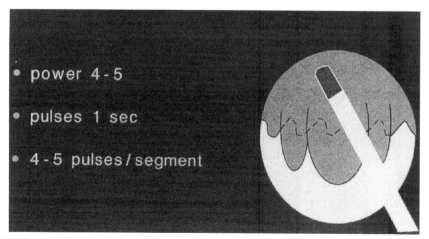

FIG 5.
Bipolar coagulation technique for the treatment of internal hemorrhoids. (From Randall GM, Jensen DM, Machicado GA, et al: *Gastrointest Endosc* 40:403–410, 1994. Used by permission.)

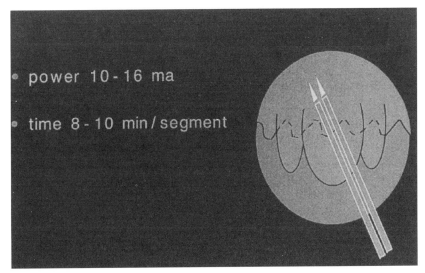

FIG 6.
Direct current coagulation technique for the treatment of internal hemorrhoids. (From Randall GM, Jensen DM, Machichado GA, et al: *Gastrointest Endosc* 40:403–410, 1994. Used by permission.)

tate line at the hemorrhoid base. Current was gradually increased in 2-mA increments for a maximum of 10 to 16 mA. Treatment time was 8 to 10 minutes, with a gradual decrease in current to zero. Two hemorrhoidal segments were treated per session, and sessions were repeated after 3 to 4 weeks. The bipolar probe was similarly positioned on the hemorrhoid base as just described. Coagulation energy was delivered in 1-second pulses for a total of four to six pulses per hemorrhoidal segment.

After the 1-year follow-up, 92% of the patients had no or mild symptoms (69% with no symptoms, 23% with mild symptoms) and 8% had severe symptoms. Bipolar treatment was significantly faster than dc coagulation, with a mean session treatment time of 24 seconds vs. 16 minutes with dc current. More recurrences but fewer complications were noted after dc treatment (P = NS). Endoscopic treatment of internal hemorrhoids with dc or bipolar coagulation appears to be safe and effective with little significant difference between the two modalities except for a faster treatment time with bipolar coagulation.

PANCREATICOBILIARY ENDOSCOPY

Cytology

Conventional endoscopic techniques for diagnosing gastrointestinal malignancy (forceps biopsy, snare polypectomy) are not of great value in diagnosing pancreaticobiliary malignancy. Although endoscopic brush cytology has been shown to be an effective means of diagnosing bile duct and pancreatic malignancy, its yield is suboptimal. Further refinement of technique or newer devices are needed to maximize the yield of ductal cytology. Ferrari et al.[44] demonstrated a 56% sensitivity of brush cytology in the diagnosis of pancreaticobiliary malignancy with an overall accuracy of 70%. Ryan and Baldauf[45] sought to determine whether flow cytometry in addition to standard cytology would increase the diagnostic yield of malignancy. They determined that the addition of flow cytometry for DNA content to routine cytology increased the sensitivity from 42% to 63%. This technique appears promising, but further validation is necessary. In an effort to maximize standard brush cytology, Baron et al.[46] examined whether salvage cytology from the brush sheath would improve the results when the brush is withdrawn from the sheath. Indeed, salvage cytology resulted in an increase in sensitivity when this technique was used. Mohandas et al.[47] studied whether dilation of malignant biliary strictures to 10 F before bile aspiration cytology resulted in an improved diagnostic yield. Sensitivity increased from 27% to 63% following dilation. These studies suggest that the 27% to 56% sensitivity of bile duct cytology can be improved with a variation in technique. Further study of the effect of dilation, salvage cytology, and flow cytometry should clarify the optimal cytologic technique to detect malignancy.

Endoscopic Retrograde Cholangiopancreatography and Laparoscopic Cholecystectomy

The emergence of laparoscopic cholecystectomy (LC) has led to the widespread use of this procedure in treating gallbladder disease. Biliary complications of LC include retained common bile duct stones, bile duct leaks, or cystic duct stump leaks. Many of these complications are now managed endoscopically. The optimal timing, success rates, and complications of diagnostic and therapeutic endoscopic retrograde cholangiopancreatography (ERCP) following LC remain an area of debate. Pencev et al.[48] evaluated 56 patients by ERCP after LC for various indications, including common duct stones, elevated aminotransferase levels with abdominal pain, and biliary duct injury. Within the first 24 hours after LC, ERCP was performed in 12 patients without complication. Twenty-three patients underwent therapeutic ERCP for common bile duct stones, 14 patients for biliary duct or cystic duct leaks, and 1 patient for gallstone pancreatitis. Leaks were treated by temporary stenting with either nasobiliary or internal stents. One patient had a common bile duct stricture, 2 patients had possible malignancy, and there were 14 normal studies. This study demonstrated that ERCP after LC can be performed successfully and safely for a wide array of biliary duct problems. Intervention can occur within the first 24 hours postoperatively without a significantly increased risk and thus preserves the advantages (shortened hospital stay) gained by a laparoscopic procedure.

Laser Lithotripsy

The majority of common duct stones can be removed endoscopically following papillotomy; however, a small percentage of stones require the use of other modalities (e.g., percutaneous approaches) for extraction. Laser lithotripsy via percutaneous T tubes or existing sphincterotomies has previously been described for the treatment of choledocholithiasis and intrahepatic lithiasis with the advantage of causing minimal biliary ductal injury. Prat et al.[49] treated 16 patients who had choledocholithiasis or intrahepatic stones with intracorporeal lithotripsy. Clearance of the bile duct was achieved in 14 of 16 patients (87.5%) with no laser-related morbidity or mortality. Although laser lithotripsy can be successfully performed, technical difficulties and a prolonged procedural time make it a technique with limited utility.

Endoscopic Sphincterotomy

Endoscopic sphincterotomy (ES) can be successfully accomplished in the vast majority of patients. The increased skill of endoscopists and the broadening of indications had led to more challenging cases. Because ES is now often performed in the setting of surgically altered anatomy and/or periampullary diverticula, the risk of complications is increased. The use of stent-guided sphincterotomy with a "needle knife" sphincterotome appears to be an effective technique in these settings and is associated with low complication rates.[50] Seigel et al. used this procedure in 229 patients for a variety of indications, including 67 patients with Bilroth II gastrectomies, 23 with periampullary diverticula, 57 with pancreas divisum, and 82 with recurrent pancreatitis. Procedure-related pancreatitis occurred in 19 patients (8.3%) and in most cases was mild (17 of 19). This technique allows precise incisions that follow the duct and, in the case of pancreatic sphincterotomy, prevents duct occlusion secondary to edema.

Stents

High–surgical risk patients (e.g., advanced liver disease, cardiopulmonary disease, or other major medical illnesses) are not considered good candidates for cholecystectomy (laparoscopic or open) for symptomatic cholelithiasis. Alternative methods of therapy for these patients are often necessary; however, such therapies are not universally successful (oral dissolution, lithotripsy, etc.). Endoscopic gallbladder stenting with a nasobiliary pigtail catheter inserted over a hydrophilic, angled guide wire may be an effective method for maintaining cystic duct patency in high-risk patients with symptomatic cholelithiasis.[51] Further study of this technique will clarify its clinical role.

Stent occlusion and the development of jaundice and/or cholangitis and major problems with biliary stents. Biofilm formation caused by bacteria adherence is the mechanism of stent occlusion. It is unclear whether the stent material, design, or both are responsible for this phenomenon. Hoffman et al.[52] compared various stent materials in in vitro studies and found that copolymer and wire mesh stents caused less biofilm development than did conventional stents. Sung et al.[53] in a randomized study compared biliary stents with and without side holes and found that omitting side holes did not reduce the rate of stent occlusion.

Stent occlusion also appears to occur frequently with pancreatic stents. Ikenberry et al.[54] found that pancreatic stents occlude more quickly than previously appreciated. Using a standardized method for measuring the flow rate, they found that 50% of the stents were occluded at 6 weeks and 100% were occluded at greater than 9 weeks. Their data suggest that the occlusion rate is nearly linear with time and that there is little difference between 5 F and 7 F stents. Thus the optimal material and design of pancreatic/biliary stents has not yet been determined. Until that time, stent changes secondary to occlusion will continue to be necessary.

Endoscopic Retrograde Cholangiopancreatography/Antibiotics

Cholangitis and sepsis are rare complications of ERCP and are more commonly seen after therapeutic or difficult diagnostic cases in which there is biliary duct obstruction. The use of preprocedural prophylactic antibiotics for ERCP remains controversial because the utility of antibiotics in preventing infection has not been uniformly demonstrated. In a randomized study, Niederau et al.[55] found that bacteremia or sepsis occurred in 8 of 50 patients (16%) without antibiotic prophylaxis vs. none of 50 patients who received a 2-g dose of cefotaxime 15 minutes before ERCP ($P < .01$). Of the 8 patients, bacteremia developed in 4 and cholangitis and/or clinical sepsis in 4. In all patients in whom cholangitis and sepsis developed, biliary obstruction was coexistent. The authors concluded that antibiotic prophylaxis does reduce the incidence of bacteremia and sepsis in patients undergoing ERCP and that the risk of sepsis is greatest with biliary obstruction. Therefore they recommend the use of antibiotic prophylaxis before ERCP only in patients in whom obstructive bile duct disease was present and in whom there was failure to decompress the obstructed biliary system.

The choice of prophylactic antibiotic to be used with biliary procedures is also controversial, with some advocating third-generation cephalosporins and others fluoroquinolones. Leung et al.[56] performed bacterologic studies on 579 patients with common bile duct stones and found 121 (21%) with bacteria. Both bile and stones were cultured, and the most common bacterial isolates were *Escherichia coli, Klebsiella, Enterobacter, Enterococcus,* and *Streptococcus.* The hepatic/biliary excretion of several antibiotics was also studied (ceftazidime, cefoperazone, imipenim, netil-micin, and ciprofloxacin). Bile samples were obtained from patients with complete biliary obstruction and analyzed for antibiotic levels. All antibiotics except ciprofloxacin had low to undetectable bile levels in this clinical setting, whereas ciprofloxacin had a concentration of 29% of the serum level. These data suggest that antibiotics need only be given in those patients with an obstructed bile duct, especially in those who cannot be decompressed. It also appears that ciprofloxacin attains the highest bile concentration and adequately covers the microbial spectrum usually encountered with these procedures and thus appears to be the drug of choice.

Pancreatitis After Endoscopic Retrograde Cholangiopancreatography

Pancreatitis is one of the major complications of diagnostic and therapeutic ERCP, with many factors contributing to its development. Whether or not the contrast agents used during ERCP play a role in post-ERCP pancreatitis was addressed by Sherman et al.[57] in a randomized, prospective, double-blind study. They compared a low-osmolality, nonionic contrast agent (Omnipaque 300; iohexol, 672 mOsm/kg water) with a high-osmolality, ionic contrast agent (Hypaque 50%; diatrizoate sodium, 1,515 mOsm/kg water) to determine whether there was a difference between the two agents in the frequency and severity of post-ERCP pancreatitis. Six hundred ninety patients undergoing diagnostic ERCP with or without sphincter of Oddi manometry or therapeutics were randomized to iohexal or diatrizoate; pancreatitis was diagnosed if serum amylase or lipase values were elevated to greater than four times normal 18 hours after the procedure and the patients had abdominal pain requiring narcotics 24 hours after the procedure. The severity of pancreatitis was determined by the need for hospitalization and the extent of medical intervention. The overall frequency (7.2% vs. 7.5%) and severity (4.3% mild, 2% moderate, 0.9% severe for diatrizoate vs. 4.3% mild, 2.6% moderate, 0.6% severe for iohexol) of post-ERCP pancreatitis was no different (P = NS). Similarly, there was no significant difference in the two groups when the data were analyzed by procedure category or by whether or not a pancreatogram was performed (P = NS). Sherman et al. concluded that routine use of the more expensive nonionic contrast agents was not warranted.

Pancreas Divisum

Pancreatic divisum is associated with recurrent pancreatitis. Coleman et al.[58] reviewed the results of endoscopic stenting of the minor papilla, with and without sphincterotomy, in 34 patients with pancreas divisum and pain or pancreatitis. They found that there was a statistically significant improvement in pain scores in patients with acute recurrent pancreatitis or chronic pancreatitis, but not in patients with pain alone (Fig 7). Sphincterotomy of the minor papilla did not change the outcome. This report suggests that we may be able to identify a subset of patients with pancreas divisum who would benefit from minor papilla stenting.

Pancreatic Duct Sphincterotomy

Biliary sphincterotomy is universally accepted and widely applied to access the biliary system and treat biliary disease. Pancreatic sphincterotomy has been rarely performed and is believed to be associated with increased complications and potentially irreversible pancreatic duct complications. Kozarek et al.[59] reported their experience on the safety of pancreatic sphincterotomy in 56 patients (54 of whom

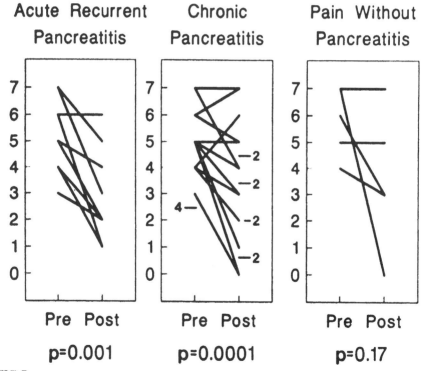

FIG 7.
Pain scores in patients with acute recurrent pancreaticis, chronic pancreatitis, and pain without pancreatitis before and after endoscopic stenting and/or sphincterotomy of the minor papilla in patients with pancreatic diseases. (From Coleman SD, Eisen GM, Troughton AB, et al: *Am J Gastroenterol* 89:1152–1156, 1994. Used by permission.)

had chronic pancreatitis). Indications were for stones (26), duct leak (18), and stricture (8). Acute complications were noted in 10% (pancreatitis in 4, cholangitis in 2). Chronic complications were noted in 30% (duct changes in 16%, sphincter stenosis in 14%). It appears that although many patients may have an improvement in pain secondary to the placement of stents, removal of calculi, or the sphincterotomy itself, the potential morbidity appears substantial. Until the clinical significance of the observed duct and sphincter changes are known, it appears prudent to avoid pancreatic sphincterotomy unless performed as a "last resort."

ENDOSCOPIC ULTRASONOGRAPHY

Endoscopic ultrasonography appears to have utility in the diagnosis and staging of the depth of invasion of various gastrointestinal malignancies such as esophageal, gastric, and rectal cancer. This expensive technology is difficult to perform, and its impact on clinical outcomes is not known.

Catalano et al.[60] evaluated the ability of EUS to assess lymph node metastasis in 100 patients with esophageal carcinoma. Endoscopic ultrasonography had a sensitivity and specificity for detecting lymph node metastasis of 89.1% and 91.7%, respectively. Several endosonographic features were predictive of malignancy, including size greater than 10 mm (most predictive), a rounded contour, sharply demarcated borders, and hypoechoic patterns (least predictive) (Figs 8 and 9). When all four features were present, malignancy was predicted with 100% accuracy. This

BENIGN   MALIGNANT

heterogeneous   **homogeneous**

hyperechoic   **hypoechoic**

FIG 8.
Endoscopic ultrasound–determined lymph node features and echotextures of benign and malignant lymph nodes. (From Catalano MF, Sivak MV, Rice T, et al: *Gastrointest Endosc* 40:442–446, 1994. Used by permission.)

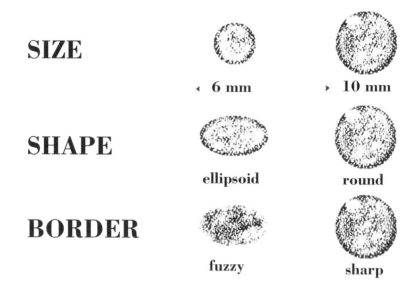

SIZE   < 6 mm   > 10 mm

SHAPE   ellipsoid   round

BORDER   fuzzy   sharp

FIG 9.
Size, shape, and border characteristic of benign and malignant lymph node features as determined by endoscopic ultrasound. (From Catalano MF, Sivak MV, Rice T, et al: *Gastrointest Endosc* 40:442–446, 1994. Used by permission.)

report suggests that EUS may also have a role in staging gastrointestinal malignancies beyond defining the depth of invasion of tumors.

Motoo et al.[61] studied the ability of EUS to differentiate extragastric compressive lesions from submucosal gastric tumors. Nineteen patients were found to have extragastric compression, 16 of which were due to normal organs and 3 were caused by extraluminal tumors. Endoscopic ultrasound correctly differentiated these lesions and identified the compressing organ with 100% accuracy. Mendis et al.[62] used EUS to determine which gastric wall layer was enlarged in patients with large gastric folds. They found that when ultrasonographic abnormalities were confined to the mucosal layer, endoscopic biopsies were diagnostic. Gastric wall layer abnormalities involving the muscularis propria without evidence of ulceration strongly suggested malignancy and warranted further workup. Gastric varices were easily indentified and prevented potentially dangerous biopsy attempts.

Endoscopic ultrasonography may also have a role in diagnosing biliary tract disease. Amouyal et al.[63] prospectively compared the accuracy of diagnosing choledocholithiasis by EUS with standard ultrasonography and computed tomography in 62 consecutive patients. Choledocholithiasis was found in 22 patients. Endoscopic ultrasonography was more sensitive (97%) than standard ultrasonography (25%; $P < .0001$) and computed tomography (75%; $P < .02$), but there was no significant difference in specificity or positive predictive value among these modalities. With improved expertise, EUS may replace standard ultrasonography and computed tomography as the procedure of choice for evaluating the biliary tree.

Endoscopic ultrasonography has also expanded our ability to acquire tissue for histologic diagnosis; EUS-guided fine-needle aspiration biopsy has successfully obtained diagnostic tissue from extraluminal, submucosal, mediastinal, and abdominal masses.[64–66] Endoscopic ultrasound–guided fine-needle aspiration is performed with small-gauge (22 to 25), 4-cm-long retractable needles that are usually housed in either metallic or Teflon catheters. Chang et al.[64] performed EUS-guided fine-needle aspiration biopsies on 38 consecutive patients with extraluminal (pancreatic, periesophageal, perigastric, liver, celiac nodes, perirectal) and submucosal (esophageal, gastric, duodenal) masses. Adequate tissue was obtained in 91% of the targeted lesions with an overall diagnostic accuracy of 87%. For malignant lesions, the sensitivity and specificity were 91% and 100%, respectively. Similarly encouraging results have been obtained by Wiersema et al.[65, 66]

As the indications for EUS expand, further improvement in the instrumentation will allow for easier and, we hope, more accurate examinations. The Olympus EU-M20, a second-generation EUS system with several technical changes that were believed to make the instrument easier to handle, was evaluated by Catalano et al.[67] Optical quality was good but not appreciably better than that of the previous-generation instruments. Endoscopic ultrasound probes have been developed and show promise with various lesions (e.g., malignant strictures) in which EUS cannot obtain adequate images.[68] Whether or not these and future technical refinements will significantly improve the accuracy or ease of use of EUS has not yet been determined.

NEW TECHNIQUES AND INSTRUMENTATION

Barkin et al.[69] reported on the effectiveness and safety of a first-generation video enteroscope in 29 patients. The mean length of insertion past the ligament of Treitz when an overtube was used was 108 cm (range, 60 to 150 cm) vs. 11 cm (range, 5 to 30 cm) without the tube. Of the patients with occult gastrointestinal bleeding, 30% were found to have small bowel disease distal to the ligament of Treitz. This instrument appears to have a significant yield in investigating small bowel disease, and performance is improved with the use of an overtube.

Shaker reported using the Olympus GIF N30 endoscope (outer diameter, 5.3 mm; working length, 925 mm) for nonsedated transnasal pharyngoesophagogastroduodenoscopy (T-EGD).[70] This technique was well tolerated by the patients and allowed for examination of the hypopharynx and laryngeal structures as well as the esophagus, stomach, and duodenum. This endoscope could become a useful, time- and cost-saving technique for evaluating the upper gastrointestinal tract, especially in an office-based setting. Comparative studies are needed to establish its diagnostic and therapeutic utility.

Hintze et al.[71] developed a new wide-channel endoscope with a 6-mm suction and accessory channel that was able to completely evacuate the stomach in 122 of 124 patients with severe upper gastrointestinal bleeding. This wide-channel endoscope may also be used for expanded nonemergent endoscopic procedures such as endosonographic probes, metallic stent placement, large-forceps biopsies, large balloons, and clipping devices as well as other applications.

Duckworth et al.[72] described a technique for placing percutaneous endoscopic gastrojejunostomy tubes (PEG/J) by using an over-the-wire approach that avoids the problem of jejunostomy tube pullback during conventional insertion of J tubes through PEG tubes. Tube placement was successful in 15 of 18 (83%) patients on the first attempt. The average procedure time was 37 minutes (range, 18 to 75 minutes). This technique may improve our ability to place a J tube when clinically necessary.

Kadakia et al.[73] compared gastrostomy tube replacement with a Foley catheter vs. a commercial gastrostomy tube and found no significant difference between the two in terms of efficacy and safety. Foley catheters are, however, considerably less expensive than commercial gastrostomy tubes and appear to be a cost-effective alternative.

Hydrocolonic sonography is a new technique in which the colon is evaluated by transabdominal ultrasonography after retrograde instillation of water. Limberg and Osswald[74] compared normal transabdominal ultrasonography and hydrocolonic ultrasonography with colonoscopy in the diagnosis of ulcerative colitis and colonic Crohn's disease. The sensitivity for detecting Crohn's disease and ulcerative colitis by hydrocolonic ultrasonography was 96% and 91%, respectively. This technique was also able to differentiate Crohn's disease from ulcerative colitis in 93% of the cases. This technique requires further validation but appears to be promising in evaluating the colon for inflammatory bowel disease.

SUMMARY

Advances in endoscopic utilization and technology continue to develop at an accelerating pace. It is likely that endoscopy itself as well as new instruments will be subjected to intense scrutiny as regards their cost-effectiveness and impact on clinical outcome. It is expected that this literature will become the most important factor in future endoscopy development and practice.

REFERENCES

1. Iwao T, Toyonaga A, Harada H, et al: Arterial oxygen desaturation during non-sedated diagnostic upper gastrointestinal endoscopy. *Gastrointest Endosc* 40:277–280, 1994.

2. Iwao T, Toyonaga A, Harada H, et al: Arterial oxygen desaturation during non-sedated diagnostic upper gastrointestinal endoscopy in patients with cirrhosis. *Gastrointest Endosc* 40:281–284, 1994.

3. Saunders BP, Fukumoto M, Halligan S, et al: Patient-administered nitrous oxide/oxygen inhalation provides effective sedation and analgesia for colonoscopy. *Gastrointest Endosc* 40:418–421, 1994.

4. Zuckerman GR, O'Brien J, Halsted R: Antibiotic prophylaxis in patients with infectious risk factors undergoing gastrointestinal endoscopic procedures. *Gastrointest Endosc* 40:538–543, 1994.

5. Mogadam M, Malhotra SK, Jackson RA: Pre-endoscopic antibiotics for the prevention of bacterial endocarditis: Do we use them appropriately? *Am J Gastroenterol* 89:832–834, 1994.

6. Raufman JP, Strauss FW: Gastrointestinal endoscopy in patients with acquired immune deficiency syndrome: An evaluation of current practices. *Gastrointest Endosc* 33:76–79, 1987.

7. Shapiro M, Brandt LJ: Endoscopy in the age of HIV: A study of current practices and attitudes. *Gastrointest Endosc* 40:477–480, 1994.

8. Church JM: Complete colonoscopy: How often? And if not, why not? *Am J Gastroenterol* 89:556–560, 1994.

9. Kundrotas LW, Clement DJ, Kubik CM, et al: A prospective evaluation of successful terminal ileum intubation during routine colonoscopy. *Gastrointest Endosc* 40:544–546, 1994.

10. Genta RM, Graham DY: Comparison of biopsy sites for the histopathologic diagnosis of Helicobacter pylori: A topographic study of H. pylori density and distribution. *Gastrointest Endosc* 40:342–345, 1994.

11. Yang R, Naritoku W, Laine L: Prospective, randomized comparison of disposable and reusable biopsy forceps in gastrointestinal endoscopy. *Gastrointest Endosc* 40:671–674, 1994.

12. Karita M, Tada M: Endoscopic and histologic diagnosis of submucosal tumors of the gastrointestinal tract using combined strip biopsy and bite biopsy. *Gastrointest Endosc* 40:749–753, 1994.

13. Margulies C, Krevsky B, Catalano MF: How accurate are endoscopic estimates of size? *Gastrointest Endosc* 40:174–177, 1994.

14. Vakil N, Smith W, Bourgeois K, et al: Endoscopic measurement of lesion size: Improved accuracy with image processing. *Gastrointest Endosc* 40:178–183, 1994.

15. DiSario JA, Fennerty MB, Tietze CC, et al: Endoscopic balloon dilation for ulcer-induced gastric outlet obstruction. *Am J Gastroenterol* 89:868–871, 1994.

16. Laine L, Freeman M, Cohen H: Lack of uniformity in evaluation of endoscopic prognostic features of bleeding ulcers. *Gastrointest Endosc* 40:411–417, 1994.

17. Yang C, Shin J, Lin X, et al: The natural history (fading time) of stigmata of recent hemorrhage in peptic ulcer disease. *Gastrointest Endosc* 40:562–566, 1994.

18. Leung FW, Wong D, Lau J, et al: Endoscopic assessment of blood flow in duodenal ulcers. *Gastrointest Endosc* 40:334–341, 1994.

19. Lai KH, Peng SN, Guo WS, et al: Endoscopic injection for the treatment of bleeding ulcers: Local tamponade or drug effect? *Endoscopy* 26:328–341, 1994.

20. Berg PL, Barina W, Born P: Endoscopic injection of fibrin glue versus polidocanol in peptic ulcer hemorrhage: A pilot study. *Endoscopy* 26:528–530, 1994.

21. Bac DJ, de Marie S, Siersema, et al: Post-sclerotherapy bacterial peritonitis: A complication of sclerotherapy or of variceal bleeding? *Am J Gastroenterol* 89:859–862, 1994.

22. Berner JS, Gaing AS, Sharma R, et al: Sequelae after esophageal variceal ligation and sclerotherapy: A prospective randomized study. *Am J Gastroenterol* 89:852–858, 1994.

23. Spinelli P, Cerrai FG, Ciuffi M, et al: Endoscopic stent placement for cancer of the lower esophagus and gastric cardia. *Gastrointest Endosc* 40:455–457, 1994.

24. Raijman I, Walden D, Kortan P, et al: Expandable esophageal stents: Initial experience with a new nitinol stent. *Gastrointest Endosc* 40:614–621, 1994.

25. Ell C, Hochberger J, May A, et al: Coated and uncoated self-expanding metal stents for malignant stenosis in the upper GI tract: Preliminary clinical experiences with Wallstents. *Am J Gastroenterol* 89:1496–1500, 1994.

26. Raijman I, Kortan P, Haber GB, et al: Contrast injection to identify tumor margins during esophageal stent placement. *Gastrointest Endosc* 40:222–224, 1994.

27. Chung SCS, Leong HT, Choi CYC, et al: Palliation of malignant oesophageal obstruction by endoscopic alcohol injection. *Endoscopy* 26:275–277, 1994.

28. Yoshikane H, Tsukamoto Y, Niwa Y, et al: Superficial esophageal carcinoma: Evaluation by endoscopic ultrasonography. *Am J Gastroenterol* 89:702–707, 1994.

29. Abid S, Champion G, Richter JE, et al: Treatment of achalasia: The best of both worlds. *Am J Gastroenterol* 89:979–985, 1994.

30. Preston KL, Peluso FE, Goldner F: Optimal bowel preparation for flexible sigmoidoscopy—are two enemas better than one? *Gastrointest Endosc* 40:474–476, 1994.

31. Schoen RE, Weissfeld JL, Kuller LH: Are women with breast, endometrial, or ovarian cancer at increased risk for colorectal cancer? *Am J Gastroenterol* 89:835–842, 1994.

32. Zarchy TM, Ershoff D: Do characteristics of adenomas on flexible sigmoidoscopy predict advanced lesions on baseline colonoscopy? *Gastroenterology* 106:1501–1504, 1994.

33. Bertoni G, Sassatelli R, Conigliaro R, et al: Visual "disappearing phenomenon" can reliably predict the nonadenomatous nature of rectal and rectosigmoid diminutive polyps at endoscopy. *Gastrointest Endosc* 40:588–591, 1994.

34. Krevsky B, Fisher RS: Yield of rescreening for colonic polyps using flexible sigmoidoscopy. *Am J Gastroenterol* 89:1165–1168, 1994.

35. Squillace S, Berggreen P, Jaffe P, et al: A normal initial conoloscopy after age 50 does not predict a polyp-free status for life. *Am J Gastroenterol* 89:1156–1159, 1994.

36. Provenzale D, Kemp JA, Arora S, et al: A guide for surveillance of patients with Barrett's esophagus. *Am J Gastroenterol* 89:670–680, 1994.

37. Kim SL, Waring JP, Spechler SJ, et al: Diagnostic inconsistencies in Barrett's esophagus. *Gastroenterology* 107:945–949, 1994.

38. Stevens PD, Lightdale CJ, Green PHR, et al: Combined magnification endoscopy with chromoendoscopy for the evaluation of Barrett's esophagus. *Gastrointest Endosc* 40:747–749, 1994.

39. Falk GW, Catalano MF, Sivak MV, et al: Endosonography in the evaluation of patients with Barrett's esophagus and high-grade dysplasia. *Gastrointest Endosc* 40:207–212, 1994.

40. McAfee JH, Katon RM: Tiny snares prove safe and effective for removal of diminutive colorectal polyps. *Gastrointest Endosc* 40:301–303, 1994.

41. McNally PR, DeAngelis SA, Rison DR, et al: Bipolar polypectomy device for removal of colon polyps. *Gastrointest Endosc* 40:489–491, 1994.

42. Shiffman ML, Farrel MT, Yee YS: Risk of bleeding after endoscopic biopsy or polypectomy in patients taking aspirin or other NSAIDs. *Gastrointest Endosc* 40:458–462, 1994.

43. Randall GM, Jensen DM, Machicado GA, et al: Prospective randomized comparative study of bipolar versus direct current electrocoagulation for treatment of bleeding internal hemorrhoids. *Gastrointest Endosc* 40:403–410, 1994.

44. Ferrari AP, Lichtenstein DR, Slivka A, et al: Bruch cytology during ERCP for the diagnosis of biliary and pancreatic malignancies. *Gastrointest Endosc* 40:140–145, 1994.

45. Ryan ME, Baldauf MC: Comparison of flow cytometry for DNA content and brush cytology for detection of malignancy in pancreaticobiliary strictures. *Gastrointest Endosc* 40:133–139, 1994.

46. Baron TH, Lee JG, Wax TD, et al: An in vitro, randomized, prospective study to maximize cellular yield during bile duct brush cytology. *Gastrointest Endosc* 40:146–149, 1994.

47. Mohandas KM, Swaroop VS, Gullar SU, et al: Diagnosis of malignant obstructive jaundice by bile cytology: Results improved by dilating the bile duct strictures. *Gastrointest Endosc* 40:150–154, 1994.

48. Pencev D, Brady PG, Pinkas H, et al: The role of ERCP in patients after laparoscopic cholecystectomy. *Am J Gastroenterol* 89:1523–1527, 1994.

49. Prat F, Fritsch J, Choury AD, et al: Laser lithotripsy of difficult biliary stones. *Gastrointest Endosc* 40:290–295, 1994.

50. Siegel JH, Cohen SA, Kasmin FE, et al: Stent-guided sphincterotomy. *Gastrointest Endosc* 40:567–572, 1994.

51. Kalloo AN, Thuluvath PJ, Pasricha PJ: Treatment of high-risk patients with symptomatic cholelithiasis by endoscopic gallbladder stenting. *Gastrointest Endosc* 40:608–610, 1994.

52. Hoffman BJ, Cunningham JT, Marsh WH, et al: An in vitro comparison of biofilm formation on various biliary stent materials. *Gastrointest Endosc* 40:581–583, 1994.

53. Sung JJY, Chung SCS, Tsui CP, et al: Omitting side-holes in biliary stents does not improve drainage of the obstructed biliary system: A prospective randomized trial. *Gastrointest Endosc* 40:321–325, 1994.

54. Ikenberry SO, Sherman S, Hawes RH, et al: The occlusion rate of pancreatic stents. *Gastrointest Endosc* 40:611–613, 1994.

55. Niederau C, Pohlmann U, Lubke H, et al: Prophylactic antibiotic treatment in therapeutic or complicated ERCP: Results of a randomized controlled clinical study. *Gastrointest Endosc* 40:533–537, 1994.

56. Leung JWC, Ling TKW, Chan RCY, et al: Antibiotics, biliary sepsis, and bile duct stones. *Gastrointest Endosc* 40:716–721, 1994.

57. Sherman S, Hawes RH, Rathgaber SW, et al: Post-ERCP pancreatitis: Randomized, prospective study comparing a low- and high-osmolality contrast agent. *Gastrointest Endosc* 40:422–427, 1994.

58. Coleman SD, Eisen GM, Troughton AB, et al: Endoscopic treatment in pancreas divisum. *Am J Gastroenterol* 89:1152–1155, 1994.

59. Kozarek RA, Ball TJ, Patterson DJ, et al: Endoscopic pancreatic duct sphincterotomy: Indications, technique, and analysis of results. *Gastrointest Endosc* 40:592–598, 1994.

60. Catalano MF, Sivak MV, Rice T, et al: Endosonographic features predictive of lymph node metastasis. *Gastrointest Endosc* 40:442–446, 1994.

61. Motoo Y, Okai T, Ohta H, et al: Endoscopic ultrasonography in the diagnosis of extra-luminal compressions mimicking gastric submucosal tumors. *Endoscopy* 26:239–242, 1994.

62. Mendis RE, Gerdes H, Lightdale CJ, et al: Large gastric folds: A diagnostic approach using endoscopic ultrasonography. *Gastrointest Endosc* 40:437–441, 1994.

63. Amouyal P, Amouyal G, Levy P, et al: Diagnosis of choledocholithiasis by endoscopic ultrasonography. *Gastroenterology* 106:1062–1067, 1994.

64. Chang KJ, Katz KD, Durbin TE, et al: Endoscopic ultrasound–guided fine-needle aspiration. *Gastrointest Endosc* 40:694–699, 1994.

65. Wiersema MJ, Kochman ML, Cramer HM, et al: Endosonography-guided real-time fine-needle aspiration biopsy. *Gastrointest Endosc* 40:700–707, 1994.

66. Weirsema MJ, Wiersema LM, Khusro Q, et al: Combined endosonography and fine-needle aspiration cytology in the evaluation of gastrointestinal lesions. *Gastrointest Endosc* 40:199–206, 1994.

67. Catalano MF, Sivak MV, Van Stolk R, et al: Initial evaluation of a new-generation endoscopic ultrasound system. *Gastrointest Endosc* 40:356–359, 1994.

68. Maruta S, Tsukamoto Y, Niwa Y, et al: Evaluation of upper gastrointestinal tumors with a new endoscopic ultrasound probe. *Gastrointest Endosc* 40:603–608, 1994.

69. Barkin JS, Chong J, Reiner DK: First-generation video enteroscope: Fourth-generation push-type small bowel enteroscopy utilizing an overtube. *Gastrointest Endosc* 40:743–747, 1994.

70. Shaker R: Unsedated trans-nasal pharyngoesophagogastroduodenoscopy (T-EGD): Technique. *Gastrointest Endosc* 40:346–348, 1994.

71. Hintze RE, Binmoeller KF, Adler A, et al: Improved endoscopic management of severe upper gastrointestinal hemorrhage using a new wide-channel endoscope. *Endoscopy* 26:613–616, 1994.

72. Duckworth PF, Kirby DF, McHenry L, et al: Percutaneous endoscopic gastrojejunostomy made easy: A new over-the-wire technique. *Gastrointest Endosc* 40:350–353, 1994.

73. Kadakia SC, Cassaday M, Shaffer RT: Comparison of Foley catheter as a replacement gastrostomy tube with commercial replacement gastrostomy tube: A prospective randomized trial. *Gastrointest Endosc* 40:188–193, 1994.

74. Limberg B, Osswald B: Diagnosis and differential diagnosis of ulcerative colitis and Crohn's disease by hydrocolonic sonography. *Am J Gastroenterol* 89:1051–1057, 1994.

Index